Handb
in Car

SIXTH EDITION

Handbook of Patient Care in Cardiac Surgery

SIXTH EDITION

John H. Lemmer, Jr., M.D.
Northwest Surgical Associates
Legacy Good Samaritan Hospital
Clinical Assistant Professor of Surgery
Oregon Health and Science University
Portland, Oregon

Wayne E. Richenbacher, M.D.
Professor
Division of Cardiothoracic Surgery
The University of Iowa Hospitals and Clinics
Iowa City, Iowa

Gus J. Vlahakes, M.D.
Associate Professor of Surgery
Harvard Medical School
Massachusetts General Hospital
Boston, Massachusetts

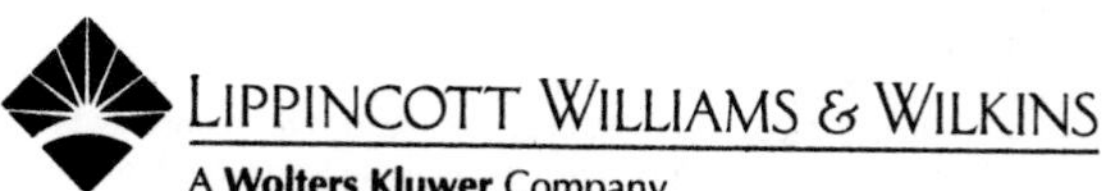

Philadelphia • Baltimore • New York • London
Buenos Aires • Hong Kong • Sydney • Tokyo

Acquisitions Editor: Lisa McAllister
Developmental Editor: Joanne Bersin
Production Editor: Emily Lerman
Manufacturing Manager: Colin J. Warnock
Cover Designer: Patricia Gast
Compositor: Circle Graphics
Printer: RR Donnelley, Crawfordsville

530 Walnut Street
Philadelphia, PA 19106 USA
LWW.com

Printed in the USA

Library of Congress Cataloging-in-Publication Data

Lemmer, John H.
Handbook of patient care in cardiac surgery.-- 6th ed. / John H. Lemmer Jr., Wayne E. Richenbacher, Gus J. Vlahakes.
p. ; cm.
Rev. ed. of: Handbook of patient care in cardiac surgery / Gus J. Vlahakes ... [et al.]. 5th ed. 1994.
Includes bibliographical references and index.
ISBN 0-7817-2906-8 (alk. paper)
1. Heart—Surgery. 2. Postoperative care. 3. Therapeutics, Surgical. I. Richenbacher, Wayne E. II. Vlahakes, Gus J. III. Title
[DNLM: 1. Cardiac Surgical Procedures—methods. 2. Perioperative Care—methods. 3. Patient Care Planning. 4. Postoperative Complications—prevention & control. WG 169 L554h2003]
RD598.B39 2003
617.4'12—dc21

2003047616

Care has been taken to confirm the accuracy of the information presented and to describe generally accepted practices. However, the authors and publisher are not responsible for errors or omissions or for any consequences from application of the information in this book and make no warranty, expressed or implied, with respect to the currency, completeness, or accuracy of the contents of the publication. Application of this information in a particular situation remains the professional responsibility of the practitioner.

The authors and publisher have exerted every effort to ensure that drug selection and dosage set forth in this text are in accordance with current recommendations and practice at the time of publication. However, in view of ongoing research, changes in government regulations, and the constant flow of information relating to drug therapy and drug reactions, the reader is urged to check the package insert for each drug for any change in indications and dosage and for added warnings and precautions. This is particularly important when the recommended agent is a new or infrequently employed drug.

Some drugs and medical devices presented in this publication have Food and Drug Administration (FDA) clearance for limited use in restricted research settings. It is the responsibility of the health care provider to ascertain the FDA status of each drug or device planned for use in their clinical practice.

10 9 8 7 6 5 4 3 2 1

Contents

Preface vii

1. Preoperative Evaluation and Management 1

2. Operative Management 25

3. Postoperative Management 65

4. Postoperative Complications Involving the Heart and Lungs 116

5. Postoperative Complications Involving Other Organ Systems 168

6. Late Postoperative Management 208

7. Management of Infants and Children 224

8. Mechanical Cardiac Support and Transplantation 253

Appendices

Appendix 1. Nomogram for Determining Body Surface Area from Height and Weight 295

Appendix 2. Recommendations for Preventing Bacterial Endocarditis 297

Appendix 3. Usual Dosages of Drugs Commonly Used in Adults 300

Appendix 4. Usual Dosages of Drugs Commonly Used in Infants and Children 310

Subject Index 315

Preface

This little book started life as a typewritten manual for house officers at the Massachusetts General Hospital in 1970. We thought it might be appropriate to publish it in the hopes that others would also find it useful. Apparently, this has been the case as it is now in its sixth edition. Each time we have been asked for a revision, we have wondered whether sufficient change had occurred in the four or five years since the previous edition to warrant the revision. Each time, as we put pen to paper, we have been surprised at the number of advances that had occurred in these brief periods. During the past thirty years, the cumulative effect of these countless small improvements in management has been a dramatic improvement in the outlook for our patients, despite their advancing age and degree of illness and the increased complexity of the operations that cardiac surgeons perform on them.

This handbook is intended to be a practical and useful guide to be carried in the pockets of those physicians, nurses, physician assistants, and others toiling "in the trenches." It is not meant to be encyclopedic. We recognize that there are many excellent ways to skin a cat, but we simply present the way this is done at the institutions in which we have worked: The Massachusetts General Hospital, The University of Iowa, The University of Michigan, The State University of Pennsylvania at Hershey, and Legacy Good Samaritan Hospital in Portland, Oregon. As time has passed and we have turned grayer of hair, we have turned the principal authorship over to those closer to the action, to ensure that the information contained remains practical and current. The references chosen include useful information for those needing this material in greater depth. These references are certainly not representative of the vast literature in our specialty; so an apology to any author of an important work that has been overlooked. Although the book contains little information about how to do operations, it will give the reader many management pointers, which, we hope, will contribute to successful outcomes. In no other specialty is patient management so complex or so interesting. Attention to detail and standardization of protocols are of paramount importance.

The topics covered in this book are arranged in chronological order. Preoperative preparation, unfortunately often slighted to the patient's detriment, comes first. Techniques are presented which can be used in the operating room to facilitate postoperative care. The postoperative protocols for patients who convalesce according to plan are detailed. Management of patients who have ventricular assist devices or operations for congenital heart disease is presented briefly, although each of these topics could easily warrant an entire book.

Just as the sailor who claims never to have run aground probably has not sailed much, the surgeon who claims never to have experienced complications either is not operating much or is not to be believed. Complications do occur frequently, but these can usually be successfully managed if anticipated, recognized promptly, and treated effectively. A substantial portion of the book is devoted to this subject.

Finally, we are very pleased that so many have found these books helpful and we are confident that this will be true of this new edition written by John H. Lemmer, Jr., Wayne E. Richenbacher, and Gus J. Vlahakes. For those who use the book, we also hope they recognize the philosophy we meant to convey when we carefully chose the title so many years ago, "Patient Care in Cardiac Surgery." That is, the secret of successful patient care is caring for the patient.

W. Gerald Austen, M.D.
Douglas M. Behrendt, M.D.

Handbook of Patient Care in Cardiac Surgery

SIXTH EDITION

1

Preoperative Evaluation and Management

Patient care in cardiac surgery begins with a thorough and precise diagnostic evaluation to define the pathophysiology, pathologic anatomy, and abnormal hemodynamics associated with the patient's heart disease. Although an evaluation has usually been performed by the referring cardiologist, it is the surgeon's responsibility to ensure that the evaluation is complete and that all information needed to plan and perform the proposed surgery is obtained. In addition to developing an operative plan, the surgeon must also identify the patient's co-existing diseases to minimize their risk to the surgical outcome. Recently, there has been the shift to outpatient preoperative management of elective cardiac surgical patients that can complicate the preoperative preparation process. Because the patient is not admitted to the hospital until the day of the operation, it is important to develop a system that ensures that all preoperative issues are addressed prior to the time of surgery. This includes the history and physical examination, laboratory and diagnostic evaluation, anesthesia evaluation, risk assessment, and patient teaching regarding the planned operation.

MEDICAL HISTORY

Obtaining a medical history begins with signs and symptoms referable to the patient's heart disease. For patients with coronary artery disease, the presence and severity of angina should be documented and characterized according to the Canadian Cardiovascular Society Functional Classification of Angina Pectoris (Table 1-1) (1,2). The patient's need for nitroglycerin tablets provides insight as to the severity of the angina. Angina severity determines the urgency of the subsequent evaluation and surgical plan. If the patient suffers from chronic stable angina, the work-up can be performed on an outpatient basis. If, however, the patient presents with accelerating angina, urgent evaluation and treatment are warranted (3). If the patient suffered a previous myocardial infarction, he or she is evaluated for signs or symptoms of congestive heart failure.

Patients with valvular heart disease often have a history of rheumatic fever or a known cardiac murmur. Such patients may describe easy fatigability or dyspnea on exertion as manifestations of congestive heart failure. Other heart failure symptoms such as dyspnea on exertion, orthopnea, paroxysmal nocturnal dyspnea, and ankle swelling may occur and should be documented. The degree of functional disability present in heart failure may be classified using the New York Heart Association Functional Classification for Heart Failure (Table 1-2) (4). For some patients, the change in activity level over time may have been quite gradual as the patient often accommodates to the limitations caused by a progressive valvular abnormality. As a result, the decline in functional capability can be insidious. Asking the patient to compare his or her activity level 1 year ago with the current status is use-

Table 1-1. Canadian Cardiovascular Society Functional Classification of Angina Pectoris

Class I	Angina resulting from strenuous exertion. Normal activity does not cause angina.
Class II	Slight limitation of normal activity. Walking more than two blocks on the level or more than one flight of stairs at a normal pace causes angina.
Class III	Marked limitation of normal activity. Walking one or two blocks on the level or climbing one flight of stairs at a normal pace causes angina.
Class IV	Angina occurs with any physical activity. Angina may be present at rest.

From Campeau L. Grading of angina pectoris. *Circulation* 1976;54:522–523, with permission.

ful. The presence of syncopal episodes or angina (both potentially associated with aortic stenosis) and arrhythmias should be noted.

Previous cardiac interventions such as coronary angioplasty or stent placement should be documented. The history of previous cardiac surgery has a major impact on a repeat operation. In such patients, the previous surgeon's dictated operative notes should be carefully reviewed. Knowledge concerning previous cannulation sites, the appearance and quality of native coronary arteries, and the location of old bypass grafts facilitates the subsequent ("redo") operation.

The complete relevant medical history includes family history (including age and cause of death of parents and siblings) and heart disease risk factors. Although the preoperative evaluation is not geared toward risk factor modification, identification of risk factors will allow targeted education during the patient's convalescence. The commonly recognized risk factors for coronary artery disease are shown in Table 1-3 (5).

The purpose of the medical history and review of systems evaluation is to identify disease processes that impact the conduct and

Table 1-2. New York Heart Association Functional Classification for Heart Failure

Class 1	No symptoms with ordinary physical activity.
Class 2	Symptoms with ordinary activity. Slight limitation of activity.
Class 3	Symptoms with less than ordinary activity. Marked limitation of activity.
Class 4	Symptoms with any physical activity or even at rest.

From Criteria Committee of the New York Heart Association. *Diseases of the heart and blood vessels: nomenclature and criteria for diagnosis of the heart and great vessels,* 6th ed. New York: New York Heart Association/Little, Brown, 1964, with permission.

Table 1-3. Risk factors for coronary artery disease

Family history of coronary artery disease
Tobacco use
Advanced age
Obesity
Male gender
Physical inactivity
Dyslipidemia
Hypertension
Diabetes mellitus and insulin resistance
Psychological factors
Hyperhomocystinemia

results of the cardiac operation. For example, patients with diabetes mellitus have increased rates of postoperative complications including renal insufficiency, stroke, and infections (6). The presence of diabetes may be a relative contraindication to the use of bilateral internal mammary artery grafts (7,8). Insulin-dependent diabetic patients may be at risk for an allergic response to protamine administration (9). Patients with hypothyroidism should be sure to receive their thyroid hormone supplementation perioperatively (10). Patients with a history of excessive bleeding (such as easy bruisability or long-lasting bleeding following a previous operation) or excessive clotting (such the history of thrombophlebitis) may be more likely to experience postoperative hemorrhagic or thrombotic complications (11). Therefore, inquiry regarding these and related topics should be made.

Patients with transient ischemic attacks or a previous stroke are at risk for neurologic complications and should undergo preoperative carotid duplex study (12). Carotid ultrasound imaging may also be indicated for patients with aortic stenosis and those with left main coronary artery disease. Patients with aortic stenosis often have a murmur that radiates to the neck that may obscure a carotid bruit. Patients with a left main stenosis may be at increased risk for carotid occlusive disease. If the carotid duplex identifies a severe internal carotid artery stenosis, carotid endarterectomy at the time of the cardiac procedure may be indicated depending on the patient's anatomy and symptoms (13).

Patients who provide a history of leg claudication or who have nonhealing foot ulcers likely suffer from arterial insufficiency. The ankle–brachial index (the ratio of the lower to upper extremity systolic blood pressure) documents the severity of the problem. Patients with lower extremity vascular disease are at increased risk for wound-healing complications following saphenous vein removal. Patients with saphenous vein varicosities, or who have undergone previous vein stripping or sclerosis, may have insufficient venous conduit for use in a coronary bypass operation. For these patients, alternative conduit choices such as bilateral internal mammary arteries and/or radial artery grafts may need to be considered.

The history of cancers that are of particular interest to the cardiac surgeon includes mediastinal tumors and breast carcinoma (14). Both may be associated with chest wall or mediastinal dissection and posttreatment radiotherapy. In such patients, the mammary arteries should be studied by angiography at the time of cardiac catheterization to rule out radiation-induced stenoses if their use in coronary revascularization is planned. Although previous mediastinal radiotherapy is not necessarily a contraindication to sternotomy, it may be associated with sternal radionecrosis, constrictive pericarditis, and significant intrapericardial adhesions (15).

MEDICATIONS

The patient's current medication list is carefully reviewed as these can impact the conduct of an open-heart operation (16). Patients undergoing coronary artery bypass grafting (CABG) are usually receiving oral *nitrate* therapy, and this is continued up to the time of surgery to avoid precipitating an ischemic event. *β-Adrenergic blocking agents* are also continued preoperatively as the patient's heart rate tends to be more controlled, particularly during the induction of anesthesia, and β-blocker treatment reduces postoperative supraventricular tachyarrhythmias. *Amiodarone* is commonly used to treat cardiac surgery patients. Because it has an extended half-life, discontinuation of this medication preoperatively will usually have no impact upon serum levels at the time of the operation and may, in fact, exacerbate the patient's underlying rhythm disorder (17). Also, preoperative prophylactic amiodarone administration may have a protective effect against postoperative atrial tachyarrhythmias (see Chapter 4) (18,19). *Calcium channel blocking agents* are generally continued until surgery because withdrawal may increase the risk of coronary artery spasm or acceleration of the ventricular response in patients with chronic atrial fibrillation (20). Generally, antihypertensive drugs, including *angiotensin-converting enzyme inhibitors* (such as *captopril* and *lisinopril*), *angiotensin II receptor antagonists* (such as *losartan* and *valsartan*), and *diuretics,* are held on the morning of surgery to avoid intraoperative hypotension (21). *Clonidine,* however, is continued until surgery as abrupt discontinuation of this medication may result in rebound hypertension. *Digitalis* preparations that are being administered for rate control in patients with atrial tachyarrhythmias are usually administered on the day of surgery.

Noncardiac medications can also impact the conduct of the open-heart operation. *Insulin*-dependent diabetic patients receive half their usual dose of insulin on the morning of surgery. This is combined with the administration of a glucose-containing parenteral fluid. Oral glucose-lowering agents (such as *glyburide, glipizide, miglitol, acarbose, nateglinide,* and *tolazamide*) are not administered on the morning of surgery. The oral hypoglycemic agent *metformin* has been associated with perioperative lactic acidosis and is held for several days before surgery, if possible (22). For the patient who takes steroids (usually *prednisone*) on a chronic basis, a supraphysiologic dose of hydrocortisone (100 mg i.v.) is given preoperatively. Patients who received bleomycin in the past and those taking amiodarone on a chronic basis may be at risk for acute respiratory distress syndrome secondary to high-level oxygen exposure. During surgery, and after, excessive oxygen administration is avoided in such patients.

Patients at risk for a *protamine* reaction include insulin-dependent diabetics and patients who have previously been exposed to protamine (9). If the patient has received *aprotinin* in conjunction with previous heart surgery, especially within the preceding 6 months, there is a small risk for allergic reaction with reexposure (23).

Patients with unstable angina are frequently maintained on intravenous *heparin* until surgery, and this generally presents no problem as the heparin is usually reversed intraoperatively by the administration of protamine. In contrast, *low molecular weight heparin* is not effectively neutralized by protamine, and preoperative treatment (within 12 to 24 hours) is associated with increased bleeding and transfusions in CABG patients (24,25). We therefore recommend that the patient be switched from low molecular weight heparin to unfractionated heparin at least 24 hours prior to surgery. Patients who receive preoperative heparin (especially unfractionated) are, however, more likely to experience a reduced response to heparin administered during surgery, so-called "heparin resistance," which is most likely the result of reduced antithrombin III activity (see Chapter 2) (26).

Patients with coronary disease are treated with platelet inhibitors, most commonly *aspirin*. Preoperative aspirin management practices vary. Some surgeons discontinue the patient's aspirin for several days prior to surgery, whereas others continue the drug up until the time of operation. Although preoperative aspirin treatment may increase postoperative bleeding, transfusion requirements, and the need for postoperative reexploration for bleeding, reports in this regard are not consistent (27–30). In fact, published results indicate preoperative aspirin treatment is associated with significantly improved outcomes, including lower mortality, in CABG patients (31,32). Generally, we do not postpone surgery because of aspirin treatment in our CABG patients, and a dose is routinely given early postoperatively (within 6 hours).

Patients suffering acute coronary syndromes such as unstable angina or who are undergoing percutaneous coronary interventions (such as stent placement) are often treated with other platelet inhibitors in addition to aspirin (33,34). The adenosine diphosphate receptor inhibitor *clopidogrel* irreversibly inhibits platelet function and has a duration of action of several days (the life of the platelet). Whenever possible, clopidogrel is discontinued prior to surgery, as preoperative treatment is associated with increased bleeding, transfusions, and the need to be returned to the operating room for excessive bleeding (35,36). The platelet IIb/IIIa glycoprotein receptor inhibitors include *abciximab, tirofiban,* and *eptifibatide.* Because abciximab has a longer duration of action, it is preferable to discontinue the drug 12 to 24 hours before surgery, if the patient's clinical status and coronary anatomy allow. If emergency surgery is required on the abciximab-treated patient, however, it can be successfully accomplished, and indicated surgery should not be denied (37). Tirofiban and eptifibatide have short durations of action and may be continued up until the time of surgery. See Chapter 3 for a further discussion of these drugs.

Warfarin is used to treat patients who have prosthetic valves, atrial fibrillation, cardiomyopathy with severe left ventricular dysfunction, venous thromboembolism, or other conditions. When these patients require elective surgery, the drug is usually discontinued approximately 4 days prior to the operation. If the patient is at high risk for thromboembolism (e.g., with a mechanical valve in place), he or she is admitted to the hospital about 2 days prior to surgery and treated with intravenous heparin while the warfarin effect wears off (38). Sometimes patients taking warfarin require urgent or emergency surgery, not an uncommon occurrence in prospective heart transplant recipient patients. In these cases, the prolonged prothrombin time may be corrected with fresh frozen plasma and/or vitamin K administration (39). Complete reversal of warfarin may not, however, be required, and preoperative warfarin treatment may, in fact, be associated with less postoperative bleeding and fewer transfusions [perhaps due to less thrombin generation during cardiopulmonary bypass (CPB)] (40). Vitamin K should not be given to patients who have an implanted mechanical valve, as rapid correction of the prothrombin time may precipitate valve thrombosis. Gradual reversal with fresh frozen plasma, however, is safe in patients with very elevated prothrombin times who must be operated on urgently. If vitamin K is used, only a small dose is indicated (1.0 to 2.5 mg), and the oral route is preferred (41). Excessive preoperative treatment with vitamin K will result in warfarin resistance postoperatively, possibly prolonging the patient's hospitalization.

Recently, nonprescription herbal supplements have gained increasing popularity (Table 1-4) (42–44). These medications have not been the subject of animal studies, premarketing controlled clinical trials, or postmarket surveillance, and their pharmacologic effects are not well studied. Garlic, ginseng, and ginkgo (the three "Gs"), in particular, have been associated with excessive bleeding. We request that patients discontinue all herbal supplements for at least 1 week prior to elective surgery.

Medication allergies, either documented or suspected, should be recorded, and nonmedication allergies should be investigated. A latex-free operating room environment is used for the patient with a latex allergy (45). Patients with an allergy to iodine are prepped with chlorhexidine rather than povidone–iodine (46).

Table 1-4. Commonly used herbal supplements

Echinacea
Ephedra
Feverfew[a]
Garlic[a]
Ginger[a]
Ginkgo biloba[a]
Ginseng[a]
Kava
Saw palmetto[a]
St. John's wort
Valerian
Vitamin E[a]

[a]Reported to increase the risk of bleeding.

PHYSICAL EXAMINATION

A thorough physical examination is warranted in all presurgical patients. Particular attention should be directed to findings that impact the proposed open-heart operation. The patient's height and weight are determined and used to calculate the body surface area using either a nomogram (Appendix 1) or a readily available hand-held computer freeware program such as MedMath (47,48). The body surface area is used in the calculation of the arterial perfusion flow rate during CPB and the thermodilution cardiac index using the pulmonary artery catheter. The patient's preoperative weight is used for comparison with the weight after surgery. The use of CPB during surgery is associated with capillary leakage, increases in interstitial fluid, and weight gain. Postoperatively, the patient is treated with diuretics to reduce his or her weight to the baseline value; thus, an accurate preoperative weight determination is important.

Examination determines the patient's heart rate and rhythm. Cardiac auscultation will identify a cardiac murmur and suggest its etiology. Patients should be evaluated for congestive heart failure. Signs of congestive heart failure include a laterally displaced cardiac apex (not to be confused with the point of maximum impulse), an S3 gallop, pulmonary rales that do not clear with coughing, peripheral edema, and jugulovenous distention. Patients with end-stage right heart failure may have a prominent, or even pulsatile, liver margin and ascites. Arterial desaturation, whether cardiac or pulmonary in origin, is demonstrated by cyanosis of the nail beds and mucous membranes.

Because atherosclerosis is a systemic disease, the patient should be carefully examined for peripheral vascular disease. The carotid arteries are auscultated. If there is a bruit or the history of cerebrovascular occlusive disease, a carotid duplex study is performed. Pulses in the upper extremities are palpated and blood pressures determined in both of the patient's arms. A differential in blood pressure between the two arms suggests a stenosis of the subclavian artery that may preclude the use of the ipsilateral internal mammary artery as an *in situ* bypass conduit. This finding is also a marker for the presence of increased carotid and proximal atherosclerotic aortic disease (49). Similarly, a patient who has a reduction in palmar perfusion or a decrease in the pulsation from the palmar arch by Doppler examination during compression of the radial artery may not be a candidate for use of the radial artery as a bypass graft. In anticipation of the use of the radial artery as conduit, the patient's nondominant hand should be identified and an Allen test and digital pulse oximetry performed. These tests will help to ensure that the ulnar artery and palmar arch are intact and that the patient's hand perfusion will not be jeopardized following removal of the radial artery (50). Femoral, posterior tibial, and dorsalis pedis pulses are palpated. If the pulses are diminished, this may prompt further investigation with determination of the ankle–brachial index. If a patient has an ankle–brachial index of <0.6, some surgeons recommend not harvesting the saphenous vein from that leg due to concerns about wound healing following saphenous venectomy (51). Others will restrict the vein removal to the thigh portion only in legs with severe vascular insufficiency. If the femoral pulse is markedly decreased, it may not be possible to insert an intraaortic balloon pump (IABP) through that vessel.

For patients undergoing CABG, evaluation of the lower extremities includes inspection of the greater and lesser saphenous veins. With the patient standing, the greater saphenous vein is located on the medial aspect of the ankle, anterior to the medial malleolus. The patient is examined for the presence of venous varicosities and for brawny edema or skin changes suggestive of chronic venous insufficiency. If the greater saphenous vein is surgically absent or of poor quality, the lesser saphenous vein (located on the posterolateral aspect of the calf) is inspected. Preoperative venous duplex mapping is helpful in CABG patients to determine the location and diameter of the greater and lesser saphenous veins (52,53). The skin overlying the located veins is marked with an indelible marker to facilitate intraoperative vein removal. This is particularly helpful in obese patients.

The patient's skin is inspected for the presence of infections or a localized rash. The presence of acne in the presternal area or groin fungal infection increases the risk of a wound infection. If indicated, elective patients are treated with antistaphylococcal or antifungal therapy prior to surgery. If the patient is to undergo valve replacement or implantation of prosthetic material, the patient's dentition is carefully inspected. Elective valve surgery patients undergo complete evaluation by their dentist to rule out occult infections. Any necessary dental work should be completed prior to surgery (with appropriate endocarditis prophylaxis) to avoid postoperative endocarditis (54).

LABORATORY TESTING

A variety of laboratory and noninvasive diagnostic studies are performed as screening tools (Table 1-5). The complete blood count identifies the patient with undiagnosed anemia or an unsuspected elevation in white blood count. The latter would initiate a further evaluation to determine the source. Serum electrolyte measurements assess the adequacy of potassium repletion in the patient on diuretic therapy, whereas the serum sodium level provides an estimate of the patient's hydration status. An elevation in serum cre-

Table 1-5. Preoperative testing

Blood studies
Complete blood count
Serum electrolytes with creatinine and BUN
Serum glucose
Liver function tests and albumin
Coagulation parameters (PT, PTT, platelet count)
Urinalysis
Chest x-ray
Electrocardiogram

BUN, serum urea nitrogen; PT, prothrombin time; PTT, partial thromboplastin time.

atinine indicates renal insufficiency that may be of a variety of etiologies including diabetic nephropathy, hypertensive nephropathy, systemic hypoperfusion in the heart failure patient, or primary renal disease. Patients with preoperative renal dysfunction will benefit from adequate hydration prior to cardiac catheterization to minimize the toxic effect of the contrast medium. If the abnormal renal function is new or worsened by the contrast agent load associated with cardiac catheterization, it is prudent to wait until the creatinine returns to baseline levels prior to proceeding with surgery. Moderate renal dysfunction (creatinine >2.5 mg/dL) is associated with an increased operative morbidity, need for postoperative dialysis, and mortality (55,56). An elevated blood glucose level may identify the previously unsuspected diabetic patient; determination of the patient's glycosylated hemoglobin (hemoglobin A1C) level may aid in the diagnosis of diabetes mellitus.

Extensive coagulation studies (such as bleeding time and measurement of platelet function) are not required for patients who have no history of bleeding or excessive bruising. For most patients, measurement of the platelet count, activated partial thromboplastin time, and prothrombin time are sufficient (57). The patient with liver dysfunction, as may occur with significant right ventricular dysfunction and systemic hypertension, may have an elevated prothrombin time.

A preoperative chest radiograph is performed. Signs of congestive heart failure include an enlarged cardiac silhouette, pulmonary interstitial edema, and pleural effusions. Although the enlarged cardiac silhouette usually suggests left ventricular enlargement secondary to volume overload as a result of congestive heart failure, it may also be seen with left ventricular hypertrophy or a large pericardial effusion. A densely calcified ascending aorta can also be identified on the chest x-ray film and suggests an increased risk of atherosclerotic embolism during surgery (58). The presence of a very severely calcified or "porcelain" aorta may necessitate a change in operative plan (avoidance of ascending aorta cannulation, all arterial conduit rather than aortocoronary bypass in the revascularization patient) or preclude operative intervention altogether. The lateral chest radiograph is of particular value in reoperative patients as it shows the proximity of the cardiac structures and internal mammary artery pedicle clips to the posterior table of the sternum (59).

The preoperative electrocardiogram (ECG) demonstrates the cardiac rate and rhythm, evidence of an old myocardial infarction, and/or ongoing myocardial ischemia. It also is the reference for comparison for postoperative ECGs.

The urinalysis will identify an occult urinary tract infection (surprisingly common in the elderly), microscopic hematuria, or poor blood glucose control. Usually, CABG patients found to have a urinary tract infection are treated immediately with an appropriate antibiotic (typically trimethoprim/sulfa or levofloxacin), and the surgery is performed as scheduled. If, however, the patient is scheduled to undergo elective placement of a foreign material (e.g., valve replacement or prosthetic patch placement), the procedure is postponed until the urinary tract infection is definitively treated, and the follow-up urinalysis is negative for infection.

For the stable patient who is being evaluated as an outpatient, some of these studies need be performed only within 30 days of surgery (such as the chest x-ray film and ECG). If new symptoms develop (such as a new cough or chest pain), then it is wise to repeat any studies that may have potentially changed. Likewise, patients with a chronic condition (such as renal insufficiency or mild anemia) should have follow-up studies performed near to the day of surgery to be sure that the condition has not worsened.

DIAGNOSTIC STUDIES

Patients who present with chronic stable angina often undergo noninvasive assessment of myocardial ischemia by the referring cardiologist prior to a cardiac catheterization. The *exercise stress test* evaluates the patient's heart rate and blood pressure responses to exercise while walking on a treadmill according to a graded protocol. Development of symptoms, ECG changes (>2-mm ST-segment depression), or a reduced or blunted blood pressure response is indicative of ischemia (60).

A more quantitative means of documenting myocardial perfusion can be accomplished with *myocardial perfusion imaging* (61). During peak exercise, thallium-201 or technetium-99m is injected. These tracers are taken up by viable myocardium, whereas irreversibly infarcted myocardium demonstrates no tracer uptake. Delayed images document the redistribution of tracer into ischemic myocardium. If the patient is unable to exercise, drugs such as adenosine, dipyridamole, or dobutamine may be administered to mimic the effect of exercise on the distribution of blood flow (62). The adenosine, dipyridamole, or dobutamine myocardial perfusion scan provides results comparable to exercise-induced ischemia.

Stress echocardiography is also used to identify patients with myocardial ischemia (63). This imaging modality is based upon the principle that exercise-induced ischemia caused by occlusive coronary artery disease results in regional wall motion abnormalities. If the patient cannot exercise, dobutamine may be used to increase myocardial oxygen demand. If the increase in myocardial oxygen demand cannot be met by an increase in blood flow, a regional wall motion abnormality results and is observed on the echocardiogram.

Cardiac catheterization with coronary angiography remains the gold standard in the preoperative evaluation of most types of cardiac disease, although it may be contraindicated in patients with an acute aortic dissection or those with aortic valve endocarditis vegetations (64). Even if the preoperative patient does not have a history or symptoms of coronary insufficiency, coronary angiography is generally performed in patients over age 40 years and in younger patients who have hyperlipidemia, diabetes, tobacco abuse, or a strong family history of coronary artery disease. The complete cardiac catheterization study usually includes a left ventriculogram to identify wall motion abnormalities or the presence of a ventricular aneurysm and to provide a gross estimate of mitral regurgitation severity. The ventriculogram catheter measures pressures within the left ventricle and provides a pull-back gradient determination when it is withdrawn into the aortic root. This allows calculation of the aortic valve area (65). The aortic root injection demonstrates aortic valve insufficiency and reveals the size and length of an ascending aortic aneurysm, if present. Coronary and bypass graft angiography defines the anatomy as well as the presence, location, and severity of obstructions. Visualization of the native internal mammary arteries is particularly important in the patient being considered for repeat CABG to confirm the suitability of these vessels for use as bypass conduits.

A right heart catheterization study is performed in patients who present with signs or symptoms of congestive heart failure, patients with low ejection fractions, and those with valvular heart disease. The purpose is to determine the patient's preoperative cardiac output and pulmonary artery pressures. The pulmonary capillary wedge pressure provides an estimate of left ventricular preload, and the reversibility of pulmonary hypertension, if present, can be assessed. Significant V waves in the pulmonary capillary wedge pressure tracing are indicative, but not diagnostic, of mitral regurgitation. Parameters derived from the right heart catheterization allow an accurate assessment of heart failure and intrinsic pulmonary hypertension and can facilitate targeted therapeutic intervention.

Echocardiography provides details about intracardiac anatomy, left ventricular function, and valve function and anatomy (66,67). Transthoracic echocardiography is noninvasive, but can provide a less-than-ideal view of the heart in an obese patient or in a patient who has undergone recent chest surgery. Transesophageal echocardiography (TEE) provides highly detailed anatomic information about the mitral valve (imperative when planning a mitral valve repair) and usually provides better views of the ascending aorta (important for diagnosing an ascending aortic dissection). TEE is, however, invasive in that it requires placement of an esophageal probe under intravenous sedation. Echocardiography is valuable in evaluating the patient with a suspected malfunction of a prosthetic heart valve as it demonstrates paravalvular leaks and abnormal leaflet motion and identifies failed bioprosthetic valves (68,69). Echocardiography effectively defines the presence and location of vegetations on valve leaflets associated with endocarditis (70,71). Thrombus within the atrial appendage associated with atrial fibrillation and intraventricular thrombus associated with a transmural myocardial infarction are readily seen by echocardiography. Echocardiography can be used to estimate valve areas and pulmonary artery pressures. Echocardiography is readily performed, is associated with little risk, and can provide highly detailed information regarding cardiac anatomy and physiology, but the utility of the study is dependent upon the quality of the equipment and the knowledge and experience of the echocardiographer.

Preoperative *myocardial viability imaging* is of great value in evaluating the patient with depressed left ventricular function who is being considered for CABG. Viability imaging can identify "hibernating myocardium" that may recover function following revascularization (72). Thallium scintigraphy, as described previously, documents the presence and location of ischemic myocardium. Further confirmation of the presence of viable myocardium in ischemic segments can be obtained from positron emission tomography (73). The positron emission tomography scan identifies metabolically active myocardium. If present in the ischemic wall segment supplied by a stenotic coronary artery, the assumption is that the patient would benefit from coronary revascularization in spite of a depressed ejection fraction.

Computed tomography is used for the diagnosis of aortic aneurysms and acute aortic dissections and has largely replaced the more invasive procedure, aortography (74). Computed tomography is also helpful in evaluating the thickness of the pericardium in patients with constrictive pericarditis. Aortography does, however, remain the diagnostic mainstay for patients with traumatic tears of the proximal descending thoracic aorta (75). *Magnetic resonance imaging* and magnetic resonance angiography are emerging technologies that hold promise for the future (76). Magnetic resonance imaging provides a quantitative evaluation of ventricular function, an accurate assessment of chamber volume and ventricular mass, and an assessment of pericardial disease. These modalities have also been used to evaluate coronary artery anatomy and myocardial perfusion.

Pulmonary function testing is not routinely performed on the cardiac surgery patient, but is of value if the patient has a history of extensive tobacco use, chronic obstructive pulmonary disease, asthma, or unexplained exertional dyspnea. In these patients, preoperative testing provides an assessment of the patient's pulmonary reserve and risk for surgery (77). The patient's response to bronchodilators can be determined, and this information is used to guide postoperative therapy. Likewise, preoperative measurement of the patient's room air arterial blood gas will identify patients suffering chronic hypoxia or hypercarbia. This information facilitates weaning the patient from mechanical ventilation following surgery.

PRESURGERY VISIT

Most elective adult cardiac surgery patients are admitted to the hospital on the day of surgery. Thus, they are seen in the clinic within a few days prior to surgery for completion of their work-up and preoperative preparation (Table 1-6). Elimination of the preoperative hospital stay has reduced costs and has improved patient satisfaction, as most patients are more comfortable in an out-of-hospital environment the night prior to surgery. However, the associated reduction in patient contact places greater emphasis upon the final clinic visit prior to surgery. It is important to ensure that all preoperative issues are addressed and that final preparations are completed at this time.

The final preoperative visit includes an interval history and physical examination to confirm that a new clinical condition has not de-

Table 1-6. Elements of the final preoperative visit

Interval history and physical examination
Laboratory studies as needed
Blood bank type and cross-match
Preoperative teaching
Anesthesia evaluation
Vein mapping, if indicated
Review consent and obtain operative permit

veloped. Patients who are to undergo CABG have vein mapping performed, if indicated. Laboratory studies, as needed, are performed. In addition, a blood sample is obtained for typing and for cross-matching packed red blood cells to be available for surgery. We obtain 2 U of packed red blood cells for "routine" operations and 4 U for repeat sternotomy procedures. Chapter 3 discusses blood conservation techniques such as preoperative autologous blood donation and directed donation.

The chest x-ray film and ECG need be checked only within 30 days of surgery. However, if there has been an intervening event or an increase in shortness of breath or angina, these studies are repeated at this time.

Preoperative teaching is performed on an outpatient basis. Interactive teaching module and videotapes facilitate patient education. These may review basic cardiac anatomy, touch on operative detail (but in no way replace an operative discussion with the surgeon), and place heavy emphasis on the postoperative issues such as tubes, catheters, pacing wires, and invasive hemodynamic monitoring lines. The patients and their families are introduced to the intensive care unit environment, as well as monitoring equipment and nursing routines. These teaching tools include interviews with dietitians and cardiac rehabilitation personnel to ensure that the patient has adequate home-going education. Emphasis is placed upon appropriate level of postoperative activity and cardiac rehabilitation, as well as dietary management. The patients are informed of likely postoperative medications. The patients are instructed in, and then asked to perform, the routine for exiting a bed or chair. They are taught how to support a sternotomy incision to ensure adequate coughing and deep breathing postoperatively and how to use the incentive spirometer.

The patient has a brief, final visit with the operating surgeon to ensure that all questions and concerns are addressed. A thorough discussion of the operative plan and potential complications is conducted. Complications to be discussed include, but are not limited to, bleeding, infection, myocardial infarction, stroke, the risks of blood transfusion, and death. For procedures involving the tissue adjacent to the cardiac conduction system (such as in valve replacement), the potential for heart block requiring a permanent cardiac pacemaker is also mentioned. The potential adverse events are not belabored, but they are outlined and listed on the operative permit. The permit is signed and witnessed.

An important aspect of the preoperative evaluation of the cardiac surgery is an assessment of the patient's operative risk. This has become increasingly important as the population of adult cardiac surgery patients becomes increasingly elderly with greater numbers of co-existing diseases and greater degrees of cardiac impairment (78). The development of large clinical practice databases has provided for evaluation of surgical results (such as nonfatal complication rates and mortality) for commonly performed procedures such as CABG and valve replacement. This allows surgeons and institutions to compare their results with those of the database and thus serves as a method of quality assessment and as a basis for quality improvement. In addition, these large databases provide the necessary data from which predictive formulas may be derived. These formulas can provide, for the individual patient, a prediction of expected operative mortality based on easily assessed preoperative risk factors. A number of different risk classification indexes are available, most of which have been developed using multiple regression analysis or Bayes theorem techniques. These risk-adjusted outcome predictive tools may utilize computer software or paper-and-pencil technique (79–83). By entering a number of preoperative clinical variables into the computer program (Table 1-7) or into a worksheet, a relatively reliable estimate of the patient's predicted chance of death is derived. This information provides a basis for a risk-versus-benefit discussion with the patient and his or her family. Such a discussion is an integral part of the decision-making process regarding the proposed cardiac surgical procedure.

The preoperative anesthesia evaluation focuses on airway management and previous anesthetic experiences (84). Obesity and a history of gastroesophageal reflux increase the potential for aspiration. The anesthesiologist reviews the patient's cardiac evaluation to determine how intensively the patient needs to be monitored during surgery. In general, if the patient has a history of congestive heart failure, a low ejection fraction, or recent myocardial infarction, a pulmonary arterial (Swan–Ganz) catheter is employed. If the patient is stable with well-preserved ventricular function and is undergoing a relatively uncomplicated procedure, the use of a pulmonary arterial catheter is optional. The neck and upper extremities are inspected by the anesthesiologist to ensure that appropriate monitoring lines can be placed. If a radial artery is to be employed as a bypass conduit, that arm is not used for intravenous catheters or blood pressure monitoring (either with a blood pressure cuff or with an arterial line). The presence, absence, and condition of the patient's teeth are documented. The anesthesiologist inquires with regard to a history of esophageal disease, especially if TEE is planned.

Table 1-7. Preoperative variables commonly used to assess surgical risk

Patient age
Left ventricular function (ejection fraction)
Nature of procedure
Gender
Previous cardiac procedure
Timing of surgery (elective, urgent, emergency)
Previous myocardial infarction
Presence of congestive heart failure
Need for preoperative IABP
Diabetes mellitus
Dialysis dependency
Chronic obstructive pulmonary disease, severe
Elevated pulmonary artery pressure (systolic >60 mm Hg)
Morbid obesity (BMI >34 kg/m^2)
Cerebrovascular disease
Hypertension

BMI, body mass index [weight (kg)/height (m^2)]; IABP, intraaortic balloon pump. See references 80 to 83.

Postoperative discharge planning begins with the preoperative visit (85). If the patient lives alone or has an inadequate social support network, a social worker sees the patient preoperatively to facilitate arrangements for postoperative placement.

SPECIAL PREOPERATIVE PROBLEMS

Depressed Left Ventricular Function

Because of advances that have been made in cardiac surgery, patients previously judged to be "inoperable" due to poor left ventricular function are now considered for operation. Likewise, patients with advanced coronary artery disease who have intractable rest pain or life-threatening coronary artery anatomy face a dismal prognosis without revascularization, and CABG surgery is often recommended. Although it is attractive to consider coronary angioplasty and stent placement as a good alternative for the high-risk surgical candidate, these patients often have severe, diffuse, multivessel coronary disease that often precludes percutaneous interventions. Thus, cardiac surgeons are frequently called on to manage these challenging patients. To the extent possible, congestive heart failure should be controlled medically before surgery in these high-risk patients.

In situations where left ventricular function is very poor (e.g., ejection fraction <25%), when revascularization may not be complete, and where operative ischemic time is likely to be long, it is useful to initiate preoperative IABP counterpulsation (86–88). This is in recognition of the higher-than-usual need for IABP support after surgery for these patients. In some patients, the IABP may be inserted 1 day prior to surgery for a short term of preoperative support prior to undergoing surgery. Typically, this is performed in the catheterization laboratory, and the balloon pump catheter is inserted over a guidewire using percutaneous techniques, usually on the side opposite from that where saphenous vein harvesting is anticipated. Alternatively, patients are taken to the catheterization laboratory during transfer to the operating room for IABP insertion. IABP placement in the catheterization laboratory may be particularly useful in patients who have peripheral vascular disease for whom fluoroscopic guidance is helpful. Under other circumstances, the IABP insertion can be performed in the operating room before the induction of anesthesia. In our experience and that of other surgeons, prophylactic preoperative use of the IABP in CABG patients with poor left ventricular function is associated with significantly improved surgical results. Further discussion regarding IABP management is found in Chapter 8.

Left Main Coronary Artery Disease

Patients with significant obstruction of the left main coronary artery will frequently present with unstable angina and are at risk for sudden death. These patients can develop arrhythmias or instability during coronary arteriography, during the induction of anesthesia, and even during the handling of the heart before CPB. Maintenance of medical therapy including nitrates, aspirin, β-blockers, and heparin is useful to maintain the patient's stability while awaiting surgery. Other antiplatelet drugs, in particular, one of the short-acting glycoprotein IIb/IIIa inhibitors, tirofiban or eptifibatide, may also be indicated. Should evidence of ischemia develop on such a regimen, immediate surgery is indicated, at times with preoperative IABP support.

Critical Aortic Valve Stenosis

Like patients with left main coronary disease, patients with critical aortic valve stenosis have the propensity to become suddenly unstable or to die unexpectedly. Unlike patients with coronary artery disease, there are no options for support with IABP and really no effective medical therapy that alters the pathophysiology of this lesion. Because of the imbalance between myocardial oxygen supply and demand, the maintenance of adequate systemic blood pressure is crucial as hypotension will further compromise coronary flow and may be disastrous. Excessive treatment with diuretics should be avoided, even though the patient may be in heart failure, because they produce volume depletion and hypotension that could reduce coronary perfusion further and result in severe instability. Likewise, vasodilator therapy is to be avoided. IABP counterpulsation does little to stabilize these patients, and in instances where aortic stenosis is accompanied by regurgitation, it may actually worsen the hemodynamic state. Thus, patients with critical aortic stenosis should undergo surgery as soon as possible. If increasing heart failure is noted, the procedure should be performed on an emergency basis. In selected patients with extenuating clinical circumstances (such as concomitant severe pneumonia), percutaneous aortic valvuloplasty can be considered for short-term stabilization. The long-term results, however, are very inferior to valve replacement.

Acute Valve Regurgitation and Malfunctioning Prosthetic Valves

Patients presenting with severe, acute mitral valve regurgitation have usually experienced a ruptured papillary muscle due to a myocardial infarction or as a complication of bacterial endocarditis. If the lesion is severe enough to produce cardiogenic shock, these patients may be stabilized temporarily by IABP counterpulsation and then undergo surgery on an emergency basis. Because ongoing cardiogenic shock may have cumulative deleterious effects on other critical organ systems, there should be no delay in instituting this sequence of therapy.

In the setting of endocarditis, cardiogenic shock is less common. These patients may be initially stabilized with antibiotic therapy, diuresis, and inotropic or afterload medications. Ideally, they should have a period of appropriate antibiotic therapy before valve replacement to sterilize the native valve, but valve replacement can be successfully carried out even if surgery is mandated due to uncontrollable heart failure, recurrent emboli, or persistent bacteremia.

Patients with acute aortic valve regurgitation usually have this lesion as a complication of aortic dissection or endocarditis. It results in wide pulse pressure with a low diastolic pressure. A natural cardiac reflex to minimize the effects of aortic regurgitation is tachycardia, which decreases the amount of time that the heart spends in diastole, during which time the regurgitation occurs. Thus, when these patients develop tachycardia, drugs such as β-blockers are contraindicated. Mechanical support with an IABP is not an option for acute aortic regurgitation, as it requires a competent aortic valve. Surgical replacement or repair of the valve is the essential treatment and should be undertaken as soon as possible.

Acutely malfunctioning prosthetic valves produce relative surgical emergencies. One situation is thrombosis of a mechanical prosthesis because of inadequate systemic anticoagulation, most commonly in the mitral position. This usually creates a clinical picture of mitral valve stenosis (± regurgitation) and severe heart failure. Preoperative management includes immediate systemic heparinization and echocardiographic evaluation. Thrombolytic therapy has been used with some success, especially in critically ill patients with a very high operative risk. There is, however, a significant risk of arterial embolization with this treatment, up to 19% (89–91). Generally, emergency valve replacement is indicated for patients who are relatively stable, patients with large thrombi visible on echocardiography, and those with thrombosed mitral prostheses (because the result of thrombolysis is not as good as for thrombosed aortic prosthetic valves). Thrombosis of aortic valve prosthesis is much less common because of the higher rate of blood flow past the prosthetic orifice. Acute prosthetic regurgitation may occur with bioprosthetic tissue valves, although much more commonly, the leakage develops over time as the valve gradually deteriorates. Rarely, a mechanical valve may experience strut or disc fracture or disc occluder escape, resulting in acute regurgitation.

Postinfarction Ventricular Septal Defect

Postinfarction ventricular septal defect (VSD) has become a less frequent occurrence since the advent of thrombolytic therapy and other treatments that limit the severity of myocardial infarctions (92). When present, however, this is a lesion that produces acute cardiogenic shock and remains associated with very high morbidity and mortality (93). Preoperative management entails placement of monitoring catheters (radial artery, central venous, pulmonary artery); coronary arteriography; and IABP support. In the past, efforts were made to maintain acute VSD patients for a number of days on IABP to allow the infarcted myocardium to mature (and therefore hold sutures better). It is now, however, generally accepted that patients with significant postinfarction VSDs and heart failure should undergo urgent surgical repair. If the patient is in cardiogenic shock with a large left-to-right shunt, emergency surgery is indicated. When a patient with a postinfarction VSD experiences a significant increase in the measured thermodilution cardiac output and/or progressive increase in serum creatinine, surgery is indicated as these show that the shunt is increasing and that peripheral perfusion is decreasing.

Failed Percutaneous Coronary Intervention

The treatment strategy for coronary artery disease changed dramatically with the introduction and growth of percutaneous coronary interventions. Although this has revolutionized the treatment of coronary artery disease, it has created a small number of patients who require emergency CABG because of immediate closure of a dilated artery or coronary artery dissection or perforation. The incidence of the need for emergency CABG as a consequence of failed percutaneous coronary intervention (coronary angioplasty and/or stent placement) has decreased, but still occurs. Preoperative management for the unstable patient includes coronary stent placement, IABP support, and/or placement of a multiholed "bail-out" catheter through the coronary artery lesion to provide distal perfusion. These patients often provide management challenges because they usually have received multidrug antithrombotic therapy that often includes aspirin, heparin, clopidogrel, and a platelet glycoprotein IIb/IIIa inhibitor. In general, however, preoperative platelet transfusion is not indicated unless significant ongoing bleeding is present. To give functional platelets prior to surgery could precipitate closure of a critically stenotic (but still open) coronary artery and would subject the transfused platelets to the effects of CPB.

Pregnancy

Pregnancy imposes a substantial stress on the cardiovascular system. Cardiac output progressively rises during pregnancy, reaching a peak nearly 1.5 times baseline during the 25th to 27th weeks. Although cardiac operations during pregnancy are rare, the usual circumstance involves a woman with underlying heart disease and limited cardiovascular reserve who develops worsening congestive heart failure. Cardiac surgery, including open procedures on CPB, may be performed on pregnant women without high maternal mortality. However, when CPB is employed, fetal mortality may be high. With respect to timing, the risk of surgery to the mother is lowest in the early stages of pregnancy, but this is also the period of critical fetal development. In preoperative consultation, the potential for fetal malformation or death and relative risks to the mother are discussed if the mother does not accept therapeutic abortion and cardiac surgery cannot be avoided. Chapter 6 discusses concerns regarding pregnancy and anticoagulation regimens.

SKIN PREPARATION AND ANTIBIOTIC PROPHYLAXIS

The patient showers with chlorhexidine the night before surgery and is asked not to eat or drink anything beginning 12 hours prior to surgery. The preoperative outpatient returns to the hospital several hours in advance of the anticipated operative time. On arrival, the patient's body hair is clipped, including the anterior chest, abdomen, and, for coronary revascularization patients, the entire legs. The clip stops at the knees for patients undergoing valve replacement or another cardiac operation. An intravenous catheter is placed and the preoperative antibiotic administered. The cephalosporin class of antibiotics is considered the agent of choice, usually cefazolin or cefuroxime (94). In addition to the preoperative dose, given 30 to 60 minutes before incision, an intraoperative cephalosporin dose is also recommended. Vancomycin is the antibiotic of choice for patients undergoing surgery at institutions that have a high rate of infections caused by methicillin-resistant *Staphylococcus aureus* and *S. epidermidis* (95). In addition, vancomycin is given to patients with penicillin or cephalosporin allergy. When administered, vancomycin must be infused slowly to avoid hypotension, which may be severe. The patient's name and identification number and operative plan are confirmed, and the patient is transported to the operating room at the appropriate time.

REFERENCES

1. Christie LG Jr, Conti CR. Systematic approach to evaluation of angina-like chest pain: pathophysiology and clinical testing with emphasis on objective documentation of myocardial ischemia. *Am Heart J* 1981;102:897–912.
2. Campeau L. Grading of angina pectoris. *Circulation* 1976;54: 522–523.
3. Yeghiazarians Y, Braunstein JB, Askari A, et al. Unstable angina pectoris. *N Engl J Med* 2000;342:101–114.
4. Criteria Committee of the New York Heart Association. *Diseases of the heart and blood vessels: nomenclature and criteria for diagnosis of the heart and great vessels,* 6th ed. New York: New York Heart Association/Little, Brown, 1964.
5. Wilson PWF, D'Agostino RB, Levy D, et al. Prediction of coronary heart disease using risk factor categories. *Circulation* 1998;97: 1837–1847.
6. Szabo Z, Hakanson E, Svedjeholm R. Early postoperative outcome and medium-term survival in 540 diabetic and 2239 nondiabetic patients undergoing coronary artery bypass grafting. *Ann Thorac Surg* 2002;74:712–719.
7. Furnary AP, Zerr KJ, Grunkemeier GL, et al. Continuous intravenous insulin infusion reduces the incidence of deep sternal wound infection in diabetic patients after cardiac surgical procedures. *Ann Thorac Surg* 1999;67:352–362.
8. Gross EA, Esposito R, Harris LJ, et al. Sternal wound infections and use of internal mammary artery grafts. *J Thorac Cardiovasc Surg* 1991;102:342–347.
9. Porsche R, Brenner ZR. Allergy to protamine sulfate. *Heart Lung* 1999;28:418–428.
10. Gomberg-Maitland M, Frishman WH. Thyroid hormone and cardiovascular disease. *Am Heart J* 1998;135:187–196.
11. Klopfenstein CE. Preoperative clinical assessment of hemostatic function in patients scheduled for a cardiac operation. *Ann Thorac Surg* 1996;62:1918–1920.
12. Puskas JD, Winston AD, Wright CE, et al. Stroke after coronary artery operation: incidence, correlates, outcome, and cost. *Ann Thorac Surg* 2000;69:1053–1056.
13. Borger MA, Fremes SE. Management of patients with concomitant coronary and carotid vascular disease. *Semin Thorac Cardiovasc Surg* 2001;13:192–198.
14. Erez E, Eldar S, Sharoni E, et al. Coronary artery operation in patients after breast cancer therapy. *Ann Thorac Surg* 1998;66: 1312–1317.
15. Handa N, McGregor CGA, Danielson GK, et al. Valvular heart operation in patients with previous mediastinal radiation therapy. *Ann Thorac Surg* 2001;71:1880–1884.
16. Mets B. The pharmacokinetics of anesthetic drugs and adjuvants during cardiopulmonary bypass. *Acta Anaesthesiol Scand* 2000;44: 261–273.
17. Rady MY, Ryan T, Starr NJ. Preoperative therapy with amiodarone and the incidence of acute organ dysfunction after cardiac surgery. *Anesth Analg* 1997;85:489–497.

18. Haan CK, Geraci SA. Role of amiodarone in reducing atrial fibrillation after cardiac surgery in adults. *Ann Thorac Surg* 2002; 73:1665–1669.
19. Daoud EG, Strickberger SA, Man KC, et al. Preoperative amiodarone as prophylaxis against atrial fibrillation after heart surgery. *N Engl J Med* 1997;337:1785–1791.
20. Murphy CE, Wechsler AS. Calcium channel blockers and cardiac surgery. *J Cardiac Surg* 1987;2:299–325.
21. Brabant SM, Bertrand M, Eyraud D, et al. The hemodynamic effects of anesthetic induction in vascular surgical patients chronically treated with angiotensin II receptor antagonists. *Anesth Analg* 1999;88:1388–1392.
22. Chan NN, Brain HPS, Feher MD. Metformin-associated lactic acidosis: a rare or very rare clinical entity? *Diabetic Med* 1999;16: 273–281.
23. Dietrich W, Späth P, Ebell A, et al. Prevalence of anaphylactic reactions to aprotinin: analysis of two hundred forty-eight reexposures to aprotinin in heart operations. *J Thorac Cardiovasc Surg* 1997;113:194–201.
24. Clark SC, Vitale N, Zacharias J, et al. Effect of low molecular weight heparin (Fragmin) on bleeding after cardiac surgery. *Ann Thorac Surg* 2000;69:762–765.
25. Jones HU, Muhlestein JB, Jones KW, et al. Preoperative use of enoxaparin compared with unfractionated heparin increases the incidence of re-exploration for postoperative bleeding after open-heart surgery in patients who present with an acute coronary syndrome. *Circulation* 2002;106(Suppl I):I19–I22.
26. Lemmer JH, Despotis GJ. Antithrombin III concentrate to treat heparin resistance in patients undergoing cardiac surgery. *J Thorac Cardiovasc Surg* 2002;123:213–217.
27. Ferraris VA, Ferraris SP, Joseph O, et al. Aspirin and postoperative bleeding after coronary artery bypass grafting. *Ann Surg* 2002;235:820–827.
28. Sethis GK, Copeland JG, Goldman S, et al. Implications of preoperative administration of aspirin in patients undergoing coronary artery bypass grafting. *J Am Coll Cardiol* 1990;15:15–20.
29. Bashein G, Nessly ML, Rice AL, et al. Preoperative aspirin therapy and reoperation for bleeding after coronary artery bypass surgery. *Arch Intern Med* 1991;151:89–93.
30. Reich DL, Patel GC, Vela-Cantos F, et al. Aspirin does not increase homologous blood requirements in elective coronary bypass surgery. *Anesth Analg* 1994;79:4–8.
31. Mongano DT, Multicenter Study of Perioperative Ischemia Research Group. Aspirin and mortality from coronary bypass surgery. *N Engl J Med* 2002;347:1309–1317.
32. Dacey LJ, Munoz JJ, Johnson ER, et al. Effect of preoperative aspirin use on mortality in coronary artery bypass grafting patients. *Ann Thorac Surg* 2000;70:1986–1990.
33. Quinn MJ, Fitzgerald DJ. Ticlopidine and clopidogrel. *Circulation* 1999;100:1667–1672.
34. Kong DF, Califf RM, Miller DP, et al. Clinical outcomes of therapeutic agents that block the platelet glycoprotein IIb/IIIa integrin in ischemic heart disease. *Circulation* 1998;98:2829–2835.
35. Hongo RH, Ley J, Dick SE, et al. The effect of clopidogrel in combination with aspirin when given before coronary artery bypass grafting. *J Am Coll Cardiol* 2002;40:231–237.

36. Yende S, Wunderink RG. Effect of clopidogrel on bleeding after coronary artery bypass surgery. *Crit Care Med* 2001;29:2271–2275.
37. Lemmer JH Jr. Clinical experience in coronary bypass surgery for abciximab-treated patients. *Ann Thorac Surg* 2000;70:S33–S37.
38. Clive K, Hirsh J. Current concepts: management of anticoagulation before and after elective surgery. *N Engl J Med* 1997;336: 1506–1511.
39. Morris CD, Vega JD, Levy JH, et al. Warfarin therapy does not increase bleeding in patients undergoing heart transplantation. *Ann Thorac Surg* 2001;72:714–718.
40. Dietrich W, Spannagl M, Schramm W, et al. The influence of preoperative anticoagulation on heparin response during cardiopulmonary bypass. *J Thorac Cardiovasc Surg* 1991;102:505–514.
41. Ansell J, Hirsh J, Dalen J, et al. Managing oral anticoagulant therapy. *Chest* 2001;119:22S–38S.
42. Ang-Lee MK, Moss J, Yuan C-S. Herbal medicines and perioperative care. *JAMA* 2001;286:208–216.
43. Norred CL, Finlayson CA. Hemorrhage after the preoperative use of complementary and alternative medicines. *AANA J* 2000;68: 217–220.
44. Valli G, Giardina E-G V. Benefits, adverse effects and drug interactions of herbal therapies with cardiovascular effects. *J Am Coll Cardiol* 2002;39:1083–1095.
45. Poley GE Jr, Slater JE. Latex allergy. *J Allergy Clin Immunol* 2000;105:1054–1062.
46. Erdmann S, Hertl M, Merk HF. Allergic contact dermatitis from povidone–iodine. *Contact Dermatitis* 1999;40:331–332.
47. Du Bois D, Du Bois EF. A formula to estimate the approximate surface area if height and weight be known. *Arch Intern Med* 1916;17:863–871.
48. Cheng PM. MedMath 1.21. *http://www.stanford.edu/~pmcheng/medmath/*.
49. Baribeau Y, Westbrook M, Charlesworth DC, et al. Brachial gradient in cardiac surgical patients. *Circulation* 2002;106(Suppl I): I11–I13.
50. Greene MA, Malias MA. Arm complications after radial artery procurement for coronary bypass operation. *Ann Thorac Surg* 2001;72:126–128.
51. Avrahami R, Haddad M, Koren A, et al. Saphenous vein harvesting for coronary artery bypass grafting. Retrospective analysis of possible causes of major wound complications in patients with peripheral arterial disease. *Eur J Vasc Endovasc Surg* 2001;21: 423–426.
52. Head HD, Brown MF. Preoperative vein mapping for coronary artery bypass operations. *Ann Thorac Surg* 1995;59:144–148.
53. Lemmer JH Jr, Meng RL, Corson JD, et al. Preoperative saphenous vein mapping for coronary artery bypass. *J Cardiac Surg* 1988;3:237–240.
54. Dajnai AS, Taubert KA, Wilson W, et al. Prevention of bacterial endocarditis. Recommendations by the American Heart Association. *JAMA* 1997;277:1794–1801.
55. Durmaz I, Büket S, Atay Y, et al. Cardiac surgery with cardiopulmonary bypass in patients with chronic renal failure. *J Thorac Cardiovasc Surg* 1999;118:306–315.

56. Penta de Peppo A, Nardi P, De Paulis R, et al. Cardiac surgery in moderate to end-stage renal failure: analysis of risk factors. *Ann Thorac Surg* 2002;74:378–383.
57. De Moerloose P. Laboratory evaluation of hemostasis before cardiac operations. *Ann Thorac Surg* 1996;62:1921–1925.
58. Mills NL, Everson CT. Atherosclerosis of the ascending aorta and coronary artery bypass. Pathology, clinical correlates, and operative management. *J Thorac Cardiovasc Surg* 1991;102:546–553.
59. Gillinov AM, Casselman FP, Lytle BW, et al. Injury to a patent left internal thoracic artery graft at coronary reoperation. *Ann Thorac Surg* 1999;67:382–386.
60. Gibbons RJ, Balady GJ, Beasley JW, et al. ACC/AHA Guidelines for Exercise Testing. A report of the American College of Cardiology/American Heart Association Task Force on Practice Guidelines (Committee on Exercise Testing). *J Am Coll Cardiol* 1997;30:260–315.
61. Ritchie JL, Gibbons RJ, Bateman TM, et al. Guidelines for Clinical Use of Cardiac Radionuclide Imaging: Report of the American College of Cardiology/American Heart Association Task Force on Assessment of Diagnostic and Therapeutic Cardiovascular Procedures (Committee on Radionuclide Imaging), developed in collaboration with the American Society of Nuclear Cardiology. *J Am Coll Cardiol* 1995;25:521–547.
62. Geleijnse ML, Elhendy A, Fioretti PM, et al. Dobutamine stress myocardial perfusion imaging. *J Am Coll Cardiol* 2000;36:2017–2027.
63. Lewis JF. Current status of stress echocardiography. *Clin Cardiol* 2000;23:242–246.
64. Remetz MS, Hennecken J. Cardiac catheterization in the evaluation of heart disease. In: Baue AE, Geha AS, Hammond GL, et al., eds. *Glenn's thoracic and cardiovascular surgery,* 6th ed. Stamford, CT: Appleton and Lange, 1996:1689–1709.
65. Gorlin R, Gorlin SG. Hydraulic formula for calculation of the area of the stenotic mitral valve, other cardiac valves, and central circulatory shunts. *Am Heart J* 1951;41:1–29.
66. Shively BK. Transesophageal echocardiographic (TEE) evaluation of the aortic valve, left ventricular outflow tract, and pulmonic valve. *Cardiol Clin* 2000;18:711–729.
67. Skiles JA, Griffin BP. Transesophageal echocardiographic (TEE) evaluation of ventricular function. *Cardiol Clin* 2000;18:681–697.
68. Daniel WG, Mügge A, Grote J, et al. Comparison of transthoracic and transesophageal echocardiography for detection of abnormalities of prosthetic and bioprosthetic valves in the mitral and aortic positions. *Am J Cardiol* 1993;71:210–215.
69. Bach DS. Transesophageal echocardiographic (TEE) evaluation of prosthetic valves. *Cardiol Clin* 2000;18:751–771.
70. Yvorchuk KJ, Chan K-L. Application of transthoracic and transesophageal echocardiography in the diagnosis and management of infective endocarditis. *J Am Soc Echocardiogr* 1994;7:294–308.
71. Ryan EW, Bolger AF. Transesophageal echocardiography (TEE) in the evaluation of infective endocarditis. *Cardiol Clin* 2000;18:773–787.
72. Perrone-Filardi P, Chiariello M. The identification of myocardial hibernation in patients with ischemic heart failure by echocardi-

ography and radionuclide studies. *Prog Cardiovasc Dis* 2001; 43:419–432.

73. Maddahi J, Schelbert H, Brunken R, et al. Role of thallium-201 and PET imaging in evaluation of myocardial viability and management of patients with coronary artery disease and left ventricular dysfunction. *J Nucl Med* 1994;35:707–715.
74. Hartnell GG. Imaging of aortic aneurysms and dissection: CT and MRI. *J Thorac Imag* 2001;16:35–46.
75. Fishman JE. Imaging of blunt aortic and great vessel trauma. *J Thorac Imag* 2000;15:97–103.
76. Sinitsyn V. Magnetic resonance imaging in coronary heart disease. *Eur J Radiol* 2001;38:191–199.
77. Durand M, Combes P, Eisele JH, et al. Pulmonary function tests predict outcome after cardiac surgery. *Acta Anaesthesiol Belg* 1993;44:17–23.
78. Ferguson TB, Hammill BG, Peterson ED, et al. A decade of change–risk profiles and outcomes for isolated coronary artery bypass grafting procedures, 1990–1999: a report from the STS National Database Committee and the Duke Clinical Research Institute. *Ann Thorac Surg* 2002;73:480–490.
79. Ferguson TB, Dziuban SW, Edwards FH, et al. The STS National Database: current changes and challenges for the new millennium. *Ann Thorac Surg* 2000;69:680–691.
80. Bernstein AD, Parsonnett V. Bedside estimation of risk as an aid for decision-making in cardiac surgery. *Ann Thorac Surg* 2000; 69:823–828.
81. Dupuis J-Y, Wang F, Nathan H, et al. The cardiac anesthesia risk evaluation score: a clinically useful predictor of mortality and morbidity after cardiac surgery. *Anesthesiology* 2001;94:194–204.
82. Scheidt S. Risk-stratification parameters in patient selection for coronary artery bypass grafting. *Am J Cardiol* 1999;83:3B–9B.
83. Jamieson WRE, Edwards FH, Schwartz M, et al. Risk stratification for cardiac valve replacement. National Cardiac Surgery Database. *Ann Thorac Surg* 1999;67:943–951.
84. Hurford WE. Techniques for endotracheal intubation. *Int Anesthesiol Clin* 2000;38:1–28.
85. Quigley RL, Reitknecht FL. A coronary artery bypass "fast-track" protocol is practical and realistic in a rural environment. *Ann Thorac Surg* 1997;64:706–709.
86. Christenson JT, Simonet F, Badel P, et al. Evaluation of preoperative intra-aortic balloon pump support in high risk coronary patients. *Eur J Cardiothorac Surg* 1997;11:1097–1103.
87. Dietl CA, Berkheimer MD, Woods EL, et al. Efficacy and cost-effectiveness of preoperative IABP in patients with ejection fraction of 0.25 or less. *Ann Thorac Surg* 1996;62:401–409.
88. Christenson JT, Simonet F, Badel P, et al. Optimal timing of preoperative intraaortic balloon pump support in high-risk coronary patients. *Ann Thorac Surg* 199;68:934–939.
89. Manteiga R, Souto JC, Altes A, et al. Short-course thrombolysis as the first line of therapy for cardiac valve thrombosis. *J Thorac Cardiovasc Surg* 1998;115:780–784.
90. Lengyel M, Fuster V, Keltai M, et al. Guidelines for management of left-sided prosthetic valve thrombosis: a role for thrombolytic therapy. *J Am Coll Cardiol* 1997;30:1521–1526.

91. Vongpatanasin W, Hillis LD, Lange RA. Prosthetic heart valves. *N Engl J Med* 1996;355:407–416.
92. Crenshaw BS, Granger CB, Birnbaum Y, et al. Risk factors, angiographic patterns, and outcomes in patients with ventricular septal defect complicating acute myocardial infarction. *Circulation* 2000; 101:27–32.
93. Labrousse L, Choukroun E, Chevalier JM, et al. Surgery for post infarction ventricular septal defect (VSD): risk factors for hospital death and long term results. *Eur J Cardiothorac Surg* 2002;21: 725–732.
94. Eagle KA, Guyton RA, Davidoff R, et al. ACC/AHA Guidelines for Coronary Artery Bypass Graft Surgery: a report of the American College of Cardiology/American Heart Association Task Force on Practice Guidelines (Committee to Revise the 1991 Guidelines for Coronary Artery Bypass Graft Surgery). *J Am Coll Cardiol* 1999; 34:1262–1346.
95. Abramowicz M, ed. Antimicrobial prophylaxis in surgery. *Med Letter Drugs Ther* 1999;41:75–80.

Operative Management

BASIC MONITORING

Continuous measurement of the arterial blood pressure is standard during cardiac surgery. Most commonly, a small catheter is inserted into a radial artery by percutaneous technique, a process that is facilitated by the use of a soft-tipped guidewire. Sometimes, particularly in pediatric patients, open exposure (cutdown) of the artery is required. In teenagers and adults, an Allen test is performed before cannulation to demonstrate adequate ulnar artery collateral flow to the hand (Fig. 2-1); if the test is positive (i.e., inadequate collateral to the hand), that radial artery should not be used (1). If a radial artery is to be used as coronary artery bypass conduit, the monitoring cannula is placed into the contralateral artery. If neither radial artery can be used for whatever reason, a femoral artery is a good second alternative, and because of the size of the artery, percutaneous insertion is usually simple. If aortoiliac disease precludes use of lower extremity arterial pressure monitoring, a brachial or axillary artery monitoring line may be used, although the complication rate may be higher (2).

Following cardiopulmonary bypass (CPB), the radial artery is usually accurate for postoperative monitoring but, at times, may underestimate the true central arterial pressure due to peripheral vasoconstriction, which may be exacerbated by hypothermia or the administration of vasoconstrictor medications (2,3). On these occasions, the femoral artery is more reliable than the smaller arteries for pressure measurement (4,5).

Complications of arterial lines are rare if proper techniques of insertion and maintenance are used. The incidence of thrombotic complications is increased by the presence of low cardiac output, hypotension, administration of vasoconstrictor agents, and long duration of use (6). Although these factors are related to the individual patient, other factors may contribute to thrombosis, such as multiple attempts at cannulation and large catheter size. The risk of infection of arterial catheters is increased by the use of cutdown rather than percutaneous technique, long duration of use, and inflammation at the catheter site. Femoral arterial catheters may be at somewhat greater risk for infection.

A large-bore cannula or multilumen catheter for central venous pressure measurement, fluid infusion, and drug administration is inserted via the jugular (internal or external) vein with the tip being advanced to the superior vena cava or right atrium. Peripherally inserted catheters (placed into basilic or cephalic veins) will yield similar measurements of central venous pressure if the catheter tip is properly located and if a continuous fluid infusion device (such as are used with intraarterial lines) is used (7). During surgery, when the chest is open, catheters may also be inserted directly into the innominate vein or right atrium. In rare circumstances where mechanical valves have been placed in the tricuspid position, a small-caliber catheter or even a Swan–Ganz catheter may be inserted into the pulmonary artery (PA) during surgery via a pursestring suture in the right ventricular outflow

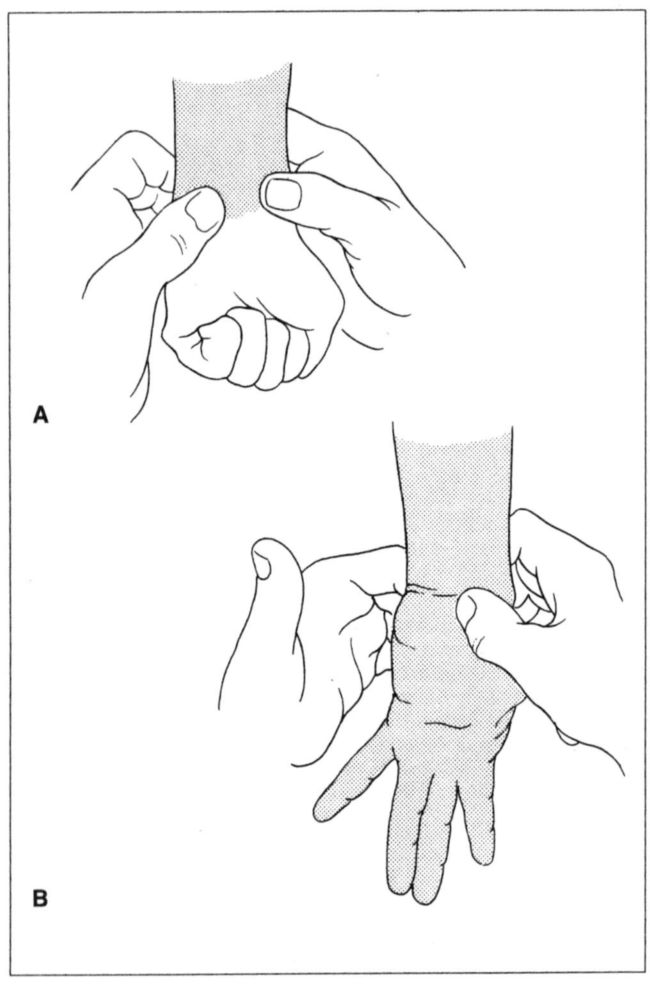

Fig. 2-1. Arterial line insertion. An Allen test is used to confirm that the collateral circulation to the hand is intact. The patient is instructed to make a fist, which results in the blanching of the palmar skin. Both ulnar and radial arteries are then manually occluded (A). The patient is instructed to open the hand, and while the radial artery is kept occluded, pressure is removed from the ulnar artery (B). If the perfusion returns to the fingers, adequate collateral circulation via the ulnar artery is intact, and a radial arterial line may be safely inserted.

tract. In such circumstances, catheter removal should be done while mediastinal chest tubes are still in place and after coagulation function has normalized.

The internal jugular vein provides safe and direct access for PA catheter insertion (Fig. 2-2). The vein is first located by puncture with a 21- or 22-gauge "exploring" needle; in this manner, an inadvertent puncture of the carotid artery can be managed by holding gentle pressure until there is no risk of hematoma formation. If the larger Swan–Ganz introducer is mistakenly inserted into the artery, the operation should be postponed unless it is an emergency or urgent, in which case this complication should be managed by open repair of the carotid artery before institution of heparinization and bypass (8). The subclavian vein is an alternative site for PA catheter insertion; the risk of pneumothorax and hemorrhage is higher, but subclavian insertion may be associated with fewer infectious complications (9). We avoid using the left-sided central veins as access routes in reoperations and other selected cases in which the innominate vein is at increased risk of injury during the surgical procedure. The technique for PA catheter insertion is outlined in Fig. 2-3. Continuous electrocardiographic (ECG) monitoring is mandatory during the insertion of PA catheters as occasional arrhythmias or conduction disturbances may complicate this procedure. These complications may be reduced by passing the catheter through the right ventricle in an expeditious manner and by avoiding redundant loops of catheter within the cardiac chambers. The development of complete heart block during passage of the PA catheter is more common in patients with left bundle branch block or in patients with *l*-looped ventricular anatomy. In these situations, a separate pacing wire can be inserted before PA catheter placement, or a PA catheter that includes a separate port for pacing wire passage can be used. Ventricular tachycardia or fibrillation is usually manageable by quickly withdrawing the catheter, defibrillation if indicated, and appropriate antiarrhythmic drugs if needed.

Complications related to PA catheters include infection, air embolism, and PA rupture. PA catheters rarely become infected if removed within 4 days of insertion (10). Air emboli are avoided by using standard techniques common to the management of all central venous lines. Rupture of a PA branch is rare but potentially catastrophic. The complication occurs in approximately 0.2% of PA catheter insertions and has a mortality rate of about 50%; it is more common in elderly women and in patients with pulmonary hypertension and in those who are anticoagulated (11). Often, the patient has a warning ("herald") bleed, specifically, an episode of hemoptysis; for the intubated patient, this would be the appearance of blood in the endotracheal tube. If this occurs in the operating room following PA catheter insertion but before surgery has begun, the operation should be postponed, the patient transferred to the intensive care unit, and management carried out as described in Chapter 3. If it occurs during the procedure, commonly during CPB, management may be difficult, especially if massive bleeding develops. Intraoperative bronchoscopy can confirm the diagnosis, and lung isolation with a bronchial blocker or double-lumen endotracheal tube may help to tamponade the bleeding and protect the

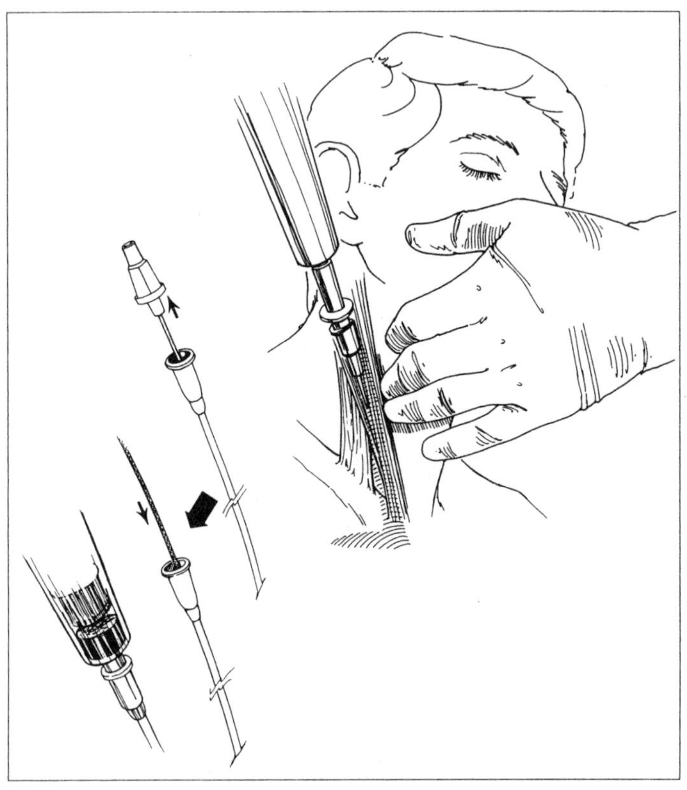

Fig. 2-2. Technique for internal jugular access. The patient is situated in the Trendelenburg position with the head turned to the side opposite line insertion. After a sterile prep and draping, the left hand is used to localize the carotid artery. A cannula with needle is then directed between the two heads of the sternocleidomastoid muscle to find the vein. After blood return is confirmed from the needle, the cannula is grasped to immobilize it, the needle is withdrawn, and a guidewire is then inserted into the internal jugular vein. The guidewire may be passed into the central venous position, which may sometimes be confirmed by observing that premature ventricular contractions have occurred when the guidewire reaches the right ventricle. The central venous catheter (or Swan–Ganz introducer sheath) may then be introduced over the guidewire. The wire is withdrawn, and central venous position is confirmed by noting that venous blood may be aspirated. If central venous pressures are low, air embolism is a potential risk, and care must be taken not to allow ingress of air when the syringe is removed from the catheter hub.

other lung. Thoracotomy and lung resection may be required to control the bleeding (12,13).

Transthoracic pressure monitoring lines, placed during the surgical procedure, are used most frequently in infants but may be necessary in older children and adults who have limited venous access. When transvenous access is not possible, insertion of a transthoracic right atrial or PA catheter will provide necessary pressure measurements. Left atrial lines may be useful when the pulmonary capillary wedge pressure does not correlate well with the true left atrial pressure (14); they may be particularly useful for managing right heart failure. A left atrial catheter also allows administration of drugs into the systemic circulation while minimizing adverse effects on the pulmonary vessels (15). Drug infusion into these lines must be performed with strict precautions to avoid air embolism. During surgery, these lines may be inserted via a pursestring suture in the right superior pulmonary vein, or if this route is used for insertion of a left ventricular vent, the resulting opening provides easy access for insertion of a left atrial line (Fig. 2-4). Left atrial catheters add the risk of complications including systemic emboli of air and particulate matter, bleeding, and interference with prosthetic mitral valves. Other catheters that are of use include right atrial lines and PA lines inserted via a pursestring suture (Fig. 2-5). This approach is particularly useful in neonates and infants for measurement of PA pressure, PA blood sampling, or insertion of thermodilution or oxygen saturation probes. This approach has proved safe, even in relatively hypertensive right ventricles (16).

Continuous measurement of the patient's temperature is routine and important. This may be accomplished via a probe on the tympanic membrane, in the nasopharynx, and/or in the esophagus. Bladder or rectal probes may also be used but are less accurate, especially in adults. A Swan–Ganz PA catheter also provides continuous determination of the PA blood temperature, but this is not of use during CPB when the lungs are excluded from the circulation. Urinary catheters are inserted after induction of anesthesia; periodic determinations of the rate of urine production are recorded before, during, and after CPB, with appropriate interventions being undertaken should the urine output fall below the volume appropriate for the size and age of the patient.

A transcutaneous oxygen saturation monitor probe is attached to the patient's finger. Although useful in detecting sudden changes in peripheral arterial oxygen saturation, it is dependent on tissue perfusion and may be unreliable in low-flow states.

Nasogastric or orogastric catheters may be inserted after induction of anesthesia, may be deferred until after the procedure is completed, or may not be used at all. If the patient is to remain intubated for a number of hours after surgery or if the abdomen is distended, then stomach drainage may be employed to prevent gastric distension and the likelihood of pulmonary aspiration. Many patients, especially those without risk factors for gastroesophageal reflux, may be managed without nasogastric tubes, and, in fact, these tubes may be associated with an increased incidence of nosocomial pneumonia (17,18). When a gastric drainage tube is used, it should always be placed to low-level suction.

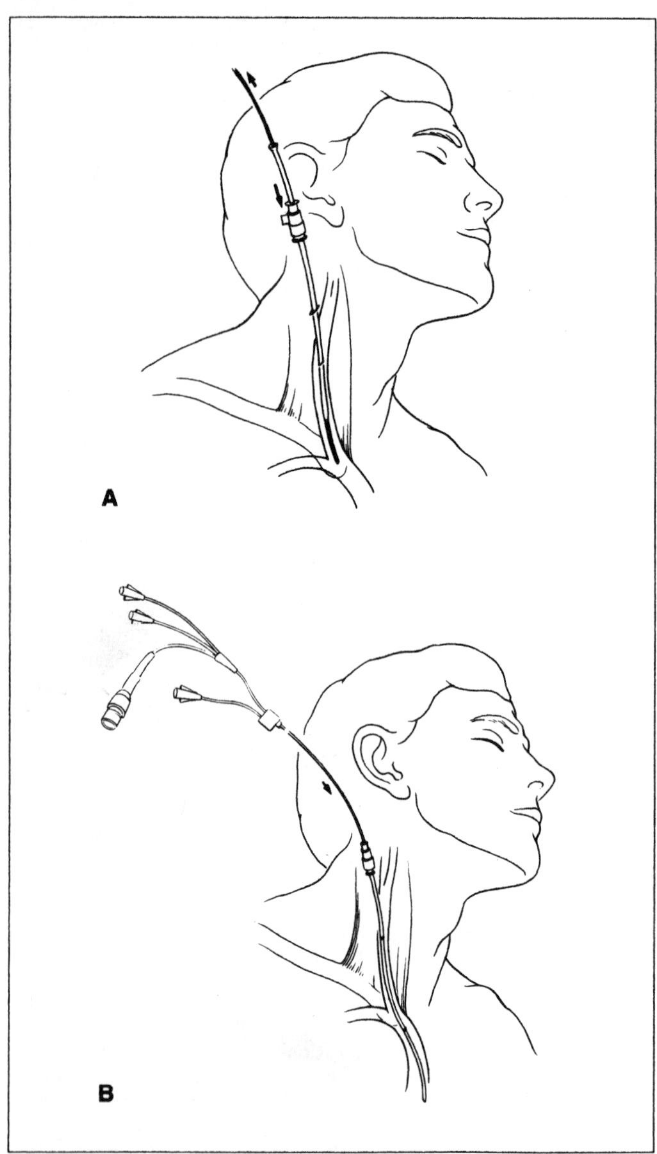

Fig. 2-3. Swan–Ganz catheter insertion. A: With use of the technique described in Fig. 2-2, an introducer sheath is placed in the internal jugular vein. Such a sheath usually contains a port for intravenous infusion and will usually contain an O ring at the end of the sheath to prevent ingress of air when the Swan–Ganz catheter is not present. B: All ports of the Swan–Ganz catheter are filled with heparinized saline, and the distal port is connected to a physiologic monitor. The Swan–Ganz catheter is inserted into the introducer sheath and advanced initially into the superior vena cava (SVC).

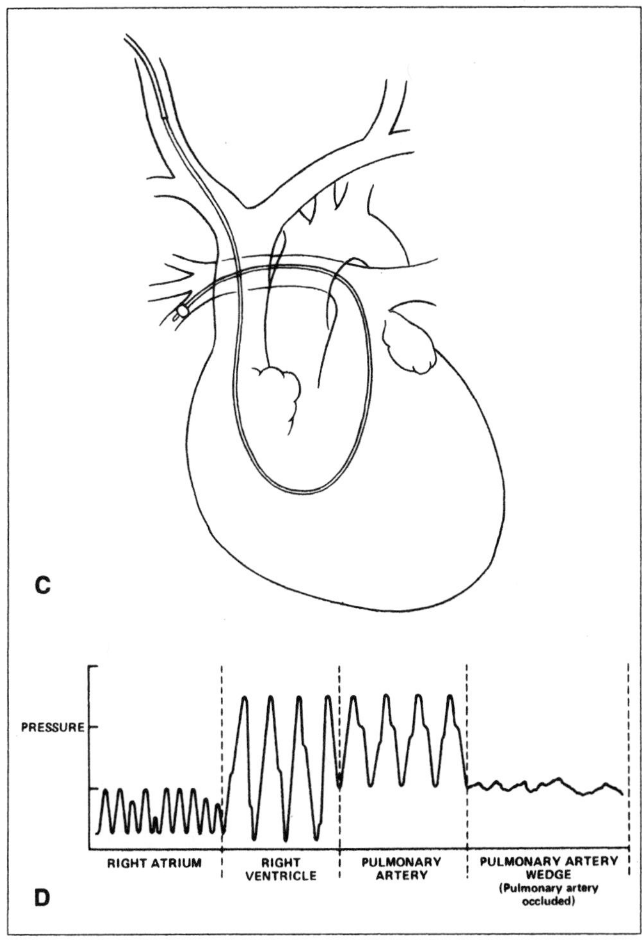

Fig. 2-3. ***Continued*** **C: Once present in the SVC, the balloon is inflated, and the catheter is advanced while the pressure monitor is continuously observed. The catheter is passed from the SVC to the right atrium and into the right ventricle. Subsequently, the catheter may be passed into the pulmonary artery and into the pulmonary capillary wedge position. Transit from right atrium to right ventricle and from right ventricle to pulmonary artery can sometimes be facilitated by having the patient take a deep inspiration, which will temporarily bring additional venous return into the heart. D: An example of the hemodynamic tracings obtained during insertion of a Swan–Ganz catheter. The difference between right atrial and right ventricular pressures is often obvious. However, when right ventricular filling pressures are elevated, it may be difficult to distinguish right ventricular from pulmonary artery pressure. A useful guide to note is that during diastole, pulmonary artery pressures will** ***decrease.***

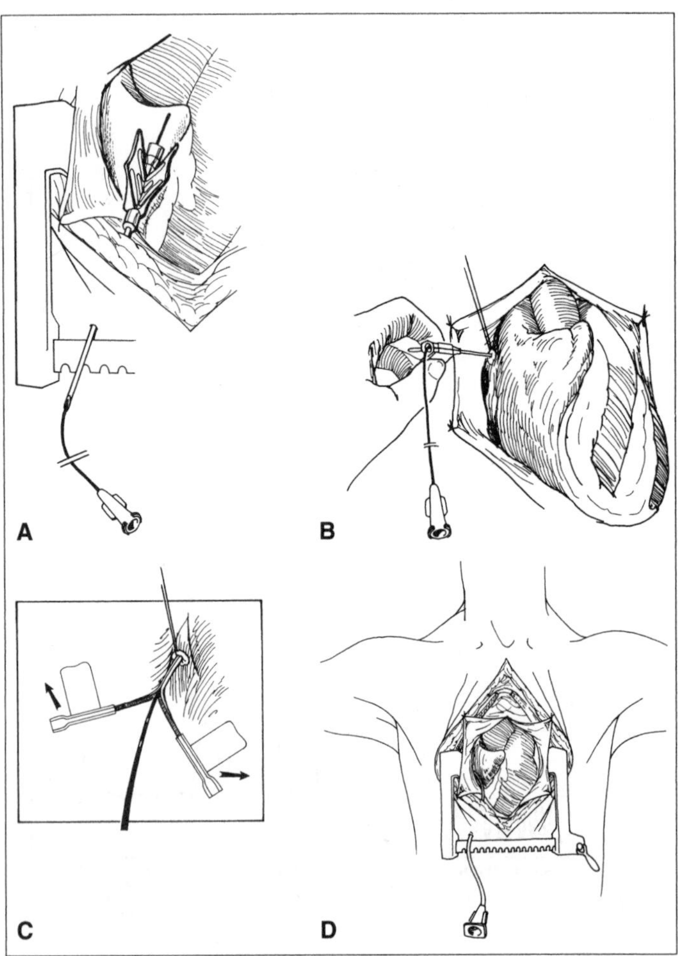

Fig. 2-4. Intraoperative technique for left atrial line insertion. A: Via a large-bore needle, inserted from inside the epigastric abdominal wall, the left atrial catheter is introduced into the chest. B: With use of a split, "break-away" needle, the end of the left atrial catheter is introduced into the left atrium via the proximal right superior pulmonary vein using a pursestring suture to secure hemostasis at the insertion site. C: The "break-away" needle is then extracted and removed. D: A gentle loop of catheter is left along the right side of the heart to prevent inadvertent extraction of the line when the chest is closed.

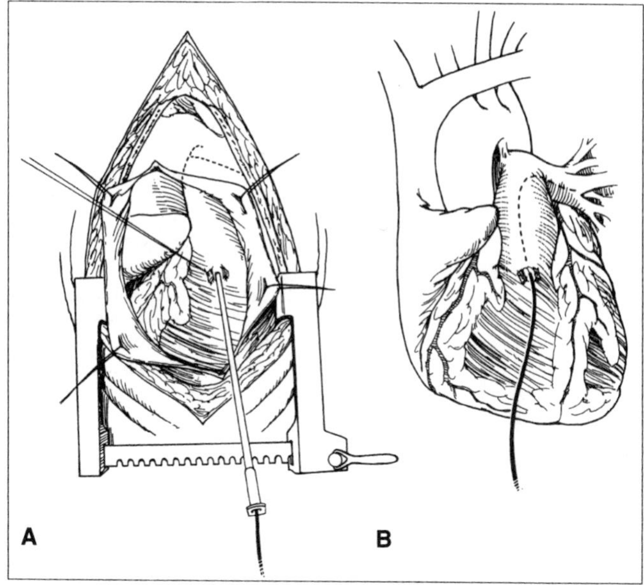

Fig. 2-5. Pulmonary artery monitoring line inserted via pursestring suture in the right ventricular outflow tract. Via a pledget-reinforced mattress suture, a catheter is introduced into the right ventricular outflow tract (A), using an introducer or a cannula-over-needle type of intravenous cannula. The introducer is withdrawn, the mattress suture is tightened, and the catheter is exteriorized through a small stab incision (B).

OTHER MONITORING TECHNIQUES

Flow-directed PA catheters, specifically the *Swan–Ganz catheter,* permit continuous measurement of central venous and PA pressures, estimation of cardiac output, and a port to withdraw blood samples for the determination of mixed venous oxygen saturation. Specially designed PA catheters (and monitors) have a distal sensor that (with a special computer and monitor) provides for continuous real-time determination of the mixed venous oxygen saturation. Other special PA catheters have built-in pacing wires to allow for temporary electrical pacing of the right ventricle. This may be particularly useful in patients with preexisting sinoatrial node dysfunction, heart block, aortic stenosis, or regurgitation or in reoperations (19). Whereas the use of PA catheters in adult cardiac surgery patients is very common, it is not universal or required. At some institutions, PA catheter use is reserved for highly selected patients with excellent results (20–22).

Intraoperative *transesophageal echocardiography* (TEE) has become a commonly performed procedure for both diagnostic and monitoring purposes. At some institutions, TEE is used in the place of a PA catheter for the purpose of monitoring cardiac function during cardiac surgery. The technique has proven to be very safe and of considerable value for both routine operations and special situations (23,24). Direct visualization of the heart with TEE allows for the identification of residual air in cardiac chambers, for the assessment of ventricular (both left and right) contractility, for the assessment of cardiac chamber filling status, and for monitoring the effects of fluid infusion and administered inotropic and vasoactive drugs (25,26). TEE is particularly useful for valve operations as it provides for direct visualization of the adequacy of native valve repair or function of the newly implanted prosthetic valve (27). Likewise, TEE is of value in diagnosing and assessing the extent of aortic dissections and for the detection of atheromatous disease in the descending aorta and aortic arch. For these reasons, the use of intraoperative TEE has become standard at our hospitals for all valve procedures and many other higher-risk operations such as coronary bypass surgery in patients with poor preoperative left ventricular function.

PACING AND ARRHYTHMIAS

Unexpected sinus bradycardia occurring during induction of anesthesia or in the earliest stages of the operation can be treated pharmacologically (see Chapter 4). Alternatively, the heart can usually be electrically paced via a pacing port Swan–Ganz catheter or via a transesophageal pacing electrode (28,29). It should be remembered that although bradycardia may be a response to anesthesia, it may also be indicative of a more serious problem such as hypoxia or myocardial ischemia.

Patients with previously placed permanent pacemakers should be evaluated before operation; the pacemaker manufacturer and model should be known, and a copy of a recent pacemaker interrogation should be available in the operating room. Electrocautery and defibrillation may affect the performance of the pacemaker in a variety of undesirable ways such as reversion to a backup mode or damage to the sensing and pulse generator circuits. Although modern pacemaker electronics permits safe and uneventful operation in most cases, certain precautions should be employed. These include placing the cautery ground plate as far from the pacemaker as possible, using the lowest possible cautery intensity, and keeping the appropriate pacemaker programmer in the operating room throughout the procedure. Pacemaker-dependent patients in whom electrocautery results in pacer suppression and bradycardia or asystole can be managed by placement of a magnet over the pacemaker generator, which will revert the generator into a fixed-rate mode. Many pacemakers implanted today are rate-responsive models that monitor and respond to physiologic parameters such as minute ventilation or muscle activity. These, in particular, have the possibility for adverse interactions (usually resulting in pacemaker-induced tachycardia). Prior to surgery, these pacemakers should be programmed to a pace-only mode to prevent the undesired rate response (30).

ANESTHESIA

Narcotics are an important component of the anesthetic management of the cardiac surgery patient because they have minimal effects on cardiac function and limited interaction with other agents. Synthetic narcotic agents such as fentanyl and sufentanil provide rapid induction and emergence from anesthesia with few effects on hemodynamics, even in patients with critical cardiac disease (31).

Narcotics alone are not always adequate to prevent hemodynamic responses to operative stimuli, particularly in children. In addition, in contemporary practice, less narcotic is being used to permit more rapid emergence and extubation following surgery. For this reason, inhalation agents (such as isoflurane, desflurane, or sevoflurane) are often added as needed, particularly during periods of greater surgical stimulation. The inhalational anesthetic agents are short acting, provide for early extubation, and are cost-effective (32). They are, however, used with care due to a mild direct negative inotropic effect (particularly at higher concentration) and a positive chronotropic effect that may increase oxygen consumption requirements. Because inhalation agents are potent vasodilators, the net effect on cardiac output may, however, be beneficial. Inhalation agents may also be added to the oxygenator gas flow during CPB; this is particularly useful for management of hypertension during bypass. Nitrous oxide is used infrequently because of its negative effects on cardiac output and blood pressure, its relative anesthetic impotency, and its ability to worsen any potential air embolism.

Intravenously administered sedatives such as the benzodiazepines are frequently added, particularly when lower doses of narcotics are used. Ketamine is used in children, particularly by intramuscular administration because of its rapidly hypnotic and analgesic effects without depression of respiratory or cardiovascular function. For this reason, ketamine may also be useful for induction of severely unstable patients such as those with tamponade or with massive pulmonary embolus. Muscle relaxants including pancuronium, vecuronium, and mivacurium are particularly useful after induction of general anesthesia to reduce the muscular rigidity associated with agents such as fentanyl that may make ventilation difficult.

At some hospitals, spinal and epidural techniques are used in conjunction with narcotic and inhalational agents for adults undergoing cardiac operations (33).

CONDUCT OF THE OPERATION

The patient should be properly positioned to allow access to all fields of interest. For coronary bypass operations, this includes adequate exposure of the saphenous vein harvest sites. A circumferential leg prep permits harvesting of greater or lesser saphenous veins, if needed. In circumstances where additional arterial conduits are desired, such as in young patients or when a lower extremity vein is not available, the radial artery can be used. If use of this conduit is a possibility, the selected extremity must be kept free of intraarterial and intravenous lines and should be included in the surgical field. In general, the radial artery is harvested from the nondominant arm. The integrity and function of the palmar arch are confirmed by the preoperative Allen test and by measuring the distal index finger oxygen saturation with an oximetry probe during manual compression of the radial pulse. In addition to a negative Allen test, fingertip oximetry should show a saturation of at least 95% during radial pulse compression in order to harvest the radial artery. We also continuously measure the index fingertip oximetry during the radial artery harvesting process.

Careful positioning of the patient is important to avoid peripheral nerve complications, which may result from hyperabduction of the shoulders or inadequate cushioning of the arms or legs. All arterial and venous lines must be secure and accessible to the anesthesiologist. Connections must be securely tightened and any stopcocks properly capped to avoid contamination. The patient's body hair is clipped (not shaved) within a few hours prior to being brought to the operating room (34). The skin is prepared with disinfectant soap by experienced personnel after all other manipulation of the patient has ceased. During the skin preparation, it is poor technique to permit members of the team to start intravenous lines, insert nasogastric tubes, attach cautery ground plates, or otherwise risk contamination.

In selected cases, including all reoperations, we apply adhesive external defibrillator pads to the lateral chest walls; these permit the transthoracic administration of direct current countershock before the heart has been adequately exposed (35). In all cases, internal defibrillator paddles must be readily available to the surgeon and should be tested at the outset to ensure proper function. The pump oxygenator is primed and present in the operating room no later than during induction of anesthesia. Sudden hemodynamic deterioration may require emergency cannulation and establishment of bypass. The perfusionist is also in attendance throughout this period.

Although the cosmetic benefits of a small incision may be appealing, it is important to make a large enough incision to perform the operation without compromising the surgical endpoint. In recent years, with the emphasis on less invasive approaches to cardiac surgery in appropriate cases, uses of alternatives to a standard full sternotomy have become more commonplace. Partial upper and lower sternotomies can be used for aortic valve surgery, mitral valve surgery, and correction of some types of congenital heart defects (36). These are illustrated in Fig. 2-6. When a lower partial sternotomy is utilized, particularly in children, access to the ascending aorta and superior vena cava can be enhanced substantially by retracting the upper sternum anteriorly, as shown in Fig. 2-7. At times, a right anterolateral thoracotomy incision can be used, particularly for mitral and tricuspid valve operations or atrial septal defects. Occasionally, coronary bypass procedures involving the left circumflex artery only are performed through a left lateral thoracotomy incision (37). A bilateral inframammary incision provides a cosmetically pleasing full median sternotomy, albeit with some compromise of exposure, although this approach is now only rarely used (38).

Operations performed on patients who have previously undergone a sternotomy incision ("redos") require special considerations (39–41). Adhesions between the heart, great vessels, sternum, and other surrounding structures can complicate reentry into the chest with risk of damage to the heart (especially the right ventricle) and/or previously placed bypass grafts (especially mammary artery grafts). The lateral chest x-ray film is reviewed to prepare

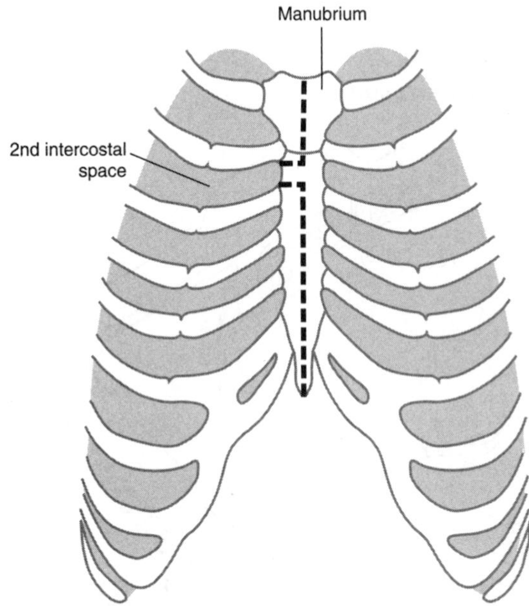

Fig. 2-6. The dotted lines indicate two options for partial sternotomy. The upper partial sternotomy may be used for procedures such as aortic valve replacement, while the lower partial sternotomy is used for operations on the mitral and tricuspid valves, as well as for congenital cardiac procedures requiring access through the atria. A vertical osteotomy is made, and in either case, a short transverse osteotomy on the right side of the second interspace completes the partial sternotomy. In most cases, retraction can be accomplished without having to divide or damage the right internal mammary artery.

for any particularly hazardous anatomy; if present, the location of the previously placed internal mammary artery pedicle is usually identifiable by the hemostatic clips that were attached to it. The surgeon should review previous operative report(s) and anesthesia records. It should be ascertained whether the patient previously received the drug aprotinin during a previous operation because reexposure to the drug has a risk of allergic reaction. The risk is very small if the prior administration was more than 6 months previously but may be as high as 4.5% if within 6 months (42). For patients previously treated with aprotinin, we delay the readministration until after the cannulas are inserted, so that CPB may be immediately initiated if an allergic reaction does occur. The patient is always given a small test dose of the drug [10,000 kallikrein inactivator units (KIU)].

For patients who do have hazardous anatomy (such as a patent internal mammary artery that appears to be hugging the posterior aspect of the sternum), we usually place a cannula into one

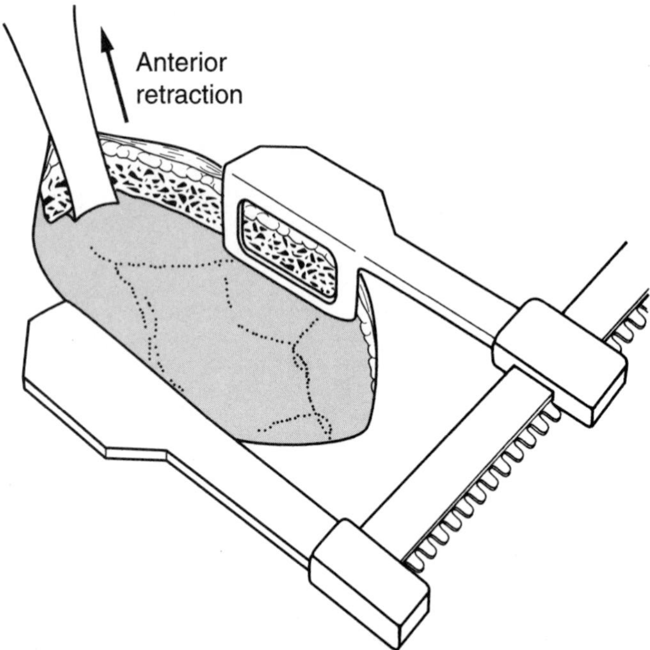

Fig. 2-7. When partial sternotomies are utilized, visibility can often be enhanced by anterior retraction on the sternum utilizing a retractor that is fixed to the side of the operating table.

of the femoral arteries to be available for access should expeditious cannulation be required. When there have been multiple previous operations, cardiomegaly, elevated right atrial pressures, or other circumstances that cause even greater concern (e.g., ascending aortic aneurysm or false aneurysm), isolation of the femoral artery and vein (via a groin cutdown incision) prior to making the sternotomy incision permits rapid cannulation if problems arise. In rare cases, bypass may be established via the femoral route before attempting posterior sternal division; this is frequently the most prudent approach in reoperations when there is severe tricuspid regurgitation with significant elevation of right atrial pressure (>20 mm Hg). Bypass may be instituted with mild hypothermia to permit continued ejection of the heart, and bypass flow can be temporarily reduced to decompress the right heart for the posterior sternotomy.

Sternal reentry is made safer by using an oscillating (cast-cutter) saw with the first assistant elevating the sternum anteriorly (Fig. 2-8). Another useful maneuver is to leave the posterior portion of the sternal wires in place while the oscillating saw is applied. In this fashion, 1 or 2 mm of additional space may be available for safe passage of the saw blade. After the sternal bone

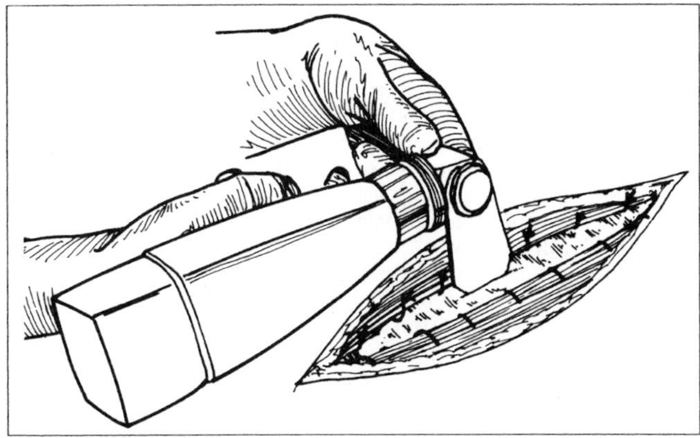

Fig. 2-8. In reoperations for cardiac surgery, the redo sternotomy is generally performed with an oscillating saw. The major concern is adherence of cardiac structures to the posterior table of the sternum. One approach to prevent injury to the aorta or right ventricle is shown: After cutting old sternal wires, they are left in place and used as a guide to the depth of penetration by the oscillating saw, thus decreasing the risk of injuring the aorta or right ventricle.

is divided, the table-mounted internal mammary artery retractor is useful for elevating the sternal half while dissecting the underlying tissues from the bone.

ANTICOAGULATION FOR CARDIOPULMONARY BYPASS

Heparin

Contact between the patient's blood and the nonendothelialized surface of the heart–lung machine is a powerful stimulus for thrombin generation and clot formation; therefore, complete anticoagulation of the blood is required for safe extracorporeal perfusion. Except for very special circumstances, this is accomplished by the administration of a large dose of unfractionated heparin. Heparin is an anionic, sulfated glycosaminoglycan derived from the mast cells of either porcine intestine or bovine lung (43). Unfractionated heparin is a heterogeneous mix of molecules with a mean molecular mass of 15,000 Da. In the United States, heparin potency is described in terms of USP units. USP units are not, however, equivalent to international units (IU). In the United States, the required potency of heparin is 140 USP U/mg of heparin (44). Thus, a dose of 3 mg/kg of body weight (a loading dose used at some institutions) is equivalent to 420 USP U/kg. Heparin acts to catalyze the rate at which the endogenous anticoagulant antithrombin III neutralizes thrombin and activated coagulation factor X (Xa). In order for heparin to be effective, therefore, sufficient antithrombin III must be present because heparin alone has little or no anticoagulant activity. There is considerable variation in responsiveness to heparin. The degree of anticoagulation may be monitored by a number of different tests, although the activated clotting time (ACT) is by far the one most commonly used (45). The patient's ACT is measured before and after administration of heparin. The ACT is a rather crude but global measure of clotting function. In the ACT tube is an activator substance, typically either celite (diatomaceous earth) or kaolin (clay), that acts to accelerate the blood coagulation. The ACT is, however, affected by other factors besides the presence of heparin, including hypothermia, extreme hemodilution, thrombocytopenia, and antithrombin III deficiency.

A commonly used heparin loading dose is 450 U/kg of body weight, although variation among institutions exists. The minimum ACT duration required to eliminate thrombin formation during CPB is not known and is likely not the same for all patients. The ACT duration of 480 seconds is a commonly used minimum threshold considered necessary for safe extracorporeal perfusion; thus, an ACT of 480 seconds is achieved before instituting CPB. The ACT is checked every 30 minutes on bypass and maintained above the selected minimum duration by additional heparin doses. Aprotinin is known to artifactually prolong the celite-activated ACT independently of heparin, and therefore, it is recommended that a celite–ACT threshold of 750 seconds be used when aprotinin is administered (46). Alternatively, and preferably, kaolin-activated tubes may be used, as they are not affected by the presence of aprotinin (47). Some institutions use the kaolin-activated ACT threshold of 600 seconds for aprotinin-treated patients.

Other methods to monitor anticoagulation for CPB are available; a common one is the heparin concentration assay, which uses an automated protamine titration method (45,48). Although quite useful, it must be remembered that measuring the direct heparin concentration may not reflect the true coagulation status of the blood. In the circumstance of antithrombin deficiency, clotting can still occur despite the presence of adequate heparin levels; therefore, concomitant measurement of the ACT is recommended even when heparin concentration assays are utilized.

Protamine

Heparin is neutralized by the administration of protamine, a strongly cationic protein derived from salmon sperm. Although generally safe, occasional adverse reactions to protamine do occur.

Not infrequently, protamine infusion produces mild hypotension by a direct vasodilation effect (49,50). This is due to the release of histamine from mast cells in response to the alkaline nature of protamine. The severity of the hypotensive response is directly related to the rate at which the protamine is infused and is increased in hypovolemic patients. Slow infusion will prevent the development of the hypotensive response to protamine.

More importantly, however, protamine may cause one of two types of hemodynamic response associated with profound systemic hypotension (51). The first type is a nonimmunologic reaction related to complement activation and thromboxane release (52). This causes severe bronchospasm and pulmonary vasoconstriction. Systemic pressure falls as a result of poor pulmonary venous return. Although this response is usually short-lived, support of the circulation sometimes requires reheparinization and placing the patient back on CPB. After several minutes of stabilization, the patient may again be separated from bypass. Because this is not a true allergic response, protamine may be safely readministered, although we prefer to infuse it into the aortic root at a very slow rate. Infusion of low-dose epinephrine may provide an extra margin of safety to prevent pulmonary vasospasm (53). The second type of protamine reaction is a true immune-mediated anaphylactic response that may be fatal (50,51). This is usually characterized by bronchospasm, pulmonary hypertension, hypoxemia, left heart failure, and complete circulatory collapse. Resumption of CPB may be lifesaving. Treatment usually requires α-adrenergic vasoconstrictor agents (norepinephrine, phenylephrine), although vasodilators (nitroglycerin, milrinone) may also be useful to combat the pulmonary hypertension. Treatment with steroids (methylprednisolone 30 mg/kg i.v.) and histamine antagonists (diphenhydramine 25 to 50 mg i.v. and cimetidine 5 mg/kg i.v.) may help prevent a second reaction on reexposure, and protamine infusion into the left side of the circulation may reduce histamine release. If the reaction was severe and life threatening, protamine should not be readministered. Risk factors for serious protamine reactions include NPH insulin use, fish allergy, and history of nonprotamine medication allergy (54).

Protamine neutralizes heparin and normalizes the ACT. The dose of protamine required for reversal of heparin may be calculated by measurement of the circulating heparin or by administering a dose based on the total dose of heparin that was administered during the procedure, followed by confirmation that the ACT has returned to baseline. A commonly used dose is 0.5 to 0.75 mg of protamine/100 U of heparin administered during the procedure. It should be administered slowly, over at least 5 minutes. The ACT is then rechecked and further protamine given if it has not returned to baseline. Excess protamine is avoided, as it is associated with impaired platelet function, prolongation of the ACT, and increased bleeding (55,56).

Heparin Resistance

Occasional patients do not achieve the ACT minimum threshold despite large doses of heparin (such as 600 U of heparin/kg of body weight). This condition of reduced heparin responsiveness or "heparin resistance" is more common in patients who have received heparin preoperatively (a common therapy for unstable angina) and patients who are on an intraaortic balloon pump before surgery (57). If the initial heparin loading dose does not achieve adequate prolongation of the ACT, an additional dose of 100 to 150 U/kg is administered. If this still does not adequately prolong the ACT, antithrombin III deficiency must be suspected and treated. Fresh frozen plasma (2 U for an adult) or antithrombin concentrate (500 to 1,000 U) is administered, and the ACT is rechecked before institution of bypass (58,59).

Heparin-Induced Thrombocytopenia

Patients treated with heparin may develop thrombocytopenia with two distinct forms of heparin-induced thrombocytopenia (HIT) being recognized. Type I is an acute and mild reduction in the platelet count that occurs as a direct agglutinating effect of heparin; this is not associated with thrombosis and resolves even with continued heparin treatment. Type II is immune-mediated. IgG antibodies react with heparin–platelet factor 4 complexes, and these complexes then bind platelets, causing platelet activation, aggregation (resulting in thrombosis), and consumption (resulting in thrombocytopenia). This subject is also discussed in Chapter 5. Patients with HIT type II who require cardiac surgery (during which heparin is to be administered) are at considerable risk for complications when reexposed to heparin. Thus, intraoperative anticoagulation is problematic (60). For this purpose, direct thrombin inhibitors such as recombinant hirudin and lepirudin and the low molecular weight heparinoid danaparoid have been used with success (61–63). The use of the platelet antagonist tirofiban, in conjunction with unfractionated heparin, has also proven to be successful for CPB in HIT patients. This combination is particularly well suited for patients with renal insufficiency as hirudin and danaparoid are excreted by the kidneys and not pharmacologically reversible (64).

TECHNIQUES OF EXTRACORPOREAL CIRCULATION (PERFUSION)

The ascending aorta is usually preferred for arterial cannulation but does carry the risk of embolization of atherosclerotic material to the head vessels. When selecting a cannulation site, the aorta should be palpated to exclude large plaques (Fig. 2-9). Intraoperative epiaortic ultrasound may be used to quickly examine the potential sites for cannulation and cross-clamp application (65). Use of this technique will, on occasion, reveal the presence of soft plaque that was not detected by palpation (Fig. 2-10). If this is encountered, the site for cannulation will need to be altered to reduce the chance of plaque embolization. The ascending aorta is cannulated, with care being taken to ensure that the cannula's flow is not directed into the innominate artery. See also the discussion of perioperative stroke in Chapter 5.

Femoral or external iliac artery access is required for a variety of aortic arch procedures, as well as for patients with severe ascending aortic disease that may make direct aortic cannulation hazardous. In patients with aortoiliac disease and ascending aortic or arch atherosclerosis, an alternative approach that is sometimes useful is cannulation of the axillary artery, as shown in Fig. 2-11 (66–69).

The technique of venous cannulation depends on the planned procedure. For operations that involve the coronary arteries, aorta, or aortic valve only, usually a dual-stage cannula placed in the right atrium provides adequate drainage. For operations involving the right heart chambers, bicaval (superior and inferior) cannulation with separate cannulas and use of caval tourniquets is required to prevent air from entering the bypass circuit. For mitral valve operations, either right atrial or bicaval cannulation may be used, although we usually use the latter method. Occasionally, the right internal jugular or innominate vein can be used for venous drainage. In children undergoing atrial septal defect repair via a partial lower sternotomy with limited access to the superior vena cava, an alternative technique for superior vena cava cannulation

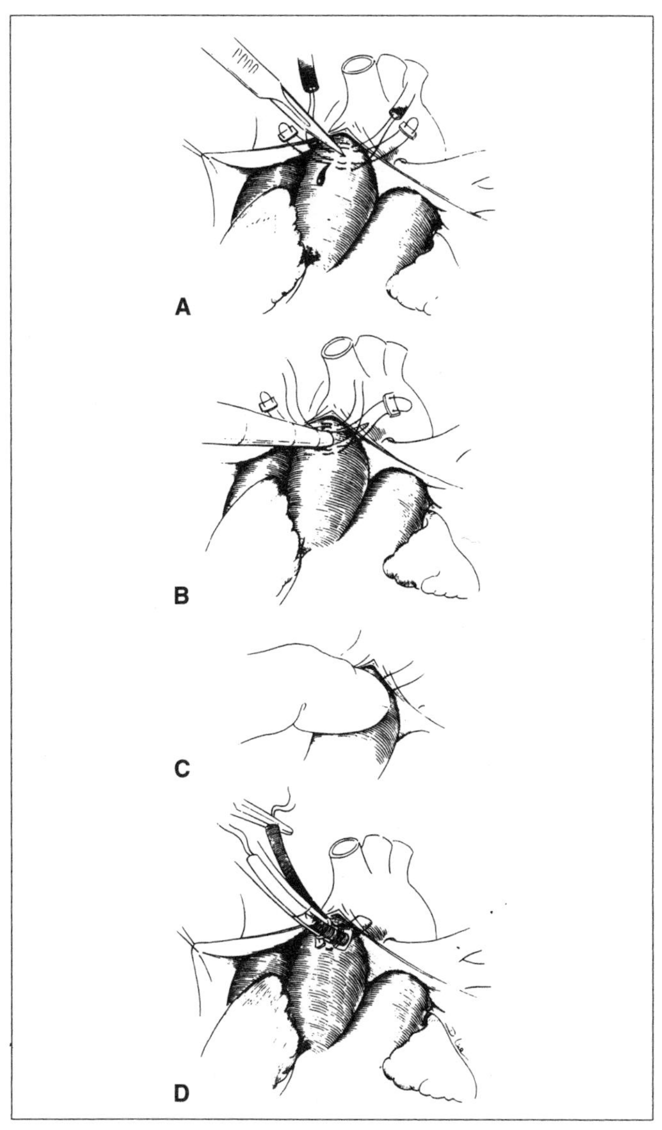

Fig. 2-9. The aorta is palpated to ensure that the site selected for cannulation does not contain palpable plaque. A: Two concentric pursestring sutures are placed around the selected site. An aortotomy is made with a no. 11 or 15 scalpel blade. B: Particularly if some aortic atherosclerosis is present, it may be necessary to dilate the aortotomy site with a tapered dilator. C: After making the aortotomy, temporary control is achieved with gentle digital pressure. D: The aortic cannula is introduced, making sure that the tip is facing downstream, aortic pursestring sutures are tightened, and the pursestring suture tourniquets are secured to the cannula using heavy silk ligatures.

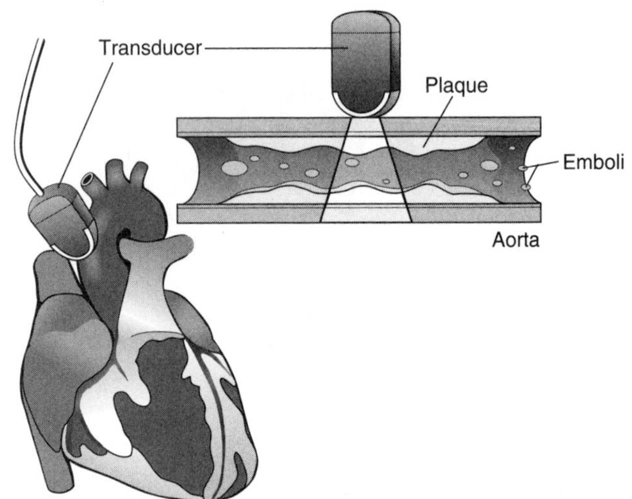

Fig. 2-10. Epiaortic and transesophageal echocardiographic scanning provides an additional level of protection to older patients who may face higher risks of brain injury due to a greater likelihood of embolization secondary to aortic atheroma. (From Hammon JW, Stump DA, Kon ND, et al. Risk factors and solutions for the development of neurobehavioral changes after coronary bypass grafting. *Ann Thorac Surg* 1997;63:1613–1618, with permission).

is to cannulate with a cuffed endotracheal tube inserted through a pursestring suture in the right atrial free wall. The cuff can be inflated in lieu of a caval tourniquet. For operations in which the right heart is not readily accessible (difficult reoperations) or in which it is desired to institute CPB prior to opening the chest (such as in the case of a substernal aortic aneurysm), then femoral vein cannulation is performed; when this is necessary, the right femoral vein usually provides the easiest access to the IVC and the atrium.

After cannulation and the institution of bypass, a sudden increase in the pressure in the arterial perfusion line associated with a decrease in the radial artery pressure should raise the suspicion of iatrogenic aortic dissection (Fig. 2-12). In this event, it is mandatory to discontinue bypass immediately, recannulate in another site, and repair the dissection. Intraoperative TEE can be very useful in making the diagnosis of aortic dissection.

Patients undergoing repair of acute ascending aortic dissection may pose additional risks and considerations regarding arterial cannulation. In these patients, there can be multiple reentry points in the descending and abdominal aorta, and retrograde (femoral artery) cannulation can result in perfusion of the false lumen and visceral branch obstruction. For this reason, upon completion of the distal aortic anastomosis, some surgeons move the perfusion site from the femoral artery to the implanted aortic graft to reestablish antegrade perfusion as early as possible.

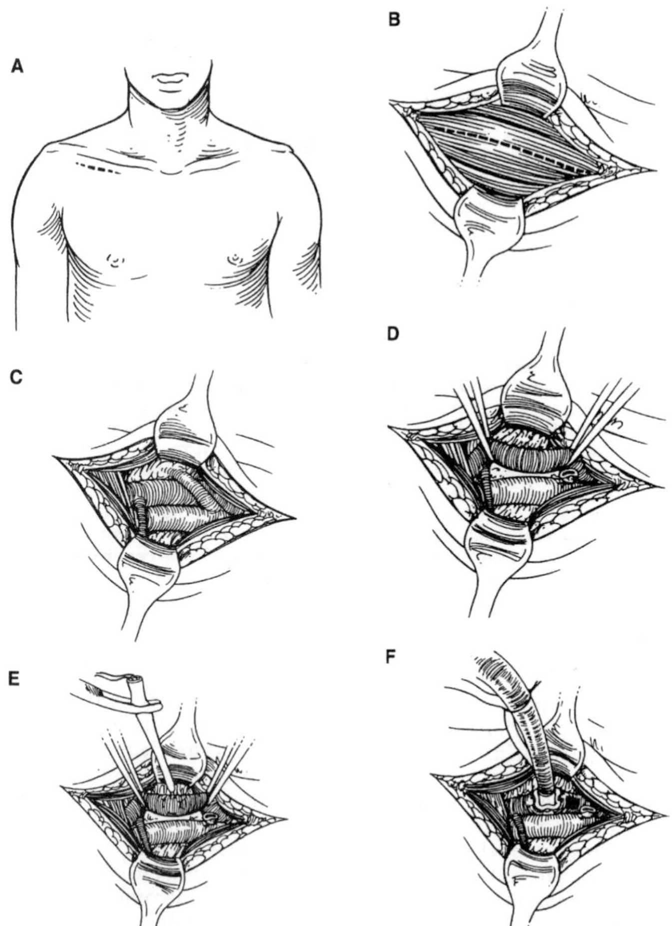

Fig. 2-11. Surgical technique of axillary artery cannulation. A: Site of incision below and parallel to clavicle. B: After incision of skin and subcutaneous tissue, before division of pectoralis major muscle in the direction of its fibers. C: After the clavipectoral fascia is incised and the pectoralis minor muscle is retracted laterally, the axillary artery is identified above the axillary vein. D: The crossing vein is divided, and proximal and distal control of the subclavian artery is obtained. E: Placement of pursestring suture and tourniquet. F: Cannulation of axillary artery with right-angled cannula. (From Sabik JF, Lytle BW, McCarthy PM, et al. Axillary artery: an alternative site of arterial cannulation for patients with extensive aortic and peripheral vascular disease. *J Thorac Cardiovasc Surg* 1995;109:885–890, with permission).

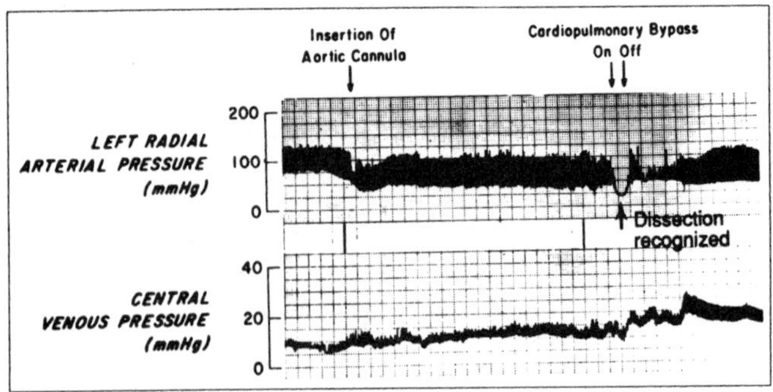

Fig. 2-12. Hemodynamic tracings from a patient in whom iatrogenic aortic dissection occurred with the aortic cannula being placed initially in a false channel. With the institution of cardiopulmonary bypass, perfusion was initiated in the false channel, resulting in loss of perfusion to the left subclavian artery. The dissection was quickly recognized, bypass was terminated, and with the cardiac output directed into the true lumen, the left radial arterial pressure was restored. The patient was recannulated using the femoral artery, bypass was instituted, and during the procedure, the iatrogenic dissection site at the ascending aortic cannulation was repaired.

Myocardial Protection

Myocardial protection is a broad concept that includes a number of measures performed to limit injury to the heart muscle. One essential component of myocardial protection is ventricular decompression. The left ventricle may become distended during CPB, most commonly during ventricular fibrillation; this may impair myocardial perfusion, particularly in the subendocardial region (70). Prevention of this complication requires venting of the left ventricle. This is accomplished by placing a cannula in one of several locations: directly into the left ventricle via the right superior pulmonary vein, in the aortic root, or into the pulmonary artery (71). If necessary, particularly when a mechanical mitral prosthesis is present, the ventricle can be vented by insertion of a small-bore cannula directly into the apex of the left ventricle. Irrespective of venting technique, in addition to metabolic protection, avoidance of distension is an important component of myocardial protection.

Cardioplegia

In the early years of this specialty, cardiac operations were performed using intermittent aortic cross-clamping or fibrillation arrest. Thus, the heart was subjected to potentially deleterious periods of ischemia, and the aorta was subjected to multiple applications of the cross-clamp that could increase the chance of plaque embolization. In contemporary practice, cardioplegia solution most frequently is used to arrest and protect the heart (72,73). A variety of cardioplegia additives have been proposed to enhance myocardial protection, including calcium channel blockers, metabolic substrates, free radical scavengers, oxygen, and red blood cells. Most often, cardioplegia solution is administered to the heart at a low temperature to reduce the myocardial oxygen consumption and to allow for total cessation of coronary blood flow between doses, thereby providing a bloodless field for the surgeon. In this fashion, the heart is arrested with cold hyperkalemic cardioplegia (usually with red blood cells), and then maintenance doses of cold normokalemic solution are given at 20- to 30-minute intervals. Alternatively, warm hyperkalemic oxygenated blood cardioplegia may be administered continuously to the heart (74–76). This technique may, however, obscure the surgeon's vision and require local coronary vessel occlusion (in order to sew the bypass grafts), thereby leading to brief periods of local ischemia. The superiority and safety of warm continuous cardioplegia over other methods have not been firmly established (73,77).

Cardioplegia may be administered by three different methods: (a) infusion into the aortic root, (b) direct cannulation of the coronary arteries and/or bypass grafts, and (c) retrograde perfusion via the coronary sinus (78). Any of these routes may be satisfactory in some cases, whereas a particular technique may be optimal in others; therefore, the surgeon should be familiar with all of these methods. Whereas some surgeons use retrograde cardioplegia routinely, others use the technique selectively for circumstances such as reoperations, when there is tight stenosis of the left main or left anterior descending coronary artery, when the left main coronary artery cannot be cannulated during aortic valve replacement, and for mitral valve procedures. Retrograde cardioplegia may not provide optimal protection of the right ventricle. Thus, if it is used, it is important that some antegrade cardioplegia is given into the right coronary artery.

Cardioplegia should be administered immediately after induction of aortic cross-clamping to reduce myocardial ischemia. Furthermore, the surgeon must be aware that standard surface ECG monitors may be an insensitive method of monitoring electrical cardiac arrest. Low-level myocardial activity (and oxygen consumption) may be occurring despite a "flat-line" ECG. Such activity during cross-clamping can compromise myocardial protection.

Hypothermia

The use of hypothermia for heart surgery may be the single most important component of myocardial protection. Hypothermia protects the myocardium by reducing its energy demands and increasing its buffering capacity (79). It also reduces the oxygen and metabolic requirements of the brain and other organs. The myocardial protection provided by systemic hypothermia is superior to that of cold cardioplegia alone, possibly due to better maintenance of myocardial cooling (80). Early in the development of cardioplegia, substantial systemic cooling was used (25°C); recent trends, however, have evolved toward using lesser degrees of cooling (28 to 32°C).

Topical cardiac hypothermia is also used in the form of cold saline or iced slush. The addition of topical hypothermia provides improved myocardial protection, particularly when coronary stenoses prevent the even distribution of cardioplegia (81). It may also be of value to supplement protection of the right ventricle, which may more be subject to rewarming in the surgical field. Care is required in the use of topical hypothermia because of the risk of phrenic nerve paresis associated with excessively cold temperatures (82). An insulation pad may help to protect the phrenic nerve when iced slush is liberally used.

Profound Hypothermia and Circulatory Arrest

Many operations in small infants and certain adult procedures, especially those involving the ascending aorta and aortic arch, are performed using profound core cooling and circulatory arrest. This provides a completely bloodless field and access to all major intrathoracic vessels. Core cooling to under 16 to 18°C is performed. Some studies have suggested that cerebral protection is optimized if deeper cooling is used and arrest times are kept to <30 minutes (83). Hemodilution is an essential part of the profound hypothermia technique to avoid red cell sludging in the capillaries, which can lead to a "no reflow" phenomenon. Rewarming is performed gradually (84). Hypothermia interferes with coagulation factors, causes platelet dysfunction, and activates vasoactive peptides (kinins). The result is impaired hemostasis, and postoperative bleeding is a frequent problem in procedures that employ deep hypothermic circulatory arrest. Aprotinin has been demonstrated to be of value in this setting, although controversy does exist (85).

Separation from Cardiopulmonary Bypass

Preparation for terminating extracorporeal circulation begins even before all technical maneuvers are completed. Among the most important considerations is removal of air from the heart. Despite great care in avoiding air embolism, there is an almost unavoidable introduction of microbubbles into the circulation, beginning with aortic cannulation (86). The use of arterial line filters may reduce this problem (87). In the case of intracardiac surgery, carbon dioxide gas, which is much more soluble than the nitrogen in air and more dense than air, can be flooded onto the surgical field during a procedure to displace air, thus helping to minimize the formation of bubbles that persist in the circulation (88). If this technique is used, additional attention must be paid to blood gas management to avoid hypercarbia from gas absorption or entrainment by cardiotomy suction (89).

Although a steep Trendelenburg position can be used at the time of aortic cross-clamp removal to minimize the passage of air into the carotid arteries, experimental evidence raises questions as to the efficacy of this maneuver (90). Additional methods of removing air from the heart include vigorous ballottement of the heart while filling it with blood before cross-clamp removal, ventilation of the lungs, and suction of the aortic root and the left ventricular vent (91).

Even after meticulous efforts to remove air, cardiac microbubbles can be detected by echocardiography in 75% of patients undergoing intracardiac operations and in 10% of coronary bypass patients (92,93). The effect of these small bubbles on postoperative neurologic status is uncertain.

Large air emboli are rare in contemporary cardiac surgery. CPB circuits incorporate multiple safety systems to avoid massive air embolism, including photoelectric blood level detectors, air-activated ball valves, and automatic shut-off devices. Nevertheless, significant air embolism may still occur. When such a catastrophe happens, the pump should be stopped and the aorta should be vented with the patient in the Trendelenburg position. Reversal of cerebral flow has been proposed by some surgeons (94). Others have advocated hypothermia, steroids (dexamethasone 10 mg i.v.), barbiturates (thiopental 10 mg/kg i.v.), and hyperbaric oxygen therapy (95,96). In general, when antegrade flow is restored in such circumstances, measures to temporarily decrease cerebral metabolic rate, such as hypothermia and use of barbiturates, may be of value to minimize ischemic injury during the transit of air through the microcirculation.

Rhythm

Separation from bypass requires a stable cardiac rhythm. In many cases, the heart must be electrically defibrillated in order to achieve this. A bolus dose of lidocaine (2 mg/kg) immediately before removal of the aortic clamp has been shown to reduce the incidence of ventricular fibrillation during reperfusion (97). Defibrillation should be accomplished with the lowest energy possible because myocardial injury can result from defibrillation, although this occurs only after multiple applications of high-energy shocks (98). Many well-perfused and well-decompressed fibrillating hearts on bypass can be successfully defibrillated with a single shock of 2.5 J, but the vast majority will be defibrillated with 10 J using conventional monophasic defibrillation (99).

Adequate coronary perfusion pressure, higher systemic vascular resistance, physiologic temperature, and serum potassium in the high-normal range facilitate defibrillation. When initial defibrillation attempts fail, increasing defibrillation energy and decreasing left ventricular volume by venting or by manual compression of the heart are two techniques to improve the results of countershock. In addition, increasing aortic perfusion pressure may help achieve successful defibrillation. For the difficult-to-defibrillate heart, we have found that a single bolus dose of esmolol (adult dose 50 to 100 mg) may be of value. For the heart that defibrillates but then repeatedly refibrillates, the use of lidocaine (1- to 2-mg/kg bolus, then infusion 1 to 2 mg/kg per minute for adults) or amiodarone (adult dose 150-mg load over 10 minutes, then 1 mg per minute for 6 hours) may help sustain normal rhythm.

Most arrhythmias that occur during cardiac operations are due to the operative manipulations, preexisting cardiac abnormalities, or myocardial ischemia. Diagnosis of arrhythmias is usually easy with the heart under direct observation. For example, whereas atrial fibrillation, atrial flutter, supraventricular tachycardia, and junctional rhythm may be difficult to distinguish using the surface ECG, they are usually readily discerned by simply inspecting the heart.

Atrial fibrillation may cause reduced cardiac performance during and after separation from CPB. When this occurs, electrical defibrillation of the atria should be attempted. To cardiovert atrial fibrillation, the defibrillator electrodes should be positioned on the atria insofar as possible. Low-level energy (2 to 5 J) should be used as a starting point. If the patient is not on bypass, the defibrillator *must be synchronized* to not discharge during the T-wave of the ECG to avoid causing ventricular fibrillation. Even in patients in whom atrial fibrillation has been present for several months preoperatively, sinus rhythm can sometimes be established for at least a portion of the early postoperative period. When sinus rhythm is established, atrial pacing may help to maintain this rhythm. If ventricular function permits and if catecholamine inotropic agents are not needed, low-level β-blockade, combined with atrial or atrioventricular pacing, not only may control atrial arrhythmias, but also may be of value in patients with ventricular irritability or recurrent ventricular fibrillation.

For patients with poor ventricular function, atrial and ventricular arrhythmias may be a serious issue following CPB and in the postoperative period. In this patient group, short-term amiodarone therapy has been used with increasing frequency (100,101). If needed, a loading dose is administered (150 to 300 mg) followed by an intravenous infusion (1 mg per minute for 6 to 12 hours, followed by 0.5 mg per minute). See Chapter 5 for further discussion of postoperative rhythm management.

Temporary pacing wires are placed on the right atrium and right ventricle (Fig. 2-13) and can be used for diagnostic or therapeutic pacing purposes. In patients receiving bicaval cannulation for CPB, atrial pacing wires can be placed under the pursestring sutures used to secure the atrial cannulation sites.

Temporary cardiac pacing is frequently helpful in maintaining an adequate heart rate, treating arrhythmias, and augmenting cardiac output. Placement of temporary pacing wires at the time of cardiac surgery is standard. Patients with normal cardiac function, as well as those with myocardial impairment benefit from the atrioventricular synchrony that a pacemaker provides (102,103). As a routine measure, we place pacing wires on the right atrium and on the right ventricle to permit sensing and pacing of the atria and ventricles (104). These wires may also be used after the chest is closed in the accurate diagnosis of postoperative arrhythmias by permitting recording of atrial electrograms (105).

Wires used most commonly for temporary postoperative pacing are made of multifilament braided or twisted stainless-steel wire with an attached needle to permit insertion into ventricular muscle. Although this type of pacing lead provides sufficient reliability for most cardiac surgical patients, if pacing, particularly ventricular pacing, is expected to be needed for more than a few days, then temporary pacing leads with discrete solitary alloy electrodes provide greater reliability over more extended periods of time (106,107). Many institutions use leads with discrete electrodes routinely rather than plain wires. Bipolar temporary pacing leads are also available that have two discrete (4-mm) electrodes that are separated by a distance thought to be optimal for electrical pacing and sensing. Bipolar lead performance is generally considered to be superior to unipolar leads, particularly in the atrium.

Contemporary external pacers are capable of atrial sensing. Thus, physiologic "tracking" of the atria is possible, resulting in

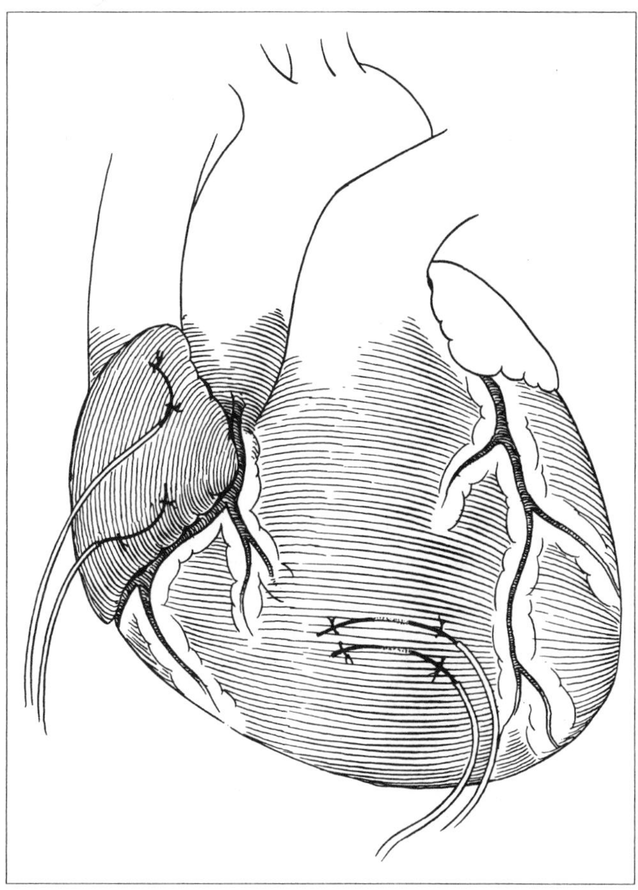

Fig. 2-13. Placement of temporary atrial and ventricular pacing wires at the end of the operation.

the benefits of atrioventricular synchrony without having to overdrive a native atrial rate such as AAI or DDD mode (see Chapter 5). The sensed atrial electrical potential is of smaller amplitude than sensed ventricular potentials, and spurious sensing and inappropriate ventricular pacing may occur because of electrical noise in the environment. To avoid this, bipolar atrial electrodes are placed 1 to 2 cm apart on the atrium, so that the amount of atrial muscle depolarizing between the two electrodes creates a signal of sufficient amplitude for the pacer to sense. If an external DDD pacer is to be used, atrial lead position should be optimized before the chest is closed to ensure that dependable atrial sensing is obtained.

Weaning From Bypass

After the placement of pacing wires, restoration of a satisfactory native or paced rhythm, and rewarming of the patient to at least 35°C, ventilation is resumed. At this point, the surgeon determines that satisfactory lung expansion occurs with ventilation, that there is no closed pneumothorax, and that ventilation compromises no structures (e.g., places tension on an internal mammary artery graft). Failure to achieve adequate ventilation may require repositioning or clearing the endotracheal tube. Mucous plugs or blood clots may create a ball-valve effect on the end of the endotracheal tube, and this may not be resolved by passage of a suction catheter. Complete endotracheal tube removal and insertion of a new tube on bypass may be required when ventilation is unsatisfactory. Rarely, bronchoscopy must be performed to establish a clear tracheobronchial tree. Pleural effusions are drained, and pleural tubes may be inserted prior to weaning from bypass, so that optimum lung expansion is ensured.

During the terminal phases of rewarming on bypass, systemic vascular resistance, and hence the systemic arterial pressure, may be low. This vasodilation is due to anesthesia, hemodilution (with resultant low blood viscosity), and preoperative use of antihypertensive and vasodilator medications. Knowledge of the prebypass cardiac output can help determine what, if any, intervention is needed to increase systemic vascular resistance prior to weaning bypass. In general, at a bypass flow equivalent to prebypass cardiac output, the desired mean blood pressure will vary according to the type of patient undergoing surgery. For example, patients with normal coronary arteries having surgery for lesions such as atrial septal defect or mitral valve pathology can be weaned from bypass with initially lower systemic pressures (e.g., mean pressure 60 to 70 mm Hg), whereas other patients such as those with coronary artery disease or with left ventricular hypertrophy may need higher systemic pressure to obtain stable hemodynamics (e.g., mean pressure 70 to 80 mm Hg or even greater). Phenylephrine and norepinephrine are two agents commonly used to increase the systemic vascular resistance.

Weaning from CPB requires adequate filling of the heart. With guidance from the surgeon, the perfusionist inhibits the venous return from the patient to the bypass apparatus and progressively transfers the fluid volume into the patient. During weaning from bypass, systemic arterial pressure and cardiac filling pressures are observed as the blood volume in the patient is gradually increased. In addition to information from invasive monitoring, adequate filling is also confirmed by observation of ventricular size and motion and by palpation of the PA and aorta. TEE can also help assess left ventricular filling and is particularly useful for this purpose in patients with left ventricular hypertrophy. Caution must be used in attempting to infer left ventricular end-diastolic pressure or left ventricular volume from PA diastolic or pulmonary capillary wedge pressures; the latter are at best unreliable guides to the former (108). Knowledge of prebypass filling pressures can often serve as a preliminary guide to filling pressures during weaning from bypass. If ventricular performance was reasonably good preoperatively and an effective operation has been performed with good myocardial protection, CPB can usually be terminated without difficulty.

If the patient does not manifest adequate perfusion after achieving adequate cardiac filling pressures, the surgeon must attempt to determine a cause. In the absence of a definable, remediable condition, poor myocardial performance may require a return to CPB for an additional period of reperfusion before a second attempt to separate. During this time, the use of inotropic agents and afterload reduction may be initiated and often make it possible to separate the patient from bypass. At this point, TEE is extremely useful to examine global and regional ventricular function and valve function. In a systematic way, TEE can evaluate the results of the surgical repair, that valve function is satisfactory, and that regional and global myocardial function is adequate. If mechanical heart valve(s) have been implanted, their function and seating can be confirmed. The information gained from TEE should be approximately consistent with that obtained by examination in the surgical field and that obtained by invasive monitoring. Residual mechanical lesions or valve dysfunction should be resolved, even if another period of aortic cross-clamping and cardioplegia is required. If the cause of failure to wean from bypass is poor ventricular function, inotropic support should be increased, with increasing doses of β-agonists (epinephrine and/or norepinephrine) and, if required, the addition of milrinone. If function is still inadequate, an intraaortic balloon pump is placed. If hemodynamics are not stable and improving after weaning a marginal patient from CPB, mechanical support should be considered, first with an intraaortic balloon pump. If this is inadequate, single-ventricle or biventricular cardiac assist may be required. Chapter 8 discusses mechanical support of the heart in more detail.

Decannulation

After separation of the patient from CPB and reinfusion of the appropriate fluid volume from the bypass circuit, the venous and arterial cannulas are removed, and the previously placed purse-string sutures are secured. Before removal of the arterial cannula, protamine administration should be started. Thus, as discussed previously, if a serious protamine reaction occurs, it is easy to readminister heparin and return to full CPB to resuscitate the patient. The protamine dose should be given slowly, and if hemodynamics are stable after the first 10% to 15% is given, decannulation can proceed. At some hospitals, removal of the arterial cannula is delayed until just after all of the protamine has been given to the patient.

After successful weaning from CPB and protamine administration, blood remaining in the bypass circuit is usually hemoconcentrated by recirculation through a hemofilter or through a cell-saver device. The concentrated product is then returned to the patient.

CARDIAC SURGERY WITHOUT CARDIOPULMONARY BYPASS

CPB results in a systemic ("whole-body") inflammatory response with resultant capillary leakage, organ edema, and coagulopathy (109–111). In recent years, the development of devices to stabilize the beating heart, combined with better pharmacologic control of hemodynamics during cardiac surgery, has led to the ability to revascularize the heart while beating and without the use of CPB ("off pump") (112–115). With use of pericardial retraction sutures, fluid administration, and control of heart rate and blood pressure, it is possible to retract the heart while it is beating so as to gain access to any myocardial territory for placement of distal anastomoses. Although practices vary widely, patients are heparinized (150 to 400 U/kg) during the procedure. Proximal and distal control is obtained of the coronary artery being grafted, usually in conjunction with a device to produce localized immobilization. Off-pump revascularization strategies usually call for placing the first bypass graft to the artery supplying the myocardial territory most at risk for ischemia, followed by the remainder of planned anastomoses. The technique is used for multivessel revascularization, including techniques that base all bypasses on the mammary arteries, thus obviating the need to place a clamp on the aorta. Although CPB is not utilized, considerable fluid administration may be required during off-pump surgery to maintain the systemic blood pressure. This may result in significant fluid gain. Practices vary widely with respect to heparin neutralization; we generally administer a full CPB dose of heparin (420 U/kg) and partially reverse the heparin with a small dose of protamine (50 to 75 mg). Aspirin is administered early after surgery. In addition, as CPB is not utilized, excessive intraoperative hypothermia can be a concern, and the operating room temperature should be increased and/or or a warming blanket should be utilized during off-pump surgery.

Theoretically, off-pump coronary bypass procedures should obviate the potential risks of CPB and may be of particular value in high-risk patients such as those with cerebrovascular disease, aortic atherosclerosis, or renal failure. Studies have demonstrated the safety and efficacy of this technique. Potential benefits include reductions in blood transfusions, stroke, and encephalopathy (116–120). The technique may be particularly useful for higher-risk patients, especially those with atherosclerosis involving the ascending aorta. Potential disadvantages include incomplete myocardial revascularization with a possible increased need for future coronary interventions (121,122).

Pericardial Closure

Some surgeons believe it is desirable to reapproximate the pericardium in patients in whom future reoperation may be possible; in practice, this includes all but the very elderly. Pericardial closure may diminish the formation of adhesions, although this point is debatable. It certainly interposes some tissue between the sternum and the anterior wall of the heart, which may increase the safety of subsequent resternotomy. When the pericardium cannot be closed, approximation of opposite pleuras may be performed instead. Other surgeons have questioned the value of pericardial closure, with some studies suggesting possible adverse hemodynamic consequences. In most practices, the pericardium is not closed if coronary bypass grafting has been performed. In other patients, it is closed if it is tolerated hemodynamically. For the patient in whom the native pericardium cannot be approximated or is absent, a variety of pericardial substitutes have been advocated, including bovine pericardium, silicone rubber, and polytetrafluoroethylene (123–126). Use of these materials has uncertain benefits; dense adhesions between the prosthesis and the epicardium, severe inflammatory reactions, pericardial effusions, and calcification have been described (127,128).

Closure of the Chest

Large tubes are positioned in the mediastinum before the chest is closed (Fig. 2-14). Conventionally, one tube lies on top of the diaphragm and another behind the sternum. Use of large (≥32 Fr) tubes may reduce the possibility of tube obstruction due to clots and consequent tamponade. Additionally, the pleural spaces

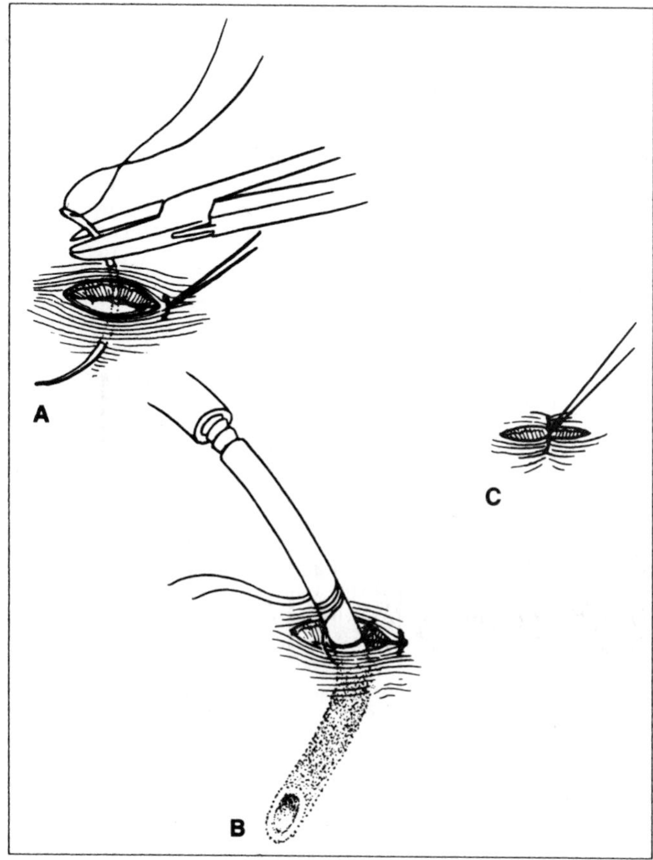

Fig. 2-14. Mediastinal tubes are secured to the skin with heavy silk suture. In addition, a heavy silk suture may be placed for subsequent closure of the chest tube insertion incision (A). The suture is not tied at the time of chest tube insertion, but the excess suture is wrapped around the chest tube (B). After chest tube removal, the suture is tied down to reapproximate the skin edges (C).

should be drained if they have been entered or if pleural effusions are present.

Closure of the chest must never be performed in a casual fashion. Lack of sternal stability is a principal cause of wound complications (129–131). The increased operative mortality associated with sternal wound infections dictates a precise and standardized approach to sternotomy closure to minimize the frequency of this dreaded complication. Excellent results have been obtained by surgeons using a wide variety of materials for sternal reapproximation, including wires, sutures, and metal bands (132). Patients at high risk for sternal instability include obese patients, patients with chronic obstructive lung disease, and patients with impaired mobility who must use crutches or significant traction with their arms to ambulate. In these situations, use of extra wires, double wires, or sternal bands may help confer additional sternal stability and integrity of the closure.

The obese patient and the cachectic patient share a common risk of sternal wound problems, the former because of the increased force applied to the line of closure and the latter because of decreased tissue strength. To a greater degree than patients of normal habitus, these individuals require particular attention to hemostasis, careful approximation of tissues, and avoidance of dead space. It is, at times, helpful to perform the "sternal weave" technique to reinforce the fragile or narrow sternum (131).

Proper closure of the abdominal fascia must not be neglected. Incisional hernia has been reported in 4% of patients undergoing median sternotomy, and up to one-third of these may be sufficiently symptomatic to require operative repair. Hernia is most common in males, obese patients, and patients with complicated postoperative courses (133).

Special Problems in Chest Closure

At times, myocardial edema, acute cardiac dilatation, or other problems may make closure of the sternum impossible. On these occasions, closure of the skin alone or coverage with a silicone rubber sheet may be performed (134). Struts may be cut from chest tubes to hold the sternal edges apart. In 1 to 4 days, the patient may be returned to the operating room for sternal approximation and complete wound closure when cardiac edema has subsided. This procedure does not increase the risk of mediastinitis or sternal osteomyelitis.

Postoperative sternotomy wound infection and mediastinitis are a major source of morbidity and mortality. These issues are discussed in detail in Chapter 5.

TRANSPORT OF THE PATIENT

Movement of the postoperative patient from the operating room to the recovery area or intensive care unit is potentially hazardous. Narcotic anesthesia minimizes hemodynamic changes during this critical period (135). Safe transport of the patient from the operating room requires careful attention to all intravascular catheters, infusion devices, and drainage tubes. The patient's ECG, blood pressure, and, ideally, oxygen saturation are monitored continuously with a battery-powered transport monitor. A portable defibrillator also accompanies the patient. Adequate ventilation and oxygenation must be ensured. If the patient is awakening, additional sedation may be necessary to avoid thrashing, which may cause disconnection of a life-supporting piece of equipment or hemodynamic instability. For our pediatric patients, we arrange for the postoperative nurse to come to the operating room to assist in transport. This measure facilitates proper organization and rapid reconnection of essential monitors and drugs on arrival in the intensive care unit.

REFERENCES

1. Cable DG, Mullany CJ, Schaff HV. The Allen test. *Ann Thorac Surg* 1999;67:876–877.
2. Bazarel MG, Welch M, Golding LAR, et al. Comparison of brachial and radial arterial pressure monitoring in patients undergoing coronary bypass surgery. *Anesthesiology* 1990;73:28–45.
3. Dorman T, Breslow MJ, Lipsett PA, et al. Radial artery pressure monitoring underestimates central artery pressure during vasopressor therapy in critically ill surgical patients. *Crit Care Med* 1998;26:1646–1649.
4. Mohr R, Lavee J, Goor DA. Inaccuracy of radial artery pressure measurement after cardiac operations. *J Thorac Cardiovasc Surg* 1987;94:286–290.
5. Augoustides J, Weiss SJ, Pochettino A. Hemodynamic monitoring of the postoperative adult cardiac surgery patient. *Semin Thorac Cardiovasc Surg* 2000;12:309–315.
6. Gardner RM, Schwartz R, Wong HC, et al. Percutaneous indwelling radial-artery catheters for monitoring cardiovascular function. Prospective study of the risk of thrombosis and infection. *N Engl J Med* 1974;290:1227–1231.
7. Black IH, Blosser SA, Murray WB. Central venous pressure measurements: peripherally inserted catheters versus centrally inserted catheters. *Crit Care Med* 2000;28:3833–3836.
8. McEnany MT, Austen WG. Life-threatening hemorrhage from inadvertent cervical arteriotomy. *Ann Thorac Surg* 1977;24:233.
9. Pearson ML, Hierholzer WJ, Garner JS, et al. Guidelines for prevention of intravascular-device-related infections. *Infect Control Hosp Epidemiol* 1996;17:438–473.
10. Kac G, Durain E, Amrein, et al. Colonization and infection of pulmonary artery catheter in cardiac surgery patients: epidemiology and multivariate analysis of risk factors. *Crit Care Med* 2001;29:971–975.
11. Mullerworth MH, Angelopoulos P, Couyant MA, et al. Recognition and management of catheter-induced pulmonary artery rupture. *Ann Thorac Surg* 1998;66:1242–1245.
12. Urschel JD, Myerowitz PD. Catheter-induced pulmonary artery rupture in the setting of cardiopulmonary bypass. *Ann Thorac Surg* 1993;56:585–589.
13. Sirivella S, Gielchinsky I, Parsonnet V. Management of catheter-induced pulmonary artery perforation: a rare complication in cardiovascular operations. *Ann Thorac Surg* 2001;72:2056–2059.
14. Raper R, Sibbald WJ. Misled by the wedge? The Swan–Ganz catheter and left ventricular preload. *Chest* 1986;89:427–434.
15. D'Ambra MN, Beller JP. Pulmonary circulation: pharmacologic management. In: Grillo HC, Austen WG, Wilkins EW Jr, et al., eds. *Current therapy in cardiothoracic surgery*. Toronto: BC Decker, 1989:278–281.

16. Gold JP, Jonas RA, Lang P, et al. Transthoracic intracardiac monitoring lines in pediatric surgical patients: a ten-year experience. *Ann Thorac Surg* 1986;42:185–191.
17. Russell GN, Ip Yam PC, Tran J, et al. Gastroesophageal reflux and tracheobronchial contamination after cardiac surgery: should a nasogastric tube be routine? *Anesth Analg* 1996;83:228–232.
18. Leal-Noval SR, Marquez-Vacaro JA, Garcia-Curiel A, et al. Nosocomial pneumonia in patients undergoing heart surgery. *Crit Care Med* 2000;28:935–940.
19. Risk CS, Brandon D, D'Ambra MN, et al. Indications for the use of pacing pulmonary artery catheters in cardiac surgery. *J Cardiothorac Anesth* 1992;6:275–279.
20. Pulmonary Artery Catheter Consensus Conference Participants. Pulmonary Artery Catheter Consensus Conference: consensus statement. *Crit Care Med* 1997;25:910–925.
21. Schwann TA, Zacharias A, Riorda CJ, et al. Safe, highly selective use of pulmonary artery catheters in coronary artery bypass grafting: an objective patient selection method. *Ann Thorac Surg* 2002;73:1394–1402.
22. Tuman KJ, McCarthy RJ, Spiess BD, et al. Effect of pulmonary artery catheterization on outcome in patients undergoing coronary artery surgery. *Anesthesiology* 1989;70:199–206.
23. Mishra M, Chauhan CR, Sharma KK, et al. Real-time intraoperative transesophageal echocardiography—how useful? Experience of 5,016 cases. *J Cardiothorac Vasc Anesth* 1998;12:625–632.
24. Bryan AJ, Barzilai B, Kouchoukos NT. Transesophageal echocardiography and adult cardiac operations. *Ann Thorac Surg* 1995;59:773–779.
25. Al-Tabbaa A, Gonzalez RM, Lee D. The role of state-of the-art echocardiography in the assessment of myocardial injury during and following cardiac surgery. *Ann Thorac Surg* 2001;72: S2214–S2219.
26. Ochiai Y, Morita S, Tanoue Y, et al. Use of transesophageal echocardiography for postoperative evaluation of right ventricular function. *Ann Thorac Surg* 1999;67:146–153.
27. Morehead AJ, Firstenberg MS, Shiota T, et al. Intraoperative echocardiographic detection of regurgitant jets after valve replacement. *Ann Thorac Surg* 2000;69:135–139.
28. Backofen JE, Schauble JF, Rogers MC. Transesophageal pacing for bradycardia. *Anesthesiology* 1984;69:595–598.
29. Buchanan D, Clements F, Reves JG, et al. Trial esophageal pacing in patients undergoing coronary artery bypass grafting: effect of previous cardiac operations and body surface area. *Anesthesiology* 1988;69:595–598.
30. Bourke M. The patient with a pacemaker or related device. *Can J Anaesth* 1996;43:R24–R41.
31. Sanford TJ Jr, Smith T, Dec-Silver H, et al. A comparison of morphine, fontanel, and sufentanyl anesthesia for cardiac surgery: induction, emergence, and extubation. *Anesth Analg* 1986;65: 259–266.
32. Engoran MC, Kraras C, Garzia F. Propofol-based versus fentanyl-isoflurane-based anesthesia for cardiac surgery. *J Cardiothorac Vasc Anesth* 1998;12:177–181.
33. Goldstein S, Dean D, Kim SJ et al. A survey of spinal and epidural techniques for adult cardiac surgery. *J Cardiothorac Vasc Anesth* 2001;15:158–168.

34. Ko W, Lazenby D, Zelano JA, et al. Effects of shaving methods and intraoperative irrigation on suppurative mediastinitis after bypass operations. *Ann Thorac Surg* 1992;53:301–305.
35. Bojar RM, Payne DD, Rastegar H, et al. Use of self-adhesive external defibrillator pads for complex cardiac surgical procedures. *Ann Thorac Surg* 1988;46:587–588.
36. Doty DB, DiRusso GB, Doty JR. Full-spectrum cardiac surgery through a minimal incision: mini-sternotomy (lower half) technique. *Ann Thorac Surg* 1998;65:573–577.
37. Pratt JW, Williams TE, Michler RE, et al. Current indications for left thoracotomy in coronary revascularization and valvular procedures. *Ann Thorac Surg* 2000;70:1366–1370.
38. Brutel de la Rieviere A, Brom GH, Nron AG. Horizontal submammary skin incision for median sternotomy. *Ann Thorac Surg* 1981;32:101–104.
39. Dobell ARC, Jain AK. Catastrophic hemorrhage during redo sternotomy. *Ann Thorac Surg* 1984;37:273–278.
40. Loop FD. Catastrophic hemorrhage during sternal reentry. *Ann Thorac Surg* 1984;37:271–272.
41. Machiraju VR. How to avoid problems in redo coronary artery bypass. *J Cardiac Surg* 2001;17:20–25.
42. Dietrich W, Spath P, Ebell A, et al. Prevalence of anaphylactic reactions to aprotinin: analysis of two hundred forty-eight reexposures to aprotinin in heart operations. *J Thorac Cardiovasc Surg* 1997;113:194–201.
43. Hirsh J, Anand SS, Halperin JL, et al. Guide to anticoagulant therapy: heparin. *Circulation* 2001;103:2994–3018.
44. McEvoy GK, ed. *AHFS drug information 2002*. Bethesda: American Society of Health-System Pharmacists, 2002:1444.
45. Despotis GJ, Gravlee G, Filos K, et al. Anticoagulation monitoring during cardiac surgery. *Anesthesiology* 1999;91:1122–1151.
46. Hunt BJ, Segal H, Yacoub M. Aprotinin and heparin monitoring during cardiopulmonary bypass. *Circulation* 1992;86(suppl II): II410–II412.
47. Kondo NI, Maddi R, Ewenstein BM, et al. Anticoagulation and hemostasis in cardiac surgical patients. *J Cardiac Surg* 1994; 9:443–461.
48. Despotis GJ, Joist JH, Hogue WCW, et al. The impact of heparin concentration and activated clotting time monitoring on blood conservation. *J Thorac Cardiovasc Surg* 1995;110:46–54.
49. Shapira N, Schaff HV, Piehler JM, et al. Cardiovascular effects of protamine sulfate in man. *J Thorac Cardiovasc Surg* 1982;84: 505–514.
50. Ravi R, Frost EAM. Cardiac surgery in patients with protamine allergy. *Heart Dis* 1999;5:289–294.
51. Porsche R, Brenner ZR. Allergy to protamine sulfate. *Heart Lung* 1999;28:418–428.
52. Morel DR, Zapol WM, Thomas SJ, et al. C5a and thromboxane generation associated with pulmonary vaso- and bronchoconstriction during protamine administration. *Anesthesiology* 1987;66:597–604.
53. Lowenstein E, Johnston WE, Lappas DG, et al. Catastrophic pulmonary vasoconstriction associated with protamine reversal of heparin. *Anesthesiology* 1983;59:470–473.

54. Kimmel SE, Sekeres MA, Berlin JA, et al. Risk factors for clinically important adverse events after protamine administration following cardiopulmonary bypass. *J Am Coll Cardiol* 1998;32: 1916–1922.
55. Despostis GJ, Joist JH. Anticoagulation and anticoagulation reversal with cardiac surgery involving cardiopulmonary bypass: an update. *J Cardiothorac Vasc Anesth* 1999;13(suppl 1):18–29.
56. Mochizuki T, Olson PJ, Szlam F, et al. Protamine reversal of heparin affects platelet aggregation and activated clotting time after cardiopulmonary bypass. *Anesth Analg* 1998;87:781–785.
57. Staples MH, Dunton RF, Karlson KJ, et al. Heparin resistance after preoperative heparin therapy or intraaortic balloon pumping. *Ann Thorac Surg* 1994;57:1211–1216.
58. Lemmer JH, Despotis GJ. Antithrombin III concentrate to treat heparin resistance in patients undergoing cardiac surgery. *J Thorac Cardiovasc Surg* 2002;123:213–217.
59. Williams MR, D'Ambra AB, Beck JR, et al. A randomized trial of antithrombin concentrate for treatment of heparin resistance. *Ann Thorac Surg* 2000;70:873–877.
60. Follis F, Schmidt CA. Cardiopulmonary bypass in patients with heparin-induced thrombocytopenia and thrombosis. *Ann Thorac Surg* 2000;70:2173–2181.
61. Koster A, Hansen R, Kuppe H, et al. Recombinant hirudin as an alternative to anticoagulation during cardiopulmonary bypass in patients with heparin-induced thrombocytopenia type II: a 1-year experience in 57 patients. *J Cardiothorac Vasc Anesth* 2000;14: 243–248.
62. Chen JL. Argatroban: a direct thrombin inhibitor for heparin-induced thrombocytopenia and other clinical applications. *Heart Dis* 2001;3:189–198.
63. Miller L, Nicest R, Magna NIH. Successful cardiopulmonary bypass surgery with Orgaran in patients with heparin induced thrombocytopenia. *Thromb Haemost* 1997;78(suppl):446.
64. Koster A, Meyer O, Fischer T, et al. One-year experience with the platelet glycoprotein IIb/IIIa antagonist tirofiban and heparin during cardiopulmonary bypass in patients with heparin-induced thrombocytopenia type II. *J Thorac Cardiovasc Surg* 2001;122:1254–1255.
65. Royse C, Royse A, Blake D, et al. Screening the thoracic aorta for atheroma: a comparison of manual palpation, transesophageal and epiaortic ultrasonography. *Ann Thorac Surg* 1998;4:347–350.
66. Leyh RG, Bartels C, Motzold A, et al. Management of the porcelain aorta during coronary artery bypass grafting. *Ann Thorac Surg* 1999;67:986–988.
67. Barbeau YR, Westbrook BM, Charlesworth DC, et al. Arterial inflow via an axillary artery graft for the severely atheromatous aorta. *Ann Thorac Surg* 1998;66:33–37.
68. Sabik JF, Lytle BW, McCarthy PM, et al. Axillary artery: an alternative site of arterial cannulation for patients with extensive aortic and peripheral vascular disease. *J Thorac Cardiovasc Surg* 1995;109:885–890.
69. Whilark JD, Goldman SM, Sutter FP. Axillary artery cannulation in acute ascending aortic dissections. *Ann Thorac Surg* 2000; 69:1127–1128.

70. Lucas SK, Schaff JT, Flaherty JT, et al. The harmful effects of ventricular distension during postischemia reperfusion. *Ann Thorac Surg* 1981;32:486–494.
71. Little AG, Lin CY, Wernly JA, et al. Use of the pulmonary artery for left ventricular venting during cardiac operations. *J Thorac Cardiovasc Surg* 1984;87:532–538.
72. Gay WA Jr, Ebert PA. Functional, metabolic, and morphologic effects of potassium-induced cardioplegia. *Surgery* 1973;74: 284–290.
73. Buckberg GD. Update on current techniques of myocardial protection. *Ann Thorac Surg* 1995;60:805–814.
74. Lichtenstein SV, Ashe KA, el Delati H, et al. Warm heart surgery. *J Thorac Cardiovasc Surg* 1991;101:269–274.
75. Salerno TA, Houck JP, Barrozo CA, et al. Retrograde continuous warm cardioplegia: a new concept in myocardial protection. *Ann Thorac Surg* 1991;51:245–247.
76. Mauney MC, Kron IL. The physiologic basis of warm blood cardioplegia (Review). *Ann Thorac Surg* 1995;60:819–823.
77. Martin TD, Craver JM, Gott JP, et al. Prospective randomized trial of retrograde warm blood cardioplegia: myocardial benefit and neurologic threat. *Ann Thorac Surg* 1994;57:298–304.
78. Solorano J, Taitelbaum G, Chiu RC. Retrograde coronary sinus perfusion for myocardial protection during cardiopulmonary bypass. *Ann Thorac Surg* 1978;25:201–208.
79. Lange R, Cavanaugh AC, Zierler M, et al. The relative importance of alkalinity, temperature, and the washout effect of bicarbonate-buffered, multidose cardioplegic solution. *Circulation* 1984;70 (suppl I):I75–I83.
80. Grover FL, Fewel JG, Ghidoni JJ, et al. Does lower systemic temperature enhance cardioplegic myocardial protection? *J Thorac Cardiovasc Surg* 1981;81:11–20.
81. Lazar HL, Rivers S. Importance of topical hypothermia during heterogeneous distribution of cardioplegic solution. *J Thorac Cardiovasc Surg* 1989;98:251–257.
82. Efthimiou J, Butler J, Woodham C, et al. Diaphragm paralysis following cardiac surgery: the rope of phrenic nerve cold injury. *Ann Thorac Surg* 1991;52:1005–1008.
83. McCollough JN, Zhang N, Reich DL, et al. Cerebral metabolic suppression during hypothermic circulatory arrest in humans. *Ann Thorac Surg* 1999;67:1895–1899.
84. Gfrigore AM, Grocott HP, Matthew JP, et al. The rewarming rate and increased peak temperature alter neurocognitive outcome after cardiac surgery. *Anesth Analg* 2002;94:4–10.
85. Smith CR, Spanier TB. Aprotinin in deep hypothermic circulatory arrest (collective review). *Ann Thorac Surg* 1999;68:278–286.
86. Padayachee TS, Parsons S, Theobold R, et al. The detection of microemboli in the middle cerebral artery during cardiopulmonary bypass: a transcranial Doppler ultrasound investigation using membrane and bubble oxygenators. *Ann Thorac Surg* 1987;44:298–302.
87. Padayachee TS, Parsons S, Theobold R, et al. The effect of arterial filtration on reduction of gaseous microemboli in the middle cerebral artery during cardiopulmonary bypass. *Ann Thorac Surg* 1988;45:647–649.

88. Frados A. Carbon dioxide field flooding: a retrospective study. *J Extracorporeal Technol* 2001;32:91–93.
89. Nadolny EM, Svensson LG. Carbon dioxide field flooding techniques for open heart surgery: monitoring and minimizing potential adverse effects. *Perfusion* 2000;15:151–153.
90. Butler BD, Laine GA, Leiman BC, et al. Effect of the Trendelenburg position on the distribution of arterial air emboli in dogs. *Ann Thorac Surg* 1988;45:198–202.
91. Oka Y, Inoue T, Hong Y, et al. Retained intracardiac air. Transesophageal echocardiography for definition of incidence and monitoring removal by improved techniques. *J Thorac Cardiovasc Surg* 1986;91:329–338.
92. Oka Y, Moriwaki KM, Hong Y, et al. Detection of air emboli in the left heart by M-mode transesophageal echocardiography following cardiopulmonary bypass. *Anesthesiology* 1985;63:109–113.
93. Topol EJ, Humphrey LS, Borkon AM, et al. Value of intraoperative left ventricular microbubbles detected by transesophageal two-dimensional echocardiography in predicting neurologic outcome after cardiac operations. *Am J Cardiol* 1985;56:773–775.
94. Mills NL, Ochsner JL. Massive air embolism during cardiopulmonary bypass. Causes, prevention, and management. *J Thorac Cardiovasc Surg* 1980;80:708–717.
95. Spampinato N, Stassano P, Gagliardi C, et al. Massive air embolism during cardiopulmonary bypass: successful treatment with immediate hypothermia and circulatory support. *Ann Thorac Surg* 1981;32:602–603.
96. Ziser A, Adir Y, Lavon H, et al. Hyperbaric oxygen therapy for massive arterial air embolism during cardiac operations. *J Thorac Cardiovasc Surg* 1999;117:818–821.
97. Fall SM, Burton NA, Graeber GM, et al. Prevention of ventricular fibrillation after myocardial revascularization. *Ann Thorac Surg* 1987;43:182–184.
98. Kerber RE, Carter J, Klein S, et al. Open chest defibrillation during cardiac surgery: energy and current requirement. *Am J Cardiol* 1980;46:393–396.
99. Lake CL, Sellers TD, Nolan SP, et al. Energy dose and other variables possibly affecting ventricular defibrillation during cardiac surgery. *Anesth Analg* 1984;63:743–751.
100. Butler J, Harriss DR, Sinclair M, et al. Amiodarone prophylaxis for tachycardias after coronary artery surgery: a randomized, double-blind, placebo controlled study. *Br Heart J* 1993;70:56–60.
101. Solomon AJ, Greenberg MD, Kilborn MJ, et al. Amiodarone versus a beta-blocker to prevent atrial fibrillation after cardiovascular surgery. *Am Heart J* 2001;142:811–815.
102. Curtis J, Walls J, Boley T, et al. Influence of atrioventricular synchrony on hemodynamics in patients with normal and low ejection fractions following open heart surgery. *Am Surg* 1986;52:93–96.
103. Hartzler GO, Maloney JD, Curtis JJ, et al. Hemodynamic benefits of atrioventricular sequential pacing after cardiac surgery. *Am J Cardiol* 1977;40:232–236.
104. Yiu P, Tansley P, Pepper JR. Improved reliability of postoperative pacing by use of bipolar temporary pacing leads. *Cardiovasc Surg* 2001;9:591–595.
105. Waldo AL, Henthorn RW, Plumb VJ. Temporary epicardial wire electrodes in the diagnosis and treatment of arrhythmias after open heart surgery. *Am J Surg* 1984;148:275–283.

106. Wigneswaran WT, Jamieson MP. Temporary pacing leads in cardiac surgery. A comparison of multifilament braided electrodes and localized solitary stainless steel electrodes. *J Cardiovasc Surg (Torino)* 1986;27:609–612.
107. Kallis P, Batrick N, Bindi F, et al. Pacing thresholds of temporary epicardial electrodes: variation with electrode type, time, and epicardial position. *Ann Thorac Surg* 1994;57:623–626.
108. Douglas PS, Edmunds LH, St. John Sutton M, et al. Unreliability of hemodynamic indexes of left ventricular size during cardiac surgery. *Ann Thorac Surg* 1987;44:31–34.
109. Edmunds LH Jr. Inflammatory response to cardiopulmonary bypass. *Ann Thorac Surg* 1998;66:S12–S16.
110. Boyle EM Jr, Morgan EN, Kovacich JC, et al. Microvascular response to cardiopulmonary bypass. *J Cardiothorac Vasc Anesth* 1999;4(suppl 1):30–37.
111. Laffey JG, Boylan JF, Cheng DCH. The systemic inflammatory response to cardiac surgery. *Anesthesiology* 2002;97:215–252.
112. Heames RM, Gill RS, Ohri SK, et al. Off-pump coronary artery surgery. *Anaesthesia* 2002;57:676–685.
113. Mack MJ. Coronary surgery: off-pump and port access (review). *Surg Clin North Am* 2000;80:1575–1591.
114. Ascione R, Caputo M, Angelini GD. Off-pump coronary artery bypass grafting: not a flash in the pan. *Ann Thorac Surg* 2003; 75:306–313.
115. Plomondon ME, Cleveland JC Jr, Ludwig ST, et al. Off-pump coronary artery bypass is associated with improved risk-adjusted outcomes. *Ann Thorac Surg* 2001;72:114–119.
116. Puskas JD, Thourani VH, Marshall JJ, et al. Clinical outcomes, angiographic patency, and resource utilization in 200 consecutive off-pump coronary bypass patients. *Ann Thorac Surg* 2001;71: 1477–1483.
117. Kshettry VR, Flavin TF, Emery RW, et al. Does multivessel, off-pump coronary bypass reduce postoperative morbidity? *Ann Thorac Surg* 2000;69:1725–1731.
118. Bull DA, Neumayer LA, Stringham JC, et al. Coronary bypass grafting with cardiopulmonary bypass versus off-pump bypass grafting: does eliminating the pump reduce morbidity and cost? *Ann Thorac Surg* 2001;71:170–175.
119. Van Dijk D, Nierich AP, Jansen EWL, et al. Early outcome after off-pump versus on-pump coronary bypass surgery: results from a randomized study. *Circulation* 2001;104:1761–1766.
120. Stamou SC, Jablonski KA, Pfister AJ, et al. Stroke after conventional versus minimally invasive coronary artery bypass. *Ann Thorac Surg* 2002;74:394–399.
121. Arom KV, Flavin TF, Emery RW, et al. Safety and efficacy of off-pump coronary bypass grafting. *Ann Thorac Surg* 2000;69: 704–710.
122. Sabik JF, Gillinov AM, Blackstone EH, et al. Does off-pump coronary surgery reduce morbidity and mortality? *J Thorac Cardiovasc Surg* 2002;124:698–707.
123. Gallo JI, Artinano E, Duran CMG. Clinical experience with glutaraldehyde-preserved heterologous pericardium for the closure of the pericardium after open heart surgery. *Thorac Cardiovasc Surg* 1982;30:306–309.

124. Opie JC, Larrieu AJ, Cornell IS. Pericardial substitutes: delayed reexploration and findings. *Ann Thorac Surg* 1987;43:383–385.
125. Laks H, Hammond G, Geha AS. Use of silicone rubber as a pericardial substitute to facilitate reoperation in cardiac surgery. *J Thorac Cardiovasc Surg* 1981;82:88–92.
126. Minale C, Hollweg G, Nikol S, et al. Closure of the pericardium using expanded polytetrafluoroethylene GORE-TEX surgical membrane: clinical experience. *Thorac Cardiovasc Surg* 1987;35: 312–315.
127. Mills SA. Complications associated with the use of heterologous bovine pericardium for pericardial closure. *J Thorac Cardiovasc Surg* 1986;92:446–454.
128. Skinner JR, Kim H, Toon RS, et al. Inflammatory epicardial reaction to processed bovine pericardium: case report. *J Thorac Cardiovasc Surg* 1984;88:789–791.
129. Labitzke R, Schramm G, Witzel U, et al. “Sleeve-rope closure” of the median sternotomy after open heart operations. *Thorac Cardiovasc Surg* 1983;31:127–128.
130. Robicsek F, Daugherty HK, Cook JW. The prevention and treatment of sternum separation following open-heart surgery. *J Thorac Cardiovasc Surg* 1977;73:267–268.
131. Sanfelippo PM, Danielson GK. Complications associated with median sternotomy. *J Thorac Cardiovasc Surg* 1972;63:419–423.
132. Losanoff JE, Richman BW, Jones JW. Disruption and infection of median sternotomy: a comprehensive review. *Eur J Cardiothorac Surg* 2002;21:831–839.
133. Davidson BR, Bailey JS. Incisional hernia following median sternotomy incisions: their incidence and aetiology. *Br J Surg* 1986;73:995–996.
134. Anderson CA, Filsoufi F, Aklog L, et al. Liberal use of delayed sternal closure for postcardiotomy hemodynamic instability. *Ann Thorac Surg* 2002;73:1484–1488.
135. Insel J, Weissman C, Kemper M, et al. Cardiovascular changes during transport of critically ill and postoperative patients. *Crit Care Med* 1986;14:539–542.
136. Hammon JW, Stump DA, Kon ND et al. Risk factors and solutions for the development of neurobehavioral changes after coronary bypass grafting. *Ann Thorac Surg* 1997;63:1613–1618.

Postoperative Management

Postoperative care of the cardiac surgical patient begins at the time of transfer from the operating room to the intensive care unit (ICU). This is a hazardous period that requires the strict attention of both the anesthesiologist and the surgeon. Electrocardiogram (ECG) and arterial pressure monitoring by a portable, battery-powered unit is essential during the transfer, and basic resuscitation medications (such as epinephrine) should be readily available for quick administration en route, if required. A portable defibrillator should accompany the patient while in transfer. Likewise, a spare endotracheal tube and a laryngoscope should be close at hand for emergency reintubation.

On arrival in the ICU, pressure monitoring lines and ECG leads are transferred to the bedside monitor without delay. Routine monitoring includes ECG, continuous arterial blood pressure, central venous pressure, pulmonary artery pressure and temperature (if a Swan–Ganz catheter is present), and arterial hemoglobin oxygen saturation using a cutaneous pulse oximeter sensor. The external pacemaker, having been attached to the patient's temporary pacing wires in the operating room, is checked to be sure it is turned on and the settings are appropriate (most often a "back-up" ventricular pacing rate appropriate for the patient's age). A verbal report of the patient's condition is given to the primary nurse by the anesthesiologist. This includes a description of the procedure performed, any problems encountered including difficulties with intubation, details regarding the filling pressure at which the patient's heart appears to function best, and any ongoing drug infusions. Blood samples should be sent *stat* for arterial blood gas analysis, hemoglobin level, and sodium and potassium concentrations. Routine measurement of platelet count and other clotting studies may be performed, but these are unnecessary for the patient who is not bleeding excessively.

The heart is auscultated to determine the presence or absence of murmurs and the loudness of the heart sounds. This baseline examination provides a reference for later examination. For example, the later development of a murmur may indicate detachment of a prosthetic valve or patch, and, similarly, muffled heart sounds later on may suggest cardiac tamponade. The chest is auscultated to determine that there are adequate breath sounds bilaterally. If not already present, an oronasogastric tube may be inserted depending on the preference of the surgeon or the presence of abdominal distension. A chest x-ray film is usually obtained, but may not be necessary for the stable patient (1). This provides verification of the position of the endotracheal tube, nasogastric tube, chest tubes, and monitoring cannulas, establishes a baseline measurement of the mediastinal silhouette, and allows one to rule out pneumothorax, hemothorax, or atelectasis. Baseline determinations of the patient's thermodilution cardiac output are obtained early after arrival in the ICU if a pulmonary artery catheter is present.

Vital signs, fluid input and output, and hemodynamic data are recorded at regular intervals on a standardized flow sheet, as shown in Fig. 3-1. The importance of a permanent staff of nurses trained in cardiac surgical care cannot be overemphasized. Such nurses can accurately record measurements, recognize ECG abnormalities, and initiate treatment for problems before they become major ones. Suggestions or concerns raised by an experienced cardiac surgical nurse should not be dismissed lightly by the physicians participating in the care of the postoperative patient.

Preprinted order sheets (Fig. 3-2) are used. These allow for individualization in differing circumstances, but also contain the common orders that are needed for most patients. This increases efficiency and helps prevent the omission of important directives. Likewise, when the patient is ready to be moved out of the ICU, preprinted transfer orders are again employed (Fig. 3-3).

MANAGEMENT OF THE HEMODYNAMIC STATE

Evaluation and Monitoring of Cardiovascular Function

Assessment of the patient's cardiovascular status after cardiac surgery begins with a physical examination. The patient with satisfactory cardiac output and blood pressure typically is alert (if not anesthetized), is warm to the touch, and has palpable pedal pulses (in the absence of lower extremity obstructive vascular disease), whereas the patient with inadequate cardiac output and blood

Date: | **24-Hour Patient Care Summary** | Weight: | Preop Weight:

		8:30	9:30	10:30	11:30	12:30 Noon	1:30	2:30	3:30 pm	8°	4:30 pm	5:30	6:30	7:30	8:30	9:30	10:30	11:30 pm	8°	12:30 MN	1:30	2:30	3:30	4:30	5:30	6:30	7:30	8°
Vital Signs	Arterial Pressure																											
	Pulse																											
	Temperature																											
	Respirations																											
	CVP																											
	PAP																											
	LAP																											
	CI																											
Intake	D_5W																											
	Oral																											
	q 1° Total																											
	Running Total In																											
	Blood Products																											
	q 1° Total																											
	Running Total In																											
Output	Urine q 1°																											
	Chest tubes																											
	Mediastinal tubes																											
	Other																											
	Running Total Out																											
Lab Values	Respirator Settings: TV																											
	FI_{O_2}																											
	Gases: Sat																											
	PO_2																											
	PCO_2																											
	PH																											
	HCO_3																											
	Na / Cl																											
	K / CO_2																											
	HCT																											
	Other																											

Fig. 3-1. Intensive care unit flow sheet for recording patient data.

DATE & TIME	LABORATORY, THERAPEUTIC & DIETARY ORDERS	
	Admit to ICU Procedure: Cardiologist:	
	Continuous monitoring: ECG, arterial, pulmonary artery, O_2 saturation	
	Vital signs per ICU protocol; weigh upon admission and then q day: Measure I & O.	
	Chest tubes to collection device @ -20cm suction. Autotransfue chest drainage when >300 ml if collection time < 4 hr. DO not give blood that had been in collection chamber > 4 hours. Nasogastric tube (if present) to low continuous suction	
	Lab studies: Electrolytes, glucose, creatinine, BUN, CBC on arrival, prn then q day for 2 days. Call MD for glucose > 150.	
	If bleeding (>200ml first hour or > 150 ml/hr for 2 hr): platelet count, PT/INR, fibrinogen level	
	CXR upon arrival, prn for bleeding > 200/hr, and then q day	
	ECG on POD #1	
	Diet: NPO until extubated. Then clear liquids and advance to cardiac and/or diabetic diet as indicated	
	Temp pacemakerL rate 80-90/min or ____; DDD or VVI (circle)	
	IV & VENTILATOR ORDERS	
	IV: D-5-W at ___ ml/hr	
	Ventilator settings: FiO_2 ____%; TV ____ml; rate ____/min Mode: AC or SIMV, PS ____; PEEP ___ MM Hg Titrate Fi O_2 to maintain O_2 saturation $\geq$ 93% Incentive spirometer – use q 1 hr when awake after extubation	
	PARAMETERS FOR DRUG & FLUID MANAGEMENT	
	SBP 90 –120 or ____ mm HG; MAP 60-90 or ____mmHg CI> 2.2 or ____; PCWP 6-16 or ____ mm HG; SVR 600–1600 or ___	
	MEDICATIONS	
	Cefazolin 1 g IV q 8 hr X 24; Pharmacy to adjust for renal function. If allergic to cephalosporin or penicillin – pharmacy to evaluate allergy and order antibiotic per protocol.	
	Nitroglycerin infusion 10 - ___ mcg/min; hold for SBP< 100	
	Aspirin 325 mg/pr qd. Begin within 6 hours of CABG if not bleeding. Do not give to valve patients.	
	Acetominophen 650 mg po/pr q 4 hr prn temp > 38.5 Limit 3 doses/24 hr.	
	Morphinie 2-5 mg IV q 1-2 hr prn OR hydromorphan 1-2 mg q 3-4 hr prn	
	Oxycodone 5-15 mg po q 3-4 hr when taking po OR acetominophen with codeine 1-2 tabs q 3-4 hr	
	Meperidine 10-25 mg IV q 1-2 hr prn shivering	
	Ondansetron 2-4 mg IV prn nausea	
	Midazolam 1-4 mg IV q 1 hr prn while intubated	
	Lorazepam 0.5-2.0 mg IV q 2-4hr prn after extubation	
	Furosemide: If PCW/PAD > 15 mm Hg and urine output < 25 ml/hr X 2 hr give 40 mg IV. May repeat 40 mg IV in 1-2 hr X1 when UO < 30 ml/hr during first 24 hr postop	
	KCl: Maintain serum K^+ 4.0 – 5.0. All KCl through central line using infusion pump; dilute KCl in 50-100 ml D5W. Repeat serum K^+ prn during replacement; If serum creatinine $\geq$ 1.5 mg/dL, give initial dose only and consult MD for repeat doses. If $K^+ \leq 4.2$; give 20 mEq over 1 hr If $K^+ \leq 3.5$; give 30 mEq over 1 hr If $K^+ \leq 3.5$; give 40 mEq over 1 hr	
	Other:	

Fig. 3-2. Typical physician's postoperative orders for adults in the intensive care unit following cardiac surgery.

DATE & TIME		
	Transfer to ____________ Procedure ____________________ POD # ________ Surgeon ____________________ Cardiologist ____________	
	Continuous telemetry ECG monitoring	
	Vital signs q 8 hr. Measure & record I & O. Weigh on transfer, then daily	
	Chest tubes to collection device @ -20cm suction if present.	
	Remove Foley catheter on POD #_____. If unable to void in 8-12 hr, may straight cath X 1.	
	Pacemaker orders:	
	Diet: progress from full liquid to cardiac diet (if indicated)	
	Fluid limit: ________ml/24 hr	
	Nasal prong O_2 _____L/min prn. Spot check O_2 saturation q shift X3 then prn. Titrate to keep saturation > 93%.	
	Incentive spirometer q 2-3 hr when awake	
	Up into chair today. Ambulate quid with assistance starting in AM.	
	Patient teaching by Cardiac Rehabilitation (Phase I/II) and by Dietician	
	Labs: 1. CBC, comprehensive panel, CXR, ECG on 3rd day after transfer or on _________ 2. Daily PT & INR if patient on warfarin Call _________________with result for warfarin order 3. Stat serum K^+ and Mg^{++} for increasing ventricular arrhythmias 4. Check serum K^+ 6 hr after IV furosemide dose	
	If serum $K^+ < 3.9$, give KCl replacement according to sliding scale: Serum K^+ — Oral KCl dose 3.8 - 3.6 — 30 mEq 3.5 - 3.0 — 40 mEq <3.0 — 50 mEq If serum $K^+ \leq 3.5$, recheck 3 hr after each dose and repeat until $K^+ \geq 3.6$ If serum creatinine > 1.5, give initial dose only. Call MD for repeat doses	
	Routine wound care.	
	For mild to moderate pain: hyrocodone/APA 5/500 to 10/1000 q 3-4 hr prn. Max 8 tabs per day	
	For moderate to severe pain: oxycodone 5-15 mg po q 3-4 hr OR morphine _____ mg, IV/IM (circle), q ______hr prn	
	Aspirin 325 mg po qd. Do not give to valve patients	
	Docusate NA 100 mg po bid; hold for loose stools	
	Acetominophen 650 mg po/pr q 4 hr prn temp > 38.5 Limit 3 doses/24 hr.	
	Ondansetron 2-4 mg IV prn nausea	
	Bisacodyl suppository prn constipation	
	Lorazepam 1-2 mg po q 6 hr prn anxiety	
	Temazepam 15 mg po qhs prn sleep	
	Other:	

Fig. 3-3. Adult postoperative cardiac surgery transfer orders.

pressure typically may be agitated or lethargic, with cool skin and slow capillary refill, and may have no palpable pedal pulses. The patient with cardiac failure, unless hypovolemic, often has jugular venous distention, but more subtle and chronic signs of heart failure such as a third heart sound or pulmonary crackles may be difficult to discern in the noisy ICU environment. The physical examination can also be confounded by the effects of hypothermia (causing peripheral vasoconstriction and cool extremities) and anesthetic agents (causing unresponsiveness). Congestive heart failure in infants is not manifested by peripheral edema or orthopnea as it is in adults. One must look instead for hepatomegaly, facial puffiness, unexplained tachycardia, weight gain, cardiac enlargement, or tachypnea.

Other parameters such as hourly urine output are taken into account, but can be misleading early after open-heart surgery. Patients with satisfactory cardiac output and blood pressure usually exhibit a relative diuresis early after surgery due to the effects of hemodilution and the osmotic agents sometimes administered during cardiopulmonary bypass (CPB). Because of these factors, even patients with poor cardiovascular performance early after surgery may continue to produce significant amounts of urine for several hours after operation. Later, when the effects of CPB have cleared, urine output becomes a more sensitive measure of cardiac output and blood pressure: A low urine output (<30 to 50 mL per hour in adults or 0.5 mL/kg per hour in infants) indicates inadequate hemodynamic performance and requires prompt investigation and treatment.

Invasive measurements provide important complementary information to these noninvasive observations (2). It must be remembered, however, that all catheters, cannulas, monitors, and tracings may be inaccurate, misread, or mislabeled. *Proper management of the cardiac surgery patient never relies on a single "number" to dictate the direction of therapy, but rather takes into account the results of all noninvasive and invasive information that is available.*

Arterial pressure is monitored continuously, usually via a cannula in the patient's radial artery. Although systolic arterial pressure reflects the systolic pressure within the left ventricle (in the absence of obstructive lesions such as aortic stenosis), arterial blood pressure is not a sensitive measure of overall hemodynamic status. The ability of the systemic circulation to vasoconstrict and maintain a relatively normal blood pressure, even in the presence of very poor cardiac function, makes this measure of hemodynamic function often the "last to fall" before total cardiovascular collapse.

Flow-directed (Swan–Ganz) pulmonary artery catheters are utilized routinely for monitoring adult patients undergoing cardiac surgery at many, but not all, hospitals or only in selected patients at other institutions. These catheters provide continuous measurement of the pulmonary artery systolic, diastolic, and mean pressures, allow for thermodilution measurements of the right heart cardiac output, and provide access for blood sampling from the pulmonary artery (mixed venous blood).

The concepts of *preload* and *afterload* are important in the care of cardiac surgical patients. For the ventricle to produce an adequate output, it first must be adequately filled. Technically, the volume of blood within the ventricle at the end of diastole is the best measure of ventricular filling and best reflects the preload of the heart, but this is difficult to measure routinely. The left ventricular end-diastolic pressure reflects the ventricular volume (ignoring the effects of compliance). However, to measure the left ventricular end-diastolic pressure, a catheter must be placed within the left ventricle, and this has the potential risks of emboli, ventricular irritability, and bleeding through the site of introduction. The mean left atrial pressure is a good measurement of left ventricular filling pressure; left atrial catheters are used for this purpose in selected patients (see Fig. 2-4). Even safer and more convenient, however, is the pulmonary capillary wedge pressure, which is obtained at the end of the pulmonary artery catheter when the vessel is occluded (or "wedged") by temporary inflation of a balloon positioned at the end of the catheter (see Fig. 2-3). The pulmonary capillary wedge pressure closely approximates left ventricular end-diastolic pressure in patients with normal hearts, although it tends to be lower than the end-diastolic pressure in many patients with cardiac disease (3).

Thermodilution cardiac output determination is based on the principle of temperature dilution. The pulmonary artery catheter has at least three lumina: one proximally opening into the right atrium, one at the catheter tip for pressure measurements, and the third for filling the balloon. The catheter and the associated computer derive the cardiac output by analysis of the decrement in temperature in the pulmonary artery produced by the dilution of a bolus of cold saline injected into the right atrial port; the temperature sensor is at the distal tip of the catheter. Thermodilution measurements of right heart cardiac output (and, normalized to body surface area, the cardiac index) provide generally reliable and useful information regarding the hemodynamic state of the patient, as the left ventricular output is usually identical. The computed cardiac output value can, however, be erroneous due to the improper injection rate or injectate volume of saline or its incorrect temperature. Thermodilution measurement of right heart output is an inaccurate measure of left heart output in the presence of a left-to-right shunt. In such instances (e.g., when the patient has an acute postinfarction ventricular septal defect), the measured thermodilution output is falsely higher than the true systemic output of the left ventricle. Tricuspid valve insufficiency may make the cardiac output determination less accurate by producing artifacts in the thermodilution curve.

Pulmonary artery catheters are not required for the successful management of heart surgery patients, in particular those at low risk for myocardial dysfunction (4,5). Risks of placing the catheter include ventricular arrhythmias and pulmonary artery rupture. Presence of pulmonary artery rupture should be suspected in any patient with a pulmonary artery catheter who experiences hemoptysis. Most commonly, the right pulmonary artery or its branch is the bleeding source. The presentation may be a small "herald" bleed, delayed recurrent hemorrhage, or exsanguination (6). Constant awareness of this rare but catastrophic complication is essential. Management of catheter-induced pulmonary artery perforation is highly individualized and involves removal of the catheter, establishment of adequate ventilation, and evaluation and intervention to achieve control of the bleeding (7,8). Depending on the amount of bleeding and other circumstances, management options include bronchoscopy, intrabronchial tamponade with a balloon catheter to protect the remaining airway, early pulmonary arteriography with embolization occlusion of the bleeding vessel, and emergency lung resection.

By measuring the arterial pressure and cardiac output, it is possible to derive the systemic vascular resistance (SVR) (Table 3-1). This parameter is also referred to as afterload. High afterload indicates vasoconstriction, whereas low afterload indicates vaso-

Table 3-1. Hemodynamic parameters

Parameter	Formula	Normal Values
Mean arterial blood pressure (MAP)	[SBP + (2 × DBP)]/3	60–105 mm Hg
Cardiac output (CO)	SV × HR	4–8 L/min
Cardiac index (CI)	CO/BSA	2.5–4.0 L/min/m^2
Stroke volume (SV)	CO/HR × 1,000	60–100 mL/beat
Systemic vascular resistance (SVR)	(MAP – RAP or CVP)/CO × 80	800–1,400 dyne-sec/m^5
Pulmonary vascular resistance (PVR)	(PAP_m – PCWP)/ CO × 80	100–150 dyne-sec/m^5
Left ventricular stroke work (LVSW)	SV/(MAP – PCWP) × 0.0136	60–80 g-m/beat

BSA, body surface area; CVP, central venous pressure; DBP, diastolic blood pressure; HR, heart rate; PAP_m, pulmonary artery pressure (mean); PCWP, pulmonary capillary wedge pressure; RAP, right atrial pressure; SBP, systolic blood pressure; SV, stroke volume.

dilatation. The magnitude of afterload is based on arterial pressure and cardiac output. A high calculated SVR indicates a high resistance to the ejection of blood from the left ventricle or a state of low cardiac output with compensatory vascular constriction to maintain the blood pressure. Pharmacologic management of the SVR is an important aspect of the management of altered hemodynamic states such as low cardiac output. It must be realized, however, that the SVR is derived from three measurements (mean aortic pressure, right atrial pressure, and cardiac output), each of which has potential sources of error and degrees of inexactness. Thus, derived vascular resistance should be considered an estimate, but not an accurate determination, of the state of constriction of the circulation. Likewise, pulmonary vascular resistance (PVR) may be derived as shown in Table 3-1.

Oxygen saturation of the pulmonary artery mixed venous blood (S_vO_2) is indicative of both oxygen delivery (cardiac output, arterial saturation, hemoglobin level) and oxygen consumption. Pulmonary artery catheters that have a built-in oxygen saturation sensor at the distal tip can continuously measure the S_vO_2, which is displayed on a bedside monitor. The normal S_vO_2 is approximately 80%. Factors that can lead to a decrease in the S_vO_2 include decreased cardiac output, hypoxia, anemia, and patient shivering. Being a continuously monitored parameter, the S_vO_2 may provide an early indication of significant hemodynamic alterations. But, being somewhat nonspecific and requiring a more expensive central catheter, the technique is not universally applied in cardiac surgery patients.

In some patients, at the time of surgery, a small catheter may be introduced into the left atrium and brought out through the chest wall to a transducer for pressure monitoring. These catheters are particularly useful for infants, who are too small for commercially available balloon-tipped pulmonary artery catheters. The left atrial catheter provides for direct continuous measurement of the filling pressure of the left ventricle. Because it provides a direct link between the inside of the left heart and the outside of the patient, extreme care must be taken to avoid air or other embolism. The left atrial catheter is sometimes used as a port for inotropic drug administration because it delivers the drug directly to the systemic circulation, thus decreasing metabolism of the agent as it passes through the lungs and decreasing its effect on the pulmonary circulation (9). Left atrial catheters are also used by some surgeons in adults at risk for postoperative low cardiac output. Inspection of the left atrial pressure waveform for the presence of tall "V" waves can serve as a guide to assess mitral valve insufficiency.

Thermodilution determination of cardiac output is usually made every 2 to 4 hours during the first 12 to 24 hours after surgery and more frequently if low cardiac output or other problems are present. In this manner, the effectiveness of therapeutic interventions such as inotropic drug therapy may be determined. For most patients who undergo uncomplicated cardiac surgery, intensive hemodynamic monitoring is employed for 12 to 24 hours after operation. If, on the day after surgery, the patient is entirely stable with satisfactory hemodynamic parameters, the pulmonary artery or left atrial catheter is removed to minimize the risks of catheter sepsis and emboli. In a patient with a left atrial line, the chest tubes remain in place until the line is removed. The left atrial catheter should not be withdrawn until confirmation of normal coagulation status has been obtained to avoid bleeding from the insertion site. After removal of the left atrial catheter, the central venous pressure should be watched closely as significant rise could indicate the development of tamponade secondary to bleeding from the left atrial insertion site. The radial artery cannula may be left in place longer (usually until the time of transfer from the ICU) to provide access for arterial blood sampling.

Management of the Cardiac Output

Cardiac surgery utilizing CPB with a period of cardioplegia-induced cardiac arrest is often associated with some degree of postoperative ventricular dysfunction. Although not usually clinically obvious, even uncomplicated procedures may result in temporary decreases in left ventricular function. This depression reaches a nadir about 4 hours after operation with recovery occurring within 1 to 3 days (10).

Low cardiac output (defined as a cardiac index of <2.0 L/min/m^2) may result from one or a combination of the following factors: decreased myocardial contractility (of the left, right, or both ventricles), abnormal heart rhythm, inadequate preload, or excessive afterload. Low cardiac output results in poor systemic perfusion and, if severe enough, ischemia of vital organs. If not successfully treated, the predictable complications include renal, hepatic, and neurologic dysfunction and further cardiac failure and eventual death. Despite careful preoperative evaluation, perfect repair of the cardiac lesion, and satisfactory intraoperative myocardial preservation, low cardiac output still may follow cardiac surgery. Early recognition of the low output state and appropriate management can lead to reversal of the situation and survival of the patient. Management of postoperative low cardiac output is detailed in Chapter 4.

Management of the Blood Pressure

Generally, it is desirable to maintain the adult patient's systolic blood pressure at 100 to 120 mm Hg (mean arterial pressure 60 to 70 mm Hg), although elderly patients with long-standing hypertension and inelastic arteries may require a higher blood pressure to adequately perfuse end-organs.

Postoperative Hypotension

Hypotension in the early period after cardiac surgery may result from reduced cardiac output (due to poor ventricular function or inadequate preload) or low vascular tone (i.e., low afterload). The management of low cardiac output is discussed in Chapter 4. Hypotension due to low afterload is characterized by elevated cardiac output confirmed by calculation of the SVR.

Hypotension secondary to low preload (as measured by the central venous pressure, pulmonary capillary wedge pressure, or left atrial pressure) usually responds to volume infusion. The choice of fluids to achieve this includes crystalloid (such as normal saline), albumin preparations (frequently a 5% solution in saline), and hydroxyethyl starch preparations (hetastarch, pentastarch). Hetastarch may interfere with platelet function and, in large doses, may cause transient prolongation of the prothrombin, partial thromboplastin, and bleeding times. Its use in CPB patients is associated with more postoperative bleeding as compared with the patients who receive albumin (11). In our practices, we limit the amount of hydroxyethyl starch solution to 1 L in the adult patient and prefer albumin solutions as the initial fluid of choice in pediatric patients.

Patients with mild to moderate hypotension with low SVR (low afterload) may respond well to dopamine infusion (2.5 to 10.0 µg/kg per minute), although tachycardia may limit the usefulness of this drug. Significant hypotension (mean arterial pressure <60 mm Hg) may require treatment with an α-adrenergic agonist agent such as phenylephrine or norepinephrine, which has both α and β-agonist actions. In fact, for the patient with normal or high cardiac output but mild hypotension and moderately low SVR, it is not uncommon to use phenylephrine infusion to "tighten up" the patient's SVR. This will cause the blood pressure to rise and helps to avoid the administration of large volumes of fluid leading to weight gain and contributing to pulmonary complications.

Occasional patients will, in the first few hours after surgery, experience severe hypotension (mean arterial pressure <60 mm Hg) with low SVR (<1,200 dyne-sec/cm^5) and normal or high cardiac output. This state of post-CPB *vasodilatory shock* may occur in adults, children, and cardiac transplant patients and is more common in patients treated preoperatively with angiotensin-converting enzyme (ACE) inhibitors (12). In this situation, the patient's blood pressure response to phenylephrine or norepinephrine is inadequate (even at high doses), and maintenance of the blood pressure may become a serious problem. Vasodilatory shock may be related to increased bradykinin and decreased plasma vasopressin levels (13). Treatment of patients in this setting with continuous arginine-vasopressin infusion results in successful elevation of the blood pressure and organ perfusion (14–16). Administered through a central venous catheter, vasopressin is started at 0.04 U per minute and titrated upward to achieve a mean arterial blood pressure of 60 to 70 mm Hg.

Postoperative Hypertension

Hypertension after cardiac surgery is common, and the incidence is high in patients undergoing coronary artery bypass procedures. Emergence from anesthesia, pain, irritation from the endotracheal tube, and disorientation all contribute to the adrenergically mediated increase in peripheral vascular resistance and tachycardia that characterizes this state. Early postoperative hypertension is associated with increased myocardial oxygen consumption, bleeding, and the potential disruption of suture lines; it may also contribute to neurologic injury. For adults, efforts to lower the blood pressure should be undertaken whenever the mean arterial pressure exceeds 90 to 100 mm Hg. In infants and children, postoperative hypertension is treated at correspondingly lower levels.

To help prevent postoperative hypertension, patients with significant preoperative hypertension under drug treatment receive their usual morning dose with a small sip of water 2 to 3 hours before going to the operating room.

Hypertension occurring early after heart surgery is treated with short-acting drugs that are administered by continuous infusion (17). A variety of drugs are available for this purpose (Table 3-2). The most popular drug, particularly for adults with coronary artery disease, is *nitroglycerin*. Nitroglycerin acts to dilate preferentially the venous capacitance vessels at low doses, affecting the resistance arteries only at higher doses. Although heart rate may increase somewhat, arterial impedance (afterload) is reduced. This results in favorable effects on myocardial metabolism. Nitroglycerin reduces the propensity of the coronary arteries to vasoconstrict (spasm) and results in improved internal mammary and radial artery flow rates (18). Nitroglycerin infusion in adults is begun at 10 to 20 μg per minute, and the rate of infusion is increased by 5 to 10 μg per minute every 5 minutes (up to 200 μg per minute) until the desired reduction in blood pressure is reached. Patients with low filling pressures may be particularly sensitive to nitroglycerin's hypotensive effect. Nitroglycerin infusion results in rapid onset, with the effect being seen in 2 to 5 minutes and rapid termination of effect when discontinued (3 to 5 minutes). Continuous measurement of the blood pressure is required when nitroglycerin is being used for blood pressure control. Side effects include headache and, rarely, methemoglobinemia (characterized by high arterial oxygen tension in the presence of relatively low oxygen saturation) when used at high doses for long periods of time (19).

Although nitroglycerin has advantages, in many patients, it is insufficiently effective in controlling hypertension and may fail to provide adequate blood pressure control in at least 15% of patients (20).

Table 3-2. Drugs for the acute treatment of early postoperative hypertension (adult intravenous doses)

Drug	Intravenous Dose	Comment
Nitroglycerin	20–300 μg/min or 0.1–5.0 μg/kg/min	Not as effective as nitroprusside, but better for coronary flow and radial artery spasm
Nitroprusside	0.10–10.0 μg/kg/min	Limit duration of use due to toxicity, especially if renal insufficiency is present
Esmolol	Load with 500 μg/kg, then 50- to 150-μg/kg/min infusion	Rapid onset and short duration of effect; easy to titrate for effect. Use with caution in presence of poor left ventricular function or bradycardia
Fenoldopam	Start with 0.025–0.3 μg/kg/min; max 1.6 μg/kg/min	For short-term use; may be useful for patient with renal insufficiency
Labetolol	Load with 5–40 mg over 2 min, then 1- to 3-mg/min infusion	Longer acting than esmolol; causes vasodilation in addition to β-blockade; do not use if ventricular function is poor
Nicardipine	2.5- to 15-mg/h infusion	Caution if cardiac conduction impaired; relatively long half-life makes titration more difficult
Enalaprilat	0.625–2.50 mg by slow infusion (>5 min); repeat every 6 h	May cause renal insufficiency in patients with renal artery stenosis

Note: For all the above drugs given intravenously, continuous blood pressure monitoring is recommended, and the drug dose should be carefully titrated to the desired result to avoid hypotension.

Nitroprusside is a highly effective agent that acts by dilating both the arterial and the venous capacitance vessels. Treatment is begun at 0.25 μg/kg per minute and titrated upward until the desired reduction in blood pressure is achieved. The maximum recommended dose is 10 μg/kg per minute. Excessively lowering the blood pressure with nitroprusside in coronary bypass patients may be deleterious for the myocardial oxygen supply–demand relationship, particularly when distal coronary arterial disease is severe. The drug may cause intracoronary steal of blood away from ischemic areas and may have detrimental effects on internal mammary artery bypass graft flow. Tachycardia is common. The use of nitroprusside should be limited to ≤12 hours and to even shorter periods of time in patients with renal insufficiency to avoid cyanogen (cyanide radical) accumulation. Cyanogen toxicity is characterized by metabolic acidosis, drug tachyphylaxis, coma, absent reflexes, dilated pupils, and pink skin color. If this occurs, the nitroprusside should be discontinued and amyl nitrate inhalations administered to induce methemoglobin formation, which binds to cyanogens and produces a nontoxic complex.

In treating coronary bypass patients with postoperative hypertension, we begin with nitroglycerin and increase the rate of infusion to a maximum of 300 μg per minute. If this is not effective, nitroprusside is added as a second agent. As the need for drug control is reduced (which usually occurs 6 to 8 hours after surgery), the nitroprusside is withdrawn first and then the nitroglycerin is removed gradually, as indicated by the patient's blood pressure.

Other types of drugs are useful for the treatment of early postoperative hypertension. Agents with short-acting β-adrenergic properties, namely, *esmolol* and *labetalol,* are effective for particular patients, especially those with both hypertension and tachycardia. Esmolol is a fast-acting β1-receptor blocking agent that has a very short half-life, allowing for rapid control of the blood pressure with rapid reversal of its effect when discontinued (21,22). As a specific β1-receptor blocker, it selectively inhibits the cardiac β-receptors (cardioselective) while having little effect on bronchial and vascular smooth muscle. Esmolol reduces the heart rate, a useful property for patients with coronary insufficiency. For adults, administration is begun with a loading dose of 0.5 to 1.0 mg/kg over 1 minute, followed by a maintenance dose of 25 to 300 μg/kg per minute. Effectiveness of esmolol in postoperative pediatric heart surgery patients has also been described (23). The patient's blood pressure and heart rate must be monitored closely to avoid overshooting the desired result. Labetalol has both β-receptor and α-receptor blocking properties. When used for postoperative hypertension control, the drug exerts moderate negative inotropic and chronotropic properties, resulting in blood pressure reduction without reflexive vasoconstriction (24). Cerebral, renal, and coronary artery blood flows are maintained (17). It should, however, be used with caution in patients with poor ventricular function. In general, β-blocker drugs should be used with care during the early postoperative period in cardiac surgery patients, especially those with bradycardia, conduction abnormalities, congenital heart defects with right-to-left shunting, reactive airway disease, diabetes, and peripheral vascular disease. In our practices, we find esmolol most often to be appropriate for younger adult patients with postoperative hypertension and tachycardia and relatively normal left ventricular function.

ACE inhibitors cause reduced SVR with generally little effect on heart rate. Patients with congestive heart failure who are treated with ACE inhibitors experience increased cardiac output and decreased pulmonary capillary wedge pressure. Thus, the postoperative use of the ACE inhibitors may be of value, particularly for the hypertensive patient with impaired ventricular function. For treatment during the early postoperative period, the intravenous form of enalapril, enalaprilat, may be particularly useful. The initial adult dose is 0.625 to 1.25 mg infused over 5 minutes, with further doses (up to 5.0 mg) every 6 hours as indicated. The use of enalaprilat in this setting results in improved cardiac output in conjunction with reduced blood pressure. When the patient is able to take oral medications, conversion to oral enalapril or another ACE inhibitor may be accomplished. When administering ACE inhibitors to patients with renal insufficiency, the serum creatinine level should be followed closely.

Calcium channel blocking drugs (nifedipine, verapamil, diltiazem, nicardipine, isradipine, and amlodipine) block transmembrane flow of calcium, resulting in peripheral vascular and coronary artery dilation, reduced myocardial contractility, and lower blood pressure (25). The calcium antagonist drugs are used extensively for the chronic treatment of patients with cardiovascular disease, in particular those with angina pectoris and/or hypertension. Verapamil and diltiazem have significant electrophysiologic effects including reduction in heart rate and prolongation of atrioventricular conduction, making them useful for the treatment of atrial fibrillation and flutter. Nicardipine has been demonstrated to be effective for the treatment of postoperative hypertension when used as continuous, titratable infusion (26,27). Although quick acting, the hypotensive effects of nifedipine cannot be closely regulated. Uncontrolled reduction in the blood pressure can occur, and this may cause cerebral, renal, and myocardial ischemia, especially in elderly patients with vascular disease. Therefore, nifedipine is not recommended for the acute treatment of severe hypertension. (17,28,29). The prophylactic administration of diltiazem (at 1 μg/kg per minute) during and after surgery using CPB has been reported to reduce ischemic and arrhythmic events in coronary bypass patients, although we do not routinely use the drug for this purpose (30). Postoperative use of calcium channel blockers such as diltiazem or verapamil has been advocated to prevent spasm of radial artery coronary bypass grafts, although the effectiveness of this treatment is unclear (31,32).

Fenoldopam is a unique drug that with selective dopamine-1-receptor agonist properties, making it useful for the treatment of hypertension, particularly in patients with renal impairment (33). When given intravenously, fenoldopam has a moderately rapid onset of action (5 to 15 minutes). The usual starting dose is 0.1 μg/kg per minute, with the drug dose increased by 0.05- to 0.1-μg/kg per minute increments until the desired blood pressure (or maximum dose of 1.6 μg/kg per minute) is reached. Reported clinical experience with fenoldopam in heart surgery has been favorable, and it may be particularly valuable in postoperative patients with hypertension and renal insufficiency (34–36). It is, however, significantly more expensive than other drugs more commonly used to treat postoperative hypertension.

PULMONARY CARE

General anesthesia, inhalation anesthetic agents, and CPB impair lung function. Contributing factors include pulmonary sequestration of activated leukocytes and platelets in pulmonary capillaries, complement activation, microemboli (gas or tissue debris), increased capillary permeability, and alveolar hypoperfusion (37,38). Furthermore, a significant proportion of cardiac surgery patients have preexisting pulmonary dysfunction as the result of either their cardiac condition or smoking-induced emphysema. Thus, postoperative pulmonary problems are not unusual in patients undergoing cardiac surgery, and appropriate perioperative management of the pulmonary system is an important aspect of the successful care of the cardiac surgery patient.

Identification of patients with compromised pulmonary function before surgery can assist in the management of the patient postoperatively. Note should be made of a history of smoking, frequent respiratory infections, episodes of wheezing, chronic sputum production, recent respiratory tract infections, and previous cardiac surgery in which damage to a phrenic nerve might have occurred. Long-term preoperative amiodarone treatment may be associated with an increased incidence of postoperative adult pulmonary insufficiency (39,40). For patients with known pulmonary disease or positive risk factors in their history, preoperative pulmonary function tests and room air arterial blood gas determinations will quantify abnormalities of ventilation and gas exchange and provide baseline information for postoperative comparison. All patients are instructed preoperatively in the use of an incentive spirometer (Fig. 3-4). Patients with chronic obstructive pulmonary disease should have their medications optimized prior to undergoing operation (41). Patients who smoke should be encouraged to stop before surgery, although the benefit of doing so is most apparent if the patient quits at least 2 months preoperatively.

Some patients, usually younger ones with little or no pulmonary disease, who have undergone an uncomplicated cardiac repair are sometimes extubated in the operating room before transfer to the ICU or soon after arrival there. Most patients who undergo cardiac surgery are, however, transported to the ICU with the endotracheal tube in place, still receiving mechanical ventilation. Expeditious weaning of the patient from the ventilator with early extubation, often within a few hours of ICU arrival, has been demonstrated to be safe and advantageous and is the goal in nearly all patients (both adult and pediatric) who have undergone uncomplicated operations (42–48). Exceptions to a "fast track" toward early extubation include patients with low cardiac output or hemodynamic instability, patients with an intraaortic balloon pump in place, patients with an apparent neurologic deficit, and those who are bleeding excessively.

Mechanical Ventilators

Mechanical ventilators provide positive pressure within the airways causing inspiration; expiration follows as a passive process. Control of ventilation may be based on volume (where the venti-

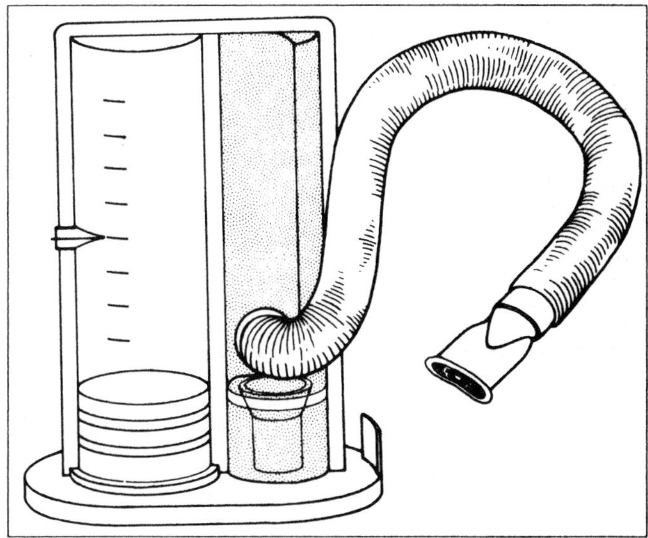

Fig. 3-4. Disposable incentive spirometer. The patient inhales deeply through the mouthpiece. The float on the left rises according to the inspiratory flow rate.

lator delivers a set volume of gas, no matter what the pressure) or based on pressure (where the ventilator delivers gas until a desired airway pressure is achieved). Most ventilators in use today have the capability of either volume or pressure control. For adults, the volume-control mode is used most frequently, and for infants, the pressure-control mode is most common. When using the volume-control mode, the operator sets the tidal volume, respiratory rate, and inspiratory gas flow. For pressure control, the settings are the ventilator rate, the inspiratory gas flow, the desired peak airway pressure, and positive end-expiratory pressure (PEEP).

For an adult patient, typical initial postoperative ventilator settings are as follows: tidal volume, 10 mL/kg; rate, 10 per minute; and F_iO_2, 0.5 (50%). This provides a minute ventilation of 100 mL/kg per minute. As the normal ratio of dead space (airways and nonperfused alveoli) to tidal volume is 0.33, the alveolar ventilation will be about 67 mL/kg per minute, or about 4.5 L per minute, a ventilation volume sufficient to remove metabolically produced carbon dioxide. For the patient with normal lungs, the inspiratory flow rate is adjusted, so that the ratio of inspiration time to expiration time (I/E ratio) is about 1:3. If the patient is experiencing high airway pressures (above 35 cm H_2O), the flow rate is decreased, so that the I/E ratio is decreased. Or, the tidal volume may be decreased, resulting in decreased plateau pressure, which is the major determinant of barotrauma to the lung. If the patient is having difficulty oxygenating, the I/E ratio is increased, although this will be at the expense of decreased CO_2 elimination. Patients with significant chronic obstructive pulmonary disease may benefit from a combination of higher ventilator rate, lower tidal volume, and higher I/E ratio (49).

Ventilators can provide various modes of ventilation (Table 3-3). For the comatose, anesthetized, or paralyzed patient, the *controlled* mechanical mode is used, in which the ventilator simply delivers breaths at set time intervals (depending on what rate has been chosen), irrespective of what the patient may do. As the patient awakens and begins to initiate breaths, the *assist-control* mode may be used. In this mode, the set breath volume (the tidal volume) is delivered every time the patient initiates a breath. The sensitivity of the assist-control mode is adjusted so as to prevent over- or underventilation, and a back-up (control) rate is specified to provide a minimum number of breaths per minute if the patient is not initiating respiration. This allows the patient to adjust his or her breathing rate to provide for normocapnia. Alternatively, the *intermittent mandatory* ventilation (IMV) mode may be used. In this mode, the patient receives a set number of breaths per minute, but may take self-initiated breaths in between those delivered by the ventilator. The tidal volume of these patient-initiated breaths is dependent upon the amount of pressure support applied, patient strength and effort, and chest compliance. The *synchronized intermittent* mandatory ventilation (SIMV) mode detects when the patient takes his or her own breath and avoids "stacking" a delivered breath on top of a spontaneous one to allow for better patient–ventilator synchrony. It is common to add some level of *pressure support* to the SIMV mode. This provides a constant small (5 to 10 cm H_2O) degree of inspiratory pressure with patient-initiated breaths so as to overcome the ventilator tubing resistance. To avoid hypoventilation with SIMV mode, the *mandatory minute ventilation* mode can be utilized. This mode monitors the patient's minute ventilation. If the patient is not breathing spontaneously at a sufficient rate to ensure that a preset minute ventilation is reached, the ventilator will deliver breaths so as to make up the difference between the patient's efforts and the preset required minute ventilation. If, however, the patient breathes at a rate and tidal volume equal to, or in excess of, the preset minute ventilation, the ventilator will not deliver additional breaths to the patient.

Table 3-3. Ventilator setting abbreviations

AV	Augmented ventilation
CMV	Continuous mechanical ventilation
CPAP	Continuous positive airway pressure
IMV	Intermittent mandatory ventilation
MMV	Mandatory minute ventilation
MV	Minute ventilation
PEEP	Positive end-expiratory pressure
PS	Pressure support
TV	Tidal volume
VR	Ventilator rate

PEEP increases the patient's functional residual capacity. This form of pressure support maintains some degree of lung inflation at all times. By decreasing the amount of atelectasis present, arterial oxygenation is increased for the same level of inspired oxygen. PEEP is therefore quite useful for the treatment of respiratory failure characterized by impaired gas exchange; however, high levels of PEEP (above 10 cm H_2O) may reduce the patient's preload, and hence cardiac output, which can limit its usefulness in some cardiac surgery patients. This may be particularly true in patients with right heart failure or after the Fontan procedure where PEEP may increase transpulmonary pressure. It can be valuable to determine the optimum PEEP for the individual patient. To construct this relationship, cardiac output determinations are made at representative levels of PEEP (e.g., 4, 8, 12, and 16 mm Hg), and the PEEP that provides improvement in oxygenation without lowering the cardiac output significantly is chosen for use.

Large tidal volumes, particularly in conjunction with high levels of PEEP, may result in overinflation of nondependent lung segments and the potential for lung injury. It is recommended that the peak airway pressure be maintained at <35 cm H_2O. A sudden increase in peak inspiratory pressures may be indicative of bronchospasm, mucous plugging of a major bronchus, pneumothorax, hemothorax, obstruction of the endotracheal tube, or compression of the ventilator circuit tubing. The sudden onset of high inspiratory pressures should be evaluated by suctioning the patient, obtaining a chest radiograph, and careful examination of the endotracheal tube and ventilator circuit tubing.

Use of Arterial Blood Gas Determination

Analysis of the arterial blood gases provides valuable information regarding gas exchange and the patient's acid–base status. Elevation of the P_{CO_2} indicates inadequate ventilation and, if severe, the need for intubation and mechanical ventilation or for a higher minute volume if the patient is already being ventilated. A diminished P_{O_2} may be caused by a ventilation–perfusion imbalance secondary to atelectasis, pneumonia, or congestive heart failure or by an unrecognized right-to-left cardiac shunt. When lung disease is present, increasing the inspired oxygen concentration (F_iO_2) will usually increase the P_{O_2}. When the P_{O_2} increases little in the presence of a high F_iO_2, there may be a fixed anatomic intracardiac right-to-left shunt or an intrapulmonary shunt. In this situation, proper therapy may include cardiac catheterization or echocardiography to define the defect, transfusion to raise the hematocrit, or, if present, shunt closure with an operation or catheter-delivered device.

The base deficit (calculated from the pH and P_{CO_2}) is usually provided as a part of the blood gas determination results. From this, the amount of sodium bicarbonate necessary to correct any metabolic acidosis can be calculated.

Weaning Ventilator Support

It is the goal to remove all patients from mechanical ventilation as soon as it is safe to do so. Adults usually retain the endotracheal tube that was placed at the time of surgery until the time of extubation. Early extubation is safe and advantageous for the patient and cost-effective for the hospital. An important factor in the development of early extubation protocols has been the application of intraoperative anesthetic techniques that reduce narcotic administration with concomitant use of inhalational anesthetic agent (43,50). This allows for the earlier attainment of consciousness and spontaneous breathing, and early weaning from the ventilator. Patient characteristics favorable for early extubation are shown in Table 3-4.

As the patient emerges from anesthesia, narcotic administration is limited to that which is necessary, at times supplemented by a nonnarcotic analgesic such as ketorolac. As the patient begins to initiate more spontaneous breaths, the ventilator setting may be changed to assist-control or, more commonly, SIMV, with gradual reductions in the ventilator rate. When the rate is <6 to 8 breaths per minute and the patient is sufficiently alert and breathing on his or her own, spontaneous breathing, usually with a low level of inspiratory pressure support, is undertaken. The pressure support lessens the work of breathing, but does not provide excessive assistance. Alternatively, the patient may be placed on a T tube and allowed to breathe on his or her own through the endotracheal tube but without mechanical assistance. After breathing 40% inspired oxygen concentration (either on pressure support or on a T tube) for 20 minutes or so, simple spirometric measurements are made (tidal volume, inspiratory force, minute ventilation), and the arterial blood gases are checked. Criteria for extubation are shown in Table 3-5; when the criteria are met, the endotracheal tube is removed.

After extubation, humidified oxygen is delivered to the patient by face mask or nasal prongs (which are more comfortable). The inspired oxygen concentration is decreased gradually over 24 to 36 hours while continuing to monitor the patient's arterial oxygen saturation. The patient is usually on nasal-prong oxygen at the time of transfer from the ICU to the postoperative care ward. Over the next few days, the nasal-prong oxygen delivery rate is gradually reduced with periodic determinations of the arterial oxygen saturation generally aiming to keep it above 92%.

Respiratory care during the early postoperative period is simple but important. At the time of surgery, the patient's chest and mediastinal tubes are connected to a commercially available three-chamber system to prevent the intrathoracic accumulation of blood and fluid (Fig. 3-5). For the intubated patient, frequent endotra-

Table 3-4. Patient characteristics for early extubation

- Uncomplicated operation with CPB time of <2.5 h
- Awake, alert, neurologically intact patient
- Adequate urine output
- No significant arrhythmias
- Hemodynamically stable
- IABP support not required
- Fully rewarmed
- Not bleeding excessively (<150 mL over 2 h)
- Satisfactory chest x-ray appearance

CPB, cardiopulmonary bypass; IABP, intraaortic balloon pump.

Table 3-5. Criteria for extubation

- Hemodynamic stability (cardiac index >2.0 L/min/m^2)
- No more than modest amount of inotropic drug support (i.e., <5 µg/kg/min dobutamine)
- Stable heart rhythm, lack of significant tachycardia
- Conscious, alert, follows commands
- Not bleeding excessively
- Measured on ventilator
  - Minute ventilation <10–15 L/min
  - Maximum inspiratory force > −20 cm H_2O
- Successful spontaneous breathing trial with
  - Respiratory rate <25 breaths per minute
  - Tidal volume >3 mL/kg
  - Vital capacity >10 mL/kg
  - P_aO_2 >70 mm Hg on F_iO_2 40%
  - P_aCO_2 <45 mm Hg

cheal suctioning, humidification of the inspired gases, and frequent changes of body position are important to prevent retained secretions and atelectasis. After extubation, the patient is encouraged to sit up, dangle his or her legs, and use the incentive spirometer. The incentive spirometer is a very effective method for preventing postoperative atelectasis (51). Early ambulation is encouraged, and the level of exertion is increased incrementally after the patient's chest tubes are removed.

Most patients are extubated within 6 hours of surgery. Some, for a variety of reasons, may be difficult to wean from the ventilator. Management of these patients is discussed in Chapter 4.

FLUIDS AND ELECTROLYTES

Postoperative Fluid Management

Patients who undergo cardiac surgery invariably gain total-body fluid. For patients undergoing surgery with CPB, this gain in predominantly extravascular fluid occurs as the result of the bypass circuit prime fluid volume, hemodilution with loss of plasma oncotic pressure, and capillary leakage during the period of CPB. The degree of hemodilution and interstitial tissue edema is proportional to the length of time on CPB and is greatest in very small children (52). For patients who undergo surgery without the use of CPB ("off pump"), intraoperative fluid loading is often necessary to prevent hypotension associated with manipulation of the beating heart. Because of these factors, at the completion of surgery, most patients are considerably fluid "long." Initial fluid orders should specify a low infusion rate: 50 mL per hour for adults and one-half of the usual maintenance rate for pediatric patients. To minimize the sodium load, 5% dextrose solution is used. Further fluid and electrolyte administration is tailored to the individual patient based on hemodynamic criteria.

Despite an increase in total-body fluid of up to 20% to 30%, the intravascular volume status of the patient during the early post-

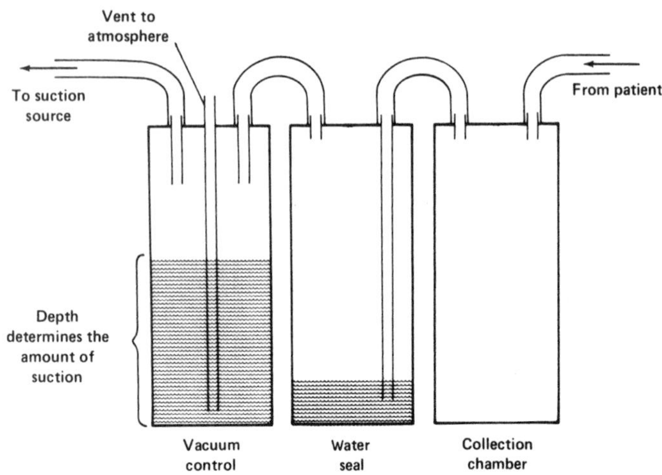

Fig. 3-5. Principles of a chest-tube suction system. The essential components of commercially available suction systems for chest-tube drainage are the following: (a) A fluid collection chamber (*right*) in which the fluid or blood draining from the chest may be collected sterilely, measured accurately, and (in some systems) detached for connection to an intravenous line, so that the shed blood can be reinfused into the patient. (b) A water seal chamber (*middle*) that functions as a one-way valve to prevent the backward flow of air into the chest and as a monitor for air leakage from the chest. Leaking air appears as bubbles from the underwater portion of the tube. The water level in this chamber is usually set at 2 cm. (c) A vacuum control chamber (*left*) in which the water level is usually set at 20 cm H_2O, the amount of negative pressure applied to the chest tubes through the other chambers. The connection to atmosphere will relieve any negative pressure in excess of this amount that is applied by the wall suction. The suction source should be adjusted to provide gentle, continuous bubbling in this chamber to ensure that the intended vacuum is being maintained. Excessive bubbling will result in a lowered water level and decreased suction.

operative period is dynamic, and volume administration may be required to maintain adequate filling (ventricular preload) of the heart. The effects of hemodilution, capillary leak with redistribution of fluid, vasodilation, and other factors may result in a decreased intravascular volume (low preload) despite the gain in total-body fluid. Monitoring the heart rate, arterial pressure, cardiac output, central venous pressure, pulmonary artery pressure, left atrial pressure (if a left atrial catheter is present), and urine output provides information to allow one to adjust colloid or crystalloid administration to the patient appropriate to the circumstances. When arterial pressure, filling pressures, and urine output are low, a trial of volume infusion should be given. Intravascular depletion usually also causes tachycardia, but this response may be blunted in patients who received β-adrenergic antagonists preoperatively. Use of a colloidal volume expander, typically 5% albumin, is customary, although a crystalloid solution (such as normal saline or lactated Ringer's solution) can also be used. The administration of blood products such as plasma or red blood cells (RBCs) for the purpose of volume expansion is not appropriate. For the patient with low preload but adequate systemic blood pressure, heart rate, and cardiac output, volume loading is not indicated. For the adult patient with low preload, hypotension, and low cardiac output (with or without tachycardia), a bolus of 250 to 500 mL of colloid solution is given over 10 minutes with monitoring of the patient's hemodynamic parameters. If the filling pressure (central venous, pulmonary artery diastolic, or left atrial) quickly rises above 15 mm Hg, the bolus infusion should be slowed and the situation reassessed. For infants, the usual trial fluid bolus is 5 to 10 mL/kg. Generally, 6 to 12 hours after surgery, the patient's volume status stabilizes and further boluses of volume-expanding solutions are not required.

Beginning the first day after surgery, to reduce interstitial edema, patients with an uncomplicated postoperative course are usually fluid restricted to approximately 50% of normal requirements. Intravenous fluid administration is minimized, and the patient is allowed to take small amounts of fluid by mouth. Diuretic therapy is usually employed to return patients to their preoperative weight. This is accomplished gradually, over 3 to 4 days following surgery. Depending on how much water weight the patient has gained, furosemide is administered either intravenously or orally, usually every 8 hours for 24 to 48 hours. Daily weights are measured, and the dose is adjusted accordingly. Frequent potassium level determinations and supplementation as needed are important. Severely fluid-overloaded patients, especially if renal and/or respiratory insufficiency is present, may benefit from continuous furosemide infusion (53). This is accomplished with a loading dose of 0.5 mg/kg followed by 0.125 to 0.5 mg/kg per hour. For adults, the typical infusion rate is 5 to 40 mg per hour. The rate of furosemide infusion is adjusted according to the urine output response. For adults who are considerably above their preoperative weight, the urine output goal is 100 to 150 mL per hour. As the patient's weight approaches the preoperative level, the furosemide infusion is slowed and then discontinued.

Potassium

Hypokalemia is the most common electrolyte abnormality that may occur after cardiac surgery. Patients on long-term preoperative diuretic therapy frequently have decreased preoperative total-body potassium stores even though their serum potassium levels may be within the normal range. When CPB is utilized, a high rate of intraoperative urine output is common, with concomitant potassium loss. This effect usually continues for several hours after the operation and will be exacerbated in hyperglycemic patients. The associated potassium loss can be considerable and may result in severe hypokalemia.

Postoperative hypokalemia is associated with nonsustained ventricular tachycardia (54). Severe hypokalemia causes muscular weakness, metabolic alkalosis, arrhythmias, ECG changes (T-wave flattening and inversion, U-wave prominence, and ST-segment depression), and increased susceptibility to digoxin toxicity. Depletion of serum potassium levels can occur quickly; therefore, frequent potassium level determinations and replacement as required are indicated. For an adult, a decrease of 1 mEq/L in the serum potassium level represents a total-body deficiency of at least 100 mEq. Thus, large amounts of potassium supplementation may be required for the severely depleted patient. When possible, oral administration is preferred (20 to 40 mEq two to three times per day for adults). For adults, intravenous potassium is administered at a rate of 10 to 20 mEq per hour. This should be mixed in 100 mL of 5% dextrose and given through a central vein catheter to prevent vein irritation. The rate of infusion must be controlled by an infusion pump to prevent inadvertent rapid delivery, which can result in serious arrhythmias. For infants, potassium chloride may be given through a central line in doses up to 0.5 mEq/kg per hour mixed in 3 to 5 mL/kg of 5% dextrose. The serum potassium level should be maintained between 4.0 and 5.0 mEq/L. After the first 24 hours, the tendency to excrete potassium will be decreased; however, administration of diuretics will continue to lower the serum concentration and supplemental potassium will need to be given.

If the patient is receiving potassium-sparing diuretics such as triamterene or spironolactone, a regularly scheduled dose of potassium *should not* be given because dangerous hyperkalemia may result. Patients who do receive potassium supplementation in addition to a potassium-sparing diuretic should have frequent potassium level determinations.

Although uncommon, hyperkalemia may occur after cardiac surgery, most frequently in patients with impaired renal function. The combination of preexisting renal insufficiency, large doses of hyperkalemic cardioplegia solution infusion, red cell damage during CPB, and (when low cardiac output is present) hypoperfusion of tissues with release of intracellular potassium can quickly result in dangerous hyperkalemia in the early postoperative period. Use of hemofiltration during operation can help lessen this problem. One maneuver useful for the patient with hyperkalemia and relatively normal renal function is to administer a moderate dose of furosemide (40 mg i.v. for the adult) and to replace the resultant urine output with a crystalloid, potassium-free solution. Severe hyperkalemia (>6.5 mEq/L) may cause weakness, paresthesia, and ECG changes (peaked T waves, atrioventricular block, and widened QRS complex) and may lead to arrhythmic death of the patient. Specific treatment is begun when the serum potassium level exceeds 5.5 mEq/L. If ECG changes are present, calcium gluconate should be administered (10 mL of 10% solution i.v. over 3 to 5 minutes); however, calcium reversal of the cardiac effects of hyperkalemia will be short-lived. Glucose (50 mL of 50% dextrose solution) with insulin (10 U of regular insulin added to the solution) may be administered over 10 minutes to drive serum potassium into the intracellular space. Definitive removal of excess potassium from the body requires the use of the cation-exchange resin sodium polystyrene sulfonate (20 to 60 g mixed with 70% sorbitol to prevent constipation) given orally or rectally. Dialysis will likely be needed to treat hyperkalemia associated with severe renal failure (see Chapter 5).

Sodium

Cardiac surgery using CPB causes a significant increase in the patient's total-body fluid volume, which is often associated with a moderate reduction in the serum sodium concentration. In this setting, hyponatremia is nearly always dilutional, the result of excess free water rather than a deficit in total-body sodium. Loss of the accumulated extra free water over the first few days after surgery, often assisted by the administration of diuretic agents, results in normalization of the sodium level. Thus, treatment of the asymptomatic mild or moderate hyponatremia in the early postoperative period by administration of sodium-containing solutions is usually not indicated. The fundamental disorder is water overload and hemodilution, not sodium deficiency; therefore, mild to moderate fluid restriction is in order.

Serious hypernatremia (serum sodium level above 160 mEq/L) is rare and is usually the result of excessive diuretic treatment and dehydration. Generally, the patient's serum blood urea nitrogen and creatinine levels will also be elevated. Less frequent causes include excessive sodium administration (often in the form of sodium bicarbonate used to treat acidosis) and diabetes insipidus. Symptoms of severe hypernatremia include restlessness, irritability, ataxia, and seizures. Treatment is the cautious administration of free water at a rate that does not correct the serum sodium level faster than 0.7 mEq/L per hour (55).

Calcium

Ionized (and total) serum calcium levels decrease during CPB and, if untreated, remain below normal during the early postoperative period largely due to hemodilution. There is no known adverse consequence of this temporary derangement when it is mild. The calcium level usually returns to normal during the first 24 hours after operation (56). The normal total plasma serum calcium level is approximately 10 mg/dL, with the physiologically active ionized fraction being about 1.1 to 1.3 mmol/L. In the patient who had normal calcium levels prior to cardiac surgery, frequent causes of postoperative ionized hypocalcemia include hemodilution and alkalosis. Whereas citrate-anticoagulated banked blood will briefly reduce the serum calcium concentration, this effect is very transient, as the citrate is cleared quickly, and for significant hypocalcemia to result, an extremely fast rate of blood infusion (>1 U every 5 minutes for an adult) is required. Thus, the administration of calcium with red cell transfusions is not recommended, even during massive transfusion, and may actually be harmful (57). Neonates may be more sensitive to the effects of citrated blood transfusion (due to liver immaturity), but calcium administration should be guided by measurement of the ionized calcium level.

In general, asymptomatic hypocalcemia does not warrant treatment. In fact, calcium overload to the recently ischemic myocardium may be injurious to the muscle and may contribute to myocardial dysfunction (58,59). Calcium administration is not generally recommended unless specifically indicated for symptomatic, documented hypocalcemia.

Symptoms of hypocalcemia may develop when the ionized calcium level falls below 0.8 mmol/L. Manifestations of hypocalcemia include low cardiac output, hypotension, arrhythmias, and ECG abnormalities (prolongation of QT and ST segments and T-wave inversion). Noncardiac effects of hypocalcemia include tetany, muscle spasms, seizures, apnea, bronchospasm, laryngospasm, and psychosis. When administered, calcium should be given intravenously. Initially, a bolus of 100 to 200 mg of elemental calcium (10 to 20 mL of 10% calcium gluconate or 4 to 8 mL of 10% calcium chloride) is given, followed by infusion of 1 to 2 mg/kg per hour. The calcium chloride form is more effective in raising the ionized serum calcium level quickly. Administration through a central line is mandatory because calcium solutions are irritating to peripheral veins. Extravasated calcium chloride causes tissue necrosis.

Severe, symptomatic hypocalcemia tends to occur most often in newborn infants undergoing operation, likely as a result of inadequate calcium stores and immature parathyroid glands. In the infant, significant hypocalcemia may be manifested by twitching, jitteriness, and seizures. Treatment is by *slow, central venous* catheter injection of 10% calcium gluconate 10 to 20 mg/kg or 10% calcium chloride 5 mg/kg.

Magnesium

Magnesium is an important intracellular element. Less than 1% of the total-body magnesium content is present in the blood. The normal adult magnesium concentration is 1.7 to 2.3 mg/dL, but the blood level may not accurately reflect intracellular stores. Normal levels may be lower in neonates and higher in infants, and preoperative hypomagnesemia is frequent in patients undergoing surgery for congenital heart disease (60).

Magnesium is important in the regulation of many cellular functions including calcium and potassium fluxes, smooth muscle tone, coronary vascular reactivity, and nitric oxide synthesis. A decrease in the patient's serum magnesium level often occurs after cardiac surgery using CPB (61). This decrease is out of proportion to that expected to occur simply due to hemodilution, and there is a gradual return to normal over a period of about 10 days. Magnesium administration to the cardiac surgery patient may have important antiarrhythmic effects and may enhance hemodynamic performance, especially for the magnesium-deficient patient (62–64). The exact role of magnesium supplementation to the cardiac surgery patient is unclear, but administration appears to be safe; in our practices, it is common to administer 2 g (adult dose) of magnesium sulfate intravenously to the patient just prior to weaning from CPB. Additionally, hypomagnesemia may be a contributor to the development of hypokalemia; both should be corrected when hypokalemia is present.

ACID–BASE BALANCE

Measurement of the arterial blood gases will determine the diagnosis of acidemia or alkalemia, although compensatory changes will occur so as to reduce the changes in the ratio of bicarbonate (HCO_3) to carbon dioxide (P_{CO_2}), thereby reducing the magnitude of the pH disturbance. Table 3-6 outlines the basic acid–base disturbances.

Table 3-6. Acid–base disturbances

	Primary			Secondary Response	
Disorder	pH	HCO_3	PCO_2	HCO_3	PCO_2
Metabolic acidosis	↓	↓			↓
Metabolic alkalosis	↑	↑			↑
Respiratory acidosis	↓		↑	↑	
Respiratory alkalosis	↑		↓	↓	

From Wait RB, Kahng Ku, Dresner LS. Fluids and electrolytes and acid base balance. In: Greenfield LJ, Mulholland MW, Oldham KT, et al., eds. *Surgery: scientific principles and practice,* 2nd ed. New York: Lippincott-Raven Publishers, 1997: 261.

Acidosis

Metabolic acidosis most often occurs when endogenous acid production exceeds bicarbonate content and production. In cardiac surgery patients, this is most often the result of low cardiac output and tissue hypoperfusion with lactate release from tissues secondary to anaerobic metabolism. Impaired renal perfusion, low filling pressures (preload), high doses of administered catecholamines, and the presence of hyperglycemia may also contribute to the accumulation of acid. Preexisting renal dysfunction and/or treatment with the oral hypoglycemic drug metformin may predispose the patient to postoperative metabolic acidosis. When possible, metformin should be discontinued for several days prior to surgery.

Hyperventilation, the respiratory response to the decreased pH, cannot be relied on as compensation for metabolic acidosis as full compensation requires 12 to 24 hours. More importantly, respiratory compensation for metabolic acidosis does not correct the underlying cause of the acidosis. Metabolic acidosis results in reduced myocardial contractility, increased PVR, peripheral arteriolar dilatation, central venous constriction, and reduced responsiveness to administered adrenergic agents such as epinephrine. The presence of β-blocker drugs may augment these adverse effects of metabolic acidosis. Other less common causes of metabolic acidosis in cardiac surgery patients include uremic acidosis due to acute or chronic renal failure and ketoacidosis secondary to insulin deficiency.

The important principle regarding the treatment of metabolic acidosis is to correct the underlying cause. For patients with lactic acidosis due to tissue hypoxia, this requires optimization of cardiac output (both myocardial function and volume status) and oxygenation. Efforts to correct the pH by the administration of alkali without correction of the underlying cause of the acidosis are generally not successful (55). When used to treat acidemia, the alkali of choice is intravenous sodium bicarbonate (65). Bicarbonate administration is generally not, however, indicated unless the pH is below 7.2, and rapid bolus infusion should be avoided, especially in infants. With use of the base deficit determined from the arterial blood gas result, the amount of sodium bicarbonate to administer may be estimated by this formula:

$NaHCO_3$ (mEq) = 0.3 × body weight (kg) × base deficit (mEq/L)

To avoid overcorrection, the initial dose should be *one-half* of this calculated dose. For example, a 70-kg patient with a base deficit of −5 would be calculated to receive 105 mEq of sodium bicarbonate; as each ampoule contains 44.6 mEq, we would begin by giving the patient a single ampoule and then recheck the arterial blood gases in 20 minutes.

Overcorrection of metabolic acidosis by excessive administration of bicarbonate must be avoided, as the resultant "overshoot" alkalosis may be detrimental to cardiac function, predispose to arrhythmias, result in increased CO_2 production, and impair oxygen delivery to the tissues by increasing hemoglobin's affinity for oxygen. Rapid correction of extracellular acidosis may actually cause worsening of intracellular acidosis (66). Because of the potential detrimental effects of administered bicarbonate, any respiratory component to the acidosis should be corrected first to lessen the need for bicarbonate. Furthermore, sodium bicarbonate administration can lead to hypernatremia and volume overload, especially in infants. *Tromethamine* (THAM) can be substituted for sodium bicarbonate, especially when the serum sodium level is above 155 mEq/L. It is an effective buffer and is sodium-free, but may have serious side effects (65). We rarely use it.

Respiratory acidosis is due to carbon dioxide accumulation as the result of inadequate ventilation. Acutely, a small compensatory increase in the plasma bicarbonate will occur, but this does not become significant unless the hypercapnia is sustained for days. Hypercarbia is associated with increases in PVR, which may result in impairment of right ventricular function (67,68). As the Pco_2 rises, a decrease in the Po_2 level may occur with hypoxia resulting, which may become the principal threat to life in this situation (65). Respiratory acidosis in the early postoperative patient who is on a mechanical ventilator is usually simple to correct: Increasing the minute ventilation by increasing the ventilator rate or delivered volume will lead toward normalization of the Pco_2, tension, and arterial pH. A portable chest x-ray will help rule out mechanical causes of compromised ventilation, such as pneumothorax or large pleural effusion. If the patient is not intubated and conservative measures fail to provide adequate ventilation and carbon dioxide excretion, the initial treatment is to secure a patent airway, administer oxygen, and institute mechanical ventilation.

Mixed metabolic and respiratory acidosis may occur in postoperative patients, especially in the setting of low cardiac output and/or renal insufficiency (metabolic causes) and chronic obstructive pulmonary disease and/or pulmonary edema (respiratory causes). Severe acidemia necessitating immediate therapy may result.

Alkalosis

Alkalosis (blood pH of >7.60) results in arteriolar constriction with the potential for reduced myocardial and cerebral perfusion, hypocalcemia, neurologic abnormalities, cardiac arrhythmias, depressed respiration with hypercapnia and hypoxemia, and difficulty weaning from mechanical ventilatory support (69).

A mild degree of *metabolic alkalosis* may develop during the first few days after uncomplicated cardiac surgery, usually the result of diuretic therapy without sufficient potassium and chloride replacement. The alkalosis is characterized by an elevated arterial bicarbonate concentration and can be induced by hypokalemia, excessive losses of gastric juice with chloride depletion, or hypovolemia (because renal retention of sodium prevails over correction of alkalosis). Some degree of respiratory compensation for metabolic alkalosis can occur in the patient who is not being ventilated mechanically. Severe hypoventilation will not usually develop because this response is limited by the hypoxic respiratory drive. The tendency to retain CO_2, to compensate for significant metabolic alkalosis, may hamper efforts to wean the patient with respiratory compromise from mechanical ventilation.

Hypokalemia-induced alkalosis will be reversed by the administration of potassium chloride with the goal of raising the serum potassium level above 4.5 mEq/dL. A mildly low serum potassium level (e.g., 3.5 mEq/dL) indicates a severe total-body depletion of potassium, and significant amounts of potassium chloride may be needed to restore the total-body reserves. In fact, patients on chronic diuretics or who are chronically overventilated may have a profound intracellular potassium deficit with a low-normal serum potassium level and significant metabolic alkalosis.

For metabolic alkalosis that is not associated with significant hypokalemia, the administration of dilute hydrochloric acid (0.15 N HCl at 0.2 mEq/kg per hour i.v. for 12 hours via a central line) may be effective.

During the early period after cardiac surgery, *respiratory alkalosis* is most often secondary to ventilator-induced hyperventilation. Typically, the arterial blood gases will exhibit a low P_{CO_2} and a decreased bicarbonate concentration. For the patient still on mechanical ventilation, this is easily corrected by decreasing the patient's minute ventilation.

USE OF BLOOD PRODUCTS IN THE PERIOPERATIVE PERIOD

Cardiac surgery results in bleeding. Tissue injury, multiple suture lines, intraoperative use of CPB, heparin administration, platelet dysfunction, and dilution of platelets and serum clotting factors all lead to significant operative blood loss and postoperative anemia. Therefore, an important part of the management of the patient undergoing cardiac surgery involves the rational use of blood products.

The Risks of Blood Transfusion

Although blood is safer than it ever has been, risks associated with blood product transfusion still exist and are a major concern of patients undergoing cardiac surgery (Table 3-7). Risks associated with blood product transfusion include the transmission of viruses (hepatitis A, B, C, human immunodeficiency virus, human T-cell lymphotrophic virus, Epstein–Barr, cytomegalovirus, and parvovirus B19), bacterial infection (more common in platelet transfu-

Table 3-7. Risks of blood product transfusion

Risk Factor	Estimated Frequency
Infection	
Viral	
Hepatitis B	1:150,000
Hepatitis C	1:1.2 million
Hepatitis A	1:1.0 million
HIV	1:1.4 million
Human T-cell leukemia virus	1:640,000
Bacterial contamination	
Red cells	1:40,000–500,000
Platelets (apheresis)	1:3,600–1:12,000
Acute hemolytic reaction	1:250,000–1:1 million
Delayed hemolytic reaction	1:1,000
Transfusion-related acute lung injury	1:5,000

From Strong DM, Latz L. Blood-bank testing for infectious diseases: how safe is blood transfusion? *Trends Mol Med* 2002;8:355–358; and Goodnough LT, Brecher ME, Kanter MH, et al. Transfusion medicine: blood transfusion. *N Engl J Med* 1999;340:438–447, with permission.

sions), acute hemolytic reaction, delayed hemolytic reaction, and transfusion-related lung injury (70). In addition to these direct risks, RBC transfusions are associated with an increased incidence of postoperative bacterial infections such as wound infection and pneumonia (71–73). This may be due to a nonspecific immunosuppressive effect, perhaps related to transfused leukocytes that are present in the standard RBC preparation. The use of leukocyte-reduced RBCs has become standard at our hospitals (74).

It is standard practice for the treating physician to discuss the indications for, and potential complications of, blood product transfusion with all cardiac surgery patients. Written permission for transfusions is obtained, usually at the time of obtaining consent for the operation.

Indications for Transfusion

Recognizing the risks (and costs) associated with blood product transfusion, cardiac surgery programs and hospitals have developed guidelines for the transfusion of blood products. Adherence to these guidelines is overseen by a hospital blood transfusion committee, and unnecessary transfusions are reviewed with the ordering clinician. Transfusion guidelines are, however, not absolute. Deviations from the guidelines are necessary to take into account individual patient characteristics (including age and co-existing diseases), but written justification in the patient's medical record for "out-of-protocol" transfusions is required. The goal of these measures is to reduce unnecessary blood product transfusions, thereby decreasing the incidence of transmission of blood-borne infections, reducing the impact of transfusion-related immunosuppression, and helping to maintain the supply of blood products. Table 3-8 lists suggested transfusion guidelines.

Reducing Postoperative Bleeding and Transfusions

Preoperative Measures to Reduce Bleeding and Transfusions

Recognition of patient and procedure characteristics that are associated with excessive postoperative bleeding, as described previously, allows for efforts to proactively prevent the complication from occurring. Preoperative methods reported to reduce bleeding and transfusions in cardiac surgery patients include preoperative autologous blood donation and preoperative erythropoietin administration.

Preoperative donation of packed RBCs may be useful for the individual patient to reduce the need for transfusion of donated RBCs, but this technique has limited applicability. In one large series of elective adult cardiac procedures, 22% of the patients were able to predonate (75). In our practices, the use of this technique is much less frequent, owing mainly to the large number of unplanned urgent and emergency operations. With this method, the patient donates a unit of blood, waits 1 to 2 weeks and donates a second unit, and then waits about 1 to 2 weeks before undergoing surgery. The predonated RBC units are transfused to the patient during or after surgery using usual criteria. Contraindications to predonation include anemia, unstable angina, severe aortic valve stenosis, bacteremia, uncontrolled heart failure, severe cyanosis, and pregnancy. Some programs prohibit predonation in the very young (under 2 years of age) and old (>80 years) and smaller adult patients (<50 kg). Although appealing, this technique of autologous predonation is not without risk to the patient and is not cost-effective, and considerable numbers of units of predonated RBCs are wasted (76,77). Widespread utilization has not been adopted.

Recombinant erythropoietin is an effective stimulator of RBC production. Preoperative administration has proven to be useful for adult and pediatric patients undergoing heart surgery, particularly when used in conjunction with autologous RBC predonation (78,79). The most effective recombinant erythropoietin dose remains to be determined, and the length of preoperative treatment (2 to 3 weeks) required to achieve erythropoiesis is generally impractical for most cardiac surgery patients. Shorter-term preoperative erythropoietin treatment courses may not be effective, and safety has not been confirmed (80). We have found this technique to be most appropriate for patients with preoperative anemia and, in this instance, usually administer a single dose (400 to 600 U/kg s.c.). Patients who receive erythropoietin must receive adequate iron supplementation and be observed closely for the development of hypertension and high hemoglobin levels (with associated increased blood viscosity), which may be particularly adverse for patients with coronary disease awaiting operation. Although potentially useful, in our practices, preoperative erythropoietin administration (with autologous predonation) has generally proven to be impractical. It is occasionally administered to postoperative, often elderly, patients who are experiencing complicated protracted recovery from surgery (as a single dose of 600 U/kg s.c.).

Table 3-8. Blood product transfusion guidelines in postoperative cardiac surgery patients

Red blood cells	
If hemoglobin <7.0 g/dL:	Most patients will require transfusion, although young healthy patients may tolerate
If hemoglobin 7–9 g/dL:	Most stable patients will tolerate without difficulty, but consider transfusion if: • Ongoing bleeding is present • Cardiovascular instability is present • Patient is symptomatic (syncope, dyspnea, angina) • Cardiovascular instability is present • Age >70 y
If hemoglobin ≥9 g/dL:	Most patients will *not* require transfusion; should be performed only if clear-cut symptoms are present or if patient is bleeding severely. At most hospitals, transfusions for hemoglobin >9 g/dL are reviewed for appropriateness.
In general, for an adult, 1 U of packed red blood cells will raise the hemoglobin by 3 g/dL.	
Platelets	
If platelet count <50,000/mm^3:	Consider transfusion, even if not bleeding, if patient is within 24 h of surgery
If platelet count ≥50,000/mm^3:	If bleeding, transfusion indicated, especially if patient recently received platelet inhibitor If *not* bleeding, transfusion *not* usually indicated

If platelet count >100,000/mm³:	If bleeding and platelet dysfunction are suspected due to recent cardiopulmonary bypass or platelet inhibitor drugs, transfusion may be indicated
Note: If heparin-induced thrombocytopenia is suspected, platelet transfusion is *not* indicated (see text). In general, for an adult, 1 platelet apheresis unit will increase the platelet count by 30,000–40,000/mm³.	
Fresh frozen plasma	
If prothrombin time is ≥16 sec (or INR ≥1.5):	If patient bleeding, transfusion indicated If patient *not* bleeding, transfusion *not* usually indicated
If prothrombin time is <16 sec (or INR <1.5):	Transfusion *not* indicated
Cryoprecipitate	
If fibrinogen level <100 mg/dL:	If patient bleeding, transfusion indicated If patient *not* bleeding, transfusion *not* indicated
If fibrinogen level >100 mg/dL:	Transfusion *not* indicated
In general, for an adult, 6 U of cryoprecipitate will increase the fibrinogen level by 100–150 mg/dL.	

INR, international normalized ratio.
Note: These are only guidelines; transfusion protocols vary among hospitals. Specific patient circumstances may require deviations. Written documentation in the patient's medical record regarding out-of-protocol transfusions is usually required.

Intraoperative Measures to Reduce Bleeding and Transfusions
For suitable coronary artery bypass surgery patients, performance of the operation without the use of CPB ("off pump") is associated with reduced bleeding and transfusions (81). This is likely due to a reduction in postoperative platelet dysfunction and depletion with a reduction in the activation of various inflammatory mediators that is caused by the use of extracorporeal circulation. The decision regarding the use of CPB for coronary surgery is based on patient characteristics and coronary anatomy.

CPB provides whole-body perfusion to replace the heart and lung functions during cardiac surgery. This extracorporeal circuit is composed of nonendothelialized tubing and oxygenator surfaces that are associated with blood activation in terms of coagulation, complement, fibrinolysis, kallikrein, leukocytes, and platelets (82). Efforts to reduce these adverse effects of CPB have included the application of bio/blood-compatible surface materials, principally through the development of heparin coating for the synthetic surfaces of the CPB circuit (83). The use of *heparin-bonded surfaces* for the extracorporeal circuit has been reported to reduce bleeding and transfusions, although the results are not consistent (84–88). Some surgeons have recommended the administration of reduced heparin doses in conjunction with the heparin-bonded tubing, but this reduced anticoagulation protocol has raised safety concerns and is not a technique currently used by our institutions (89,90).

For children and small adults, especially if anemic, reducing the volume of prime solution present in the CPB circuit helps to reduce the degree of hemodilution that occurs. This may be accomplished by removing excess tubing (and the contained prime solution) at the time of cannulation. Despite this, most infants will require the addition of blood to the prime solution to prevent excessive hemodilution and profound anemia on bypass.

Intraoperative blood salvage may be performed in several ways. The technique of *intraoperative autologous donation* involves the withdrawal of blood from the patient, storing it during the period of CPB, and then returning it to the patient after protamine administration. Following the induction of anesthesia and placement of monitoring cannulas, the blood (5 to 10 mL/kg of patient weight) may be withdrawn by the anesthesiologist via a central line and stored in anticoagulant-containing blood bags. Or blood may be "backed out" of the patient via the venous cannula by the perfusionist after cannulation, although this does expose the blood to heparin. The blood is maintained in a sterile state and stored at room temperature. The patient's volume loss is corrected by the infusion of the appropriate amount of normal saline. After the patient is weaned from CPB and protamine is administered, the blood is reinfused. This method of intraoperative hemodilution has been used for many years, is safe, and results in a reduction in transfusions as it preserves RBCs, clotting factors, and platelets (91). It cannot, however, be used in unstable or anemic patients.

During surgery, it is customary to use a *cell salvage* device that provides for suctioning of blood shed from the pericardium and thoracic cavities, washing and filtering of the blood, and then reinfusion of the washed red cells. Clotting factors and platelets are lost by this technique, but RBCs are retained. In addition, after weaning from bypass and removal of the arterial and venous cannulas from the patient, the blood remaining in the pump tubing and oxygenator is processed through the cell saver for reinfusion into the patient. The use of such cell salvage techniques is standard at most hospitals.

Drugs to Reduce Bleeding and Transfusions

During surgery, one of a number of drugs may be administered for the purpose of reducing postoperative bleeding and the need for transfusions.

Aprotinin is a naturally occurring inhibitor of the serine protease enzymes. This class of enzymes includes several that are involved in inflammation, in particular the systemic inflammatory response to CPB. When administered during CPB, aprotinin is associated with improved anticoagulation and reduced thrombin formation, reduced fibrinolysis, reduced kallikrein activity, lower plasma bradykinin levels, reduced leukocyte activation, increased plasma levels of antiinflammatory cytokine inhibitors, and reduced production of proinflammatory cytokine levels in alveolar lavage fluid (92,93). The hemostatic benefits of aprotinin administration are likely the result of reduced postoperative fibrinolysis, improved post-CPB platelet function with preservation of the platelet glycoprotein Ib receptors, and a reduced inflammatory response to the CPB stimulus (94,95).

Multiple investigations have shown aprotinin to reduce bleeding, transfusions of blood products, and the need for exploration for postoperative bleeding, each by approximately 50%, as compared with no treatment (93,96). Aprotinin administration is associated with reduced operative mortality and stroke rates (94,96,97). In the United States, aprotinin is approved for use in patients undergoing coronary artery bypass surgery using CPB. The drug is, however, often used for patients who have an increased risk of perioperative bleeding, including those who have recently received aspirin or other platelet inhibitors, patients with coagulopathy, those undergoing repeat sternotomy operations, patients with endocarditis, patients undergoing complex combined procedures expected to require prolonged durations of CPB, and patients suffering dialysis-dependent renal failure. The role of aprotinin in pediatric heart surgery and in patients undergoing deep hypothermic arrest are less well defined, but use under these conditions has been shown to be safe (52,98).

Aprotinin may be administered by either a high-dose (full) or a low-dose (half) regimen; potency is measured in kallikrein inhibitor units (KIU; 10,000 KIU = 1.4 mg of aprotinin). The dosage protocols used for aprotinin administration are shown in Table 3-9. Maintenance of adequate intraoperative anticoagulation for CPB is important for the safe and effective use of aprotinin. It is important to be aware that aprotinin artifactually prolongs the activated clotting time (ACT) when measured using test tubes containing the activator celite. This may result in overestimation of the ACT and, hence, the administration of subtherapeutic amounts of heparin during CPB with the potential for inadequate anticoagulation. Use of kaolin-activated ACT tubes avoids this problem because kaolin removes the aprotinin effect and reflects the true degree of heparin effect that is present (99). Anticoagulation protocol options for the

Table 3-9. Aprotinin dosing regimens

Regimen	Loading Dose	Added to CPB Pump Prime	Maintenance Dose
High (full) dose	2 million KIU (280 mg)	2 million KIU (280 mg)	0.5 million KIU/h (70 mg/h)
Low (half) dose	1 million KIU (140 mg)	1 million KIU (140 mg)	0.25 million KIU/h (35 mg/h)

CPB, cardiopulmonary bypass; KIU, kallikrein inactivator unit.

aprotinin treated include the use of kaolin-activated ACT tubes, the use of a fixed-dose heparin regimen (based on patient weight and duration of CPB), direct measurement of the heparin concentration in conjunction with ACT measurement, and the use of celite tubes with a longer ACT threshold (>750 seconds) (93).

Aprotinin is a small protein and has the potential to cause allergic reactions. For first-time administration, allergic reactions (including anaphylaxis) are rare. For patients who receive aprotinin for a second time within 6 months of the first administration, the incidence is considerably higher (5% in one report), but if >6 months has intervened between exposures, the incidence of allergic response is again very low (about 1%) (100). A tiny aprotinin test dose (10,000 KIU) is given to the patient (who is anesthetized and monitored) prior to infusion of the aprotinin loading dose. If the patient has received aprotinin before, we delay giving the test dose (and adding the aprotinin to the pump prime solution) until the cannulation pursestring sutures are in place. Thus, if a reaction does occur, the patient can be quickly cannulated and CPB may be instituted. Patients being reexposed to aprotinin may also benefit from pretreatment with H1 and H2 blockers (e.g., diphenhydramine 25 mg and cimetidine 300 mg i.v.).

Because of aprotinin's effectiveness in promoting postoperative hemostasis, concern has been raised regarding its potential for adverse effects such as premature bypass graft closure and renal toxicity. The majority of studies have, however, confirmed the safety of aprotinin administration, and, in fact, aprotinin is associated with reduced risks of stroke and mortality in adult cardiac surgery patients. There may be a weak trend toward more early vein graft closures in aprotinin-treated patients, although reports are conflicting in this regard, and issues regarding the adequacy of intraoperative anticoagulation exist (93,101,102). At low and high dose, however, there is no increase in perioperative myocardial infarction in aprotinin-treated patients. Mild, reversible increases in postoperative creatinine levels may occur in occasional aprotinin-treated coronary bypass patients, but there is no increase in the incidence of clinically significant renal failure (103).

The benefit-to-risk ratio for aprotinin is very favorable, and clinical experience is extensive. At our institutions, aprotinin is frequently administered, using either the high-dose (full) or the low-dose (half) regimen to patients who are at increased risk of bleeding complications. Opinion exists that the high-dose regimen is preferable to the low-dose protocol (97).

Aminocaproic acid and *tranexamic acid* are lysine analogues that specifically block the lysine binding site on plasminogen, thereby preventing plasminogen from converting fibrin to fibrin degradation products, thus inhibiting the process of fibrinolysis. Both drugs are administered prophylactically during cardiac procedures using CPB, although the indicated use is for the treatment of documented hyperfibrinolysis. Aminocaproic acid is commonly used during adult cardiac surgery, and studies indicate reductions in chest tube drainage, although reductions in transfusions have not been consistently demonstrated (104,105). Likewise, tranexamic acid has been shown to be clinically superior to placebo in terms of reduction of blood loss, although the data regarding proportions of patients requiring transfusions are not as consistent (106). Safety data for aminocaproic and tranexamic drugs are not as extensive as those available for aprotinin, and reports of abnormal clot formation and other complications exist (107,108). A variety of dosage regimens have been reported, with no standard protocol currently being universally preferred. Generally, for aminocaproic acid, a loading dose of 5 to 10 g is administered before CPB, with further similar doses being added to the pump prime solution and given after protamine administration. Alternatively, a constant infusion may be employed. Hypotension may result from too rapid infusion, anaphylaxis can occur, and renal failure associated with aminocaproic acid has been described (109,110). Aminocaproic acid *should not* be used when there is a possibility of ongoing disseminated intravascular coagulation. Being much less costly than aprotinin, aminocaproic acid and tranexamic acid have both been reported to be more cost advantageous for use in patients at low risk of bleeding complications (111,112).

Aminocaproic acid is commonly administered prophylactically in our practices for adult patients who are at low risk for bleeding. For patients at increased risk of bleeding complications, aprotinin is the drug of choice (93,94).

Desmopressin (an arginine vasopressin analogue) likely increases plasma levels of von Willebrand's factor and appears to be useful in reducing postoperative bleeding in patients with identified platelet dysfunction after surgery (113). Desmopressin is administered as a single intravenous infusion of 0.3 μg/kg.

Postoperative Reinfusion of Shed Mediastinal Blood

Following surgery, blood, which has been shed via the mediastinal tubes into a sterile receptacle, may be filtered and reinfused to the patient. This method of postoperative autotransfusion has produced conflicting results, with some studies showing reductions in the need for homologous transfusions, but others reporting either no effect or even adverse consequences of the technique (114–117).

PAIN CONTROL

Besides the obvious discomfort, postoperative pain can cause the patient to experience tachycardia, hypertension, splinting with resultant small tidal volumes, and ineffective cough. During the early postoperative period, morphine is usually the drug of choice. Mechanically ventilated adults are given 2 to 10 mg by slow intravenous bolus at 1 mg per minute; the infant bolus dose is 0.1 to 0.5 mg/kg at a rate of 0.1 mg per minute. Redosing every hour may be required in some patients. The main hemodynamic effect of morphine is vasodilation, thereby reducing ventricular preload and afterload with favorable effects on myocardial oxygen consumption. If the patient is hypovolemic, however, significant hypotension may result. Thus, morphine is given slowly with careful monitoring of the patient's arterial blood pressure and filling pressures. Small, frequent intravenous doses are preferable to larger, less frequent intramuscular injections during the early postoperative period because of the variability in absorption when the intramuscular route is used. For infants and children, we often employ a continuous morphine infusion (0.05 to 0.1 mg/kg per hour). Patients who are allergic to morphine receive oxymorphone or hydromorphan intravenously.

After extubation, care must be used to avoid excess narcotic administration, which may result in respiratory depression. Conversely, insufficient pain relief will result in failure of the patient to cough and clear secretions. For adults, we generally administer hydromorphan or hydrocodone orally or, for more severe pain, oxycodone. If the patient's pain is not relieved with oral agents, intramuscularly administered morphine (4 to 10 mg every 4 hours as needed) may be administered. As oral intake is resumed, most patients find relief with combination codeine and acetaminophen preparations taken orally. Another less potent but often effective agent is propoxyphene with acetaminophen. This drug seems to be particularly useful for older, frail patients who do not tolerate the stronger agents and suffer nausea from codeine. For patients who become too sedated with narcotics, we have found ketorolac 15 to 30 mg i.v. every 6 hours or 10 mg by mouth every 4 to 6 hours to be very useful. This nonsteroidal antiinflammatory drug provides good pain relief and does not inhibit respiratory drive (118). Important potential side effects of ketorolac include inhibition of platelet function with prolongation of the bleeding time, gastrointestinal symptoms including nausea, pain, and bleeding, and renal toxicity with hyperkalemia. This latter effect appears to be more likely in patients undergoing diuretic treatment and may lead to severe renal failure. While useful for pain control in narcotic-intolerant patients, ketorolac should not be used in patients with renal insufficiency; frequent creatinine determinations should be performed, and the drug is discontinued if the creatinine rises significantly. Commonly used analgesic agents are listed in Table 3-10.

Patients may require sedation during the early postoperative period to prevent dangerous agitation and fighting the ventilator. For this purpose, *midazolam* is used in small intravenous doses (0.01- to 0.05-mg/kg load over several minutes). Midazolam has a relatively short duration of action; thus, to provide continuous sedation of the ventilated patient, a continuous intravenous infusion is useful (0.02 to 0.1 mg/kg per hour for adults) (119). When administered to intubated neonatal patients, midazolam may be initiated at a rate of 30 μg/kg per hour without a loading dose. In general, midazolam should be administered at the lowest possible dose that pro-

Table 3-10. Commonly used pain medications

Drug	Representative Brand Name	Pain Level Indicated For	Adult Oral Dose	Parenteral Adult Dose	Pediatric Dose
Ketolorac	Toradol	Mild–moderate	Not recommended	15–30 mg i.m./i.v. q 6 h; max 120 mg q.d. limit to 5 d	1 mg/kg/i.v. q 6 h; limit to 48 h
Propoxyphene	Darvocet N-100 (100 mg with acetaminophen 650 mg)	Mild–moderate	1–2 tabs q 4–6 h	NA	NA
Codeine (30 mg) and acetaminophen (300 mg)	Tylenol #3	Mild–moderate	1–2 tabs q 4–6 h	NA	NA
Hydrocodone (5 mg) with acetaminophen (500 mg)	Vicodin	Moderate	1–2 tabs q 4–6 h	NA	NA

Continued

Table 3-10. *Continued*

Drug	Representative Brand Name	Pain Level Indicated For	Adult Oral Dose	Parenteral Adult Dose	Pediatric Dose
Hydromorphone	Dilaudid	Moderate	2–4 mg q 4–6 h p.r.n.	1–4 mg i.m./i.v./ s.c. q 4–6 h	NA
Meperidine	Demerol	Moderate–severe	150–300 mg q 3–4 h	50–150 mg i.m./ i.v. q 3–4 h	1.0–1.75 mg/kg p.o./i.m./i.v.
Oxycodone	Roxicodone	Moderate–severe	5–30 mg q 4–6 h	NA	NA
Morphine sulfate	—	Severe	30–60 mg q 4–6 h	1–10 mg i.v. q 1–2 h p.r.n.	0.1–0.2 mg/kg i.v./ i.m. q 2–4 h
Oxymorphone	Numorphan	Severe	NA	0.5–1.5 mg q 1–3 h p.r.n.	NA
Fentanyl	Sublimaze	Severe	NA	50–100 μg q 1–2 h p.r.n. or 0.5 to 1.5-μg/kg/h infusion	0.5–2.0 μg/kg q 1–4 h p.r.n. or 0.5 to 1.0-μg/kg/h infusion

vides the desired level of sedation. Another drug of use for sedation of the severely agitated, intubated patient is propofol. This short-acting anesthetic is administered as a continuous infusion (0.05 to 0.2 mg/kg per minute) and, when discontinued, is rapidly cleared. As propofol induces a state of general anesthesia, controlled ventilation of the patient is required. For the less agitated patient who requires a less sedating and longer-acting anxiolytic agent, lorazepam is useful.

Rarely, a patient, usually with severe respiratory and/or cardiac failure, will require total immobilization by a muscle relaxant. This is usually in the setting of severe hemodynamic instability, often with an intraaortic balloon pump in place, in a patient for whom satisfactory ventilation is difficult due to high peak airway pressures. For this purpose, vecuronium (0.08 to 1.0 mg/kg i.v.) and the longer-acting pancuronium (0.04 to 0.1 mg/kg i.v.) are used. As the muscle-relaxing agents do not provide analgesia or amnesia, concomitant administration of other agents (such as morphine) is required.

Haloperidol is an antipsychotic agent that is of value in the treatment of adult cardiac surgery patients suffering severe acute delirium (such as may occur with alcohol withdrawal and other medical conditions). In this setting, rapid treatment of the agitated delirious patient may be required to prevent injury to the patient and to others. Haloperidol may be given orally, but the intravenous route (1.0 to 5.0 mg i.v. every 2 to 4 hours) is preferred for a quick result. Frequently, in this setting, consultation with a neurologist will aid in the management of the patient. Care should be taken in the administration of haloperidol; extrapyramidal reactions, QT-interval prolongation, and torsade de pointes (a form of ventricular tachycardia) may occur during treatment.

For patients who are taking oral agents but still require sedation, diazepam is of use. Diazepam has a longer duration of action than midazolam, and therefore, less frequent dosing is required. Side effects of both of these benzodiazepines include hypotension and respiratory depression.

In the evaluation of the agitated patient, it must be remembered that the *patient who becomes restless or apprehensive may actually be hypoxic, acidotic, or in a low cardiac output state.* If this is the case, the administration of analgesics or sedatives will be hazardous. Evaluation of a possible metabolic abnormality by blood gas and electrolyte determination should be performed.

DIURETIC THERAPY

Patients who require cardiac surgery often suffer preoperative congestive heart failure and/or hypertension and are being treated with diuretic drugs prior to surgery. After surgery, most patients have acquired total-body excesses of sodium and water, and therefore, diuretics are frequently prescribed on a temporary basis. The mechanism of action of the commonly used diuretic agents is to inhibit sodium reabsorption in the kidney tubules, resulting in increased sodium excretion. The major groups of diuretic drugs used clinically are (a) loop diuretics (furosemide, ethacrynic acid, and bumetanide); (b) thiazide diuretics (hydrochlorothiazide, chlorthalidone, and metolazone); (c) potassium-sparing diuretics (spironolactone, triamterene, and amiloride); and (d) combination products (hydrochlorothiazide plus either spironolactone, triamterene, or amiloride).

On the first morning after uncomplicated open-heart surgery, when cardiac function has returned toward the preoperative level and the patient is fully rewarmed, a dose of a loop diuretic (most commonly furosemide 10 to 40 mg i.v. for adults, 0.5 to 1.0 mg/kg i.v. for infants) is often given to promote diuresis. Patients with cardiac failure, high filling pressures, and pulmonary edema are treated with higher doses of intravenous furosemide with careful monitoring of the ventricular filling pressures and serum potassium levels. Patients on preoperative diuretic therapy may require higher doses after surgery, particularly if they were receiving high doses for a long period of time. After extubation, when the patient is able to take medications orally, it is common practice to administer either furosemide or a combination diuretic (such as triamterene 50 mg plus hydrochlorothiazide 25 mg) for several days. The combination diuretic helps prevent hypokalemia, although the patient's potassium level should still be checked regularly. Concurrent administration of a daily dose of potassium with a combination diuretic containing a potassium-sparing agent is contraindicated because of the possibility of dangerous hyperkalemia. The patient is weighed daily; when the preoperative weight is approached, the diuretic is discontinued. Important diuretic drug interactions include potassium-sparing diuretics plus ACE inhibitors such as captopril (may cause dangerous hyperkalemia), spironolactone plus digoxin (raises digoxin levels), and furosemide plus ketorolac (may cause hyperkalemia or renal insufficiency) (53).

DIABETES MANAGEMENT

Patients with diabetes mellitus have an increased incidence of coronary artery disease, and therefore, a significant proportion (25% to 30%) of patients undergoing coronary revascularization procedures are diabetic. Patients with diabetes mellitus have an increased incidence of postoperative complications including wound infections, stroke, and death (120). Diabetic patients (insulin dependent, on oral agents, or diet controlled), as well as previously unrecognized "borderline diabetics," may become very hyperglycemic during the early postoperative period due to the stress of surgical trauma and the use of catecholamine support medications. Untreated hyperglycemia may result in osmotic diuresis with intravascular volume depletion. The renal threshold for spilling glucose into the urine with concomitant loss of water and electrolytes is a serum glucose level of approximately 200 mg/dL. On rare occasions, hyperglycemic hyperosmolar coma or ketoacidosis results from uncontrolled hyperglycemia. Close monitoring of glucose levels and the use of insulin to prevent hyperglycemia are associated with improved outcome in critically ill patients and with reduced rates of sternal infection in cardiac surgery patients (121,122).

Management of insulin-dependent diabetic patients in the perioperative period employs the administration of both glucose and insulin. On the morning of surgery, the insulin-dependent diabetic patient is begun on a constant infusion of 5% dextrose (at 25 to 50 mL per hour) and a separately controlled infusion of insulin. The patient's glucose level is checked frequently before and during surgery, and the rate of insulin infusion is adjusted to maintain the serum glucose level between 80 and 120 mg/dL. The physiologic response to surgery, use of CPB, and administration of catecholamine drugs may all contribute to marked intraoperative elevations in the patient's glucose level, and occasional bolus doses of intravenous regular insulin (2 to 10 U) may be required in addition to a continuous infusion. Postoperatively, an intravenous insulin infusion protocol may be used (Fig. 3-6).

Patients who are not taking insulin preoperatively receive no insulin before surgery. Again, intensive intraoperative monitoring of the patient's glucose level is performed; if it becomes elevated, 5% dextrose and insulin infusions may be used for control. For both groups, an intravenous infusion of 5% dextrose is infused whenever continuous intravenous insulin is being administered.

1. Use intravenous drug pump

2. If blood glucose (BG) is < 300, infuse 5% Dextrose at______ (50 – 100) ml/hr.

3. Prepare insulin as follows:

Mix 50 units of U-100 Human Regular Insulin into 250 CC normal saline (1 Unit insulin per 5 ml).

OR,

Mix 50 units of U-100 Human Regular Insulin into 250 CC normal saline (1 Unit insulin per 10 ml).

4. Do Chemstrip glucose determination q ______(1-4) hours and prn.

5. Parameters

Chemstrip	Insulin units per hour	IV Solution Speed (ml/hr)
> 80	________	________
>120	________	________
> 180	________	________
>240	________	________
> 300	________	________
	and recheck in 1 hr; proceed with schedule	
> 400	CALL PHYSICIAN	
< 80	STOP INSULIN; wait 1 hour; repeat Chemstrip and proceed	

6. If any questions, call physician.

Fig. 3-6. Intravenous insulin infusion protocol. The ordering physician fills in the blanks for the insulin concentration and units per hour based on the patient's diabetic history and previous insulin regimen. Whenever the patient's glucose level is <300 mg/dL, 5% dextrose solution is administered simultaneously with the insulin infusion.

When the patient begins to receive enteral caloric support (in the form of either oral intake or tube feedings), conversion to longer-acting preparations may be accomplished. During this transition phase, subcutaneous insulin is administered on a sliding-scale basis with frequent blood glucose measurements (every 4 to 6 hours) and charting of the results and doses of insulin. Most patients are discharged to home on the same diabetic drug regimen they were taking when they were admitted, although some oral agent-dependent diabetics may require conversion to insulin during the hospitalization to improve their glucose control.

Hypoglycemia in adult patients is unusual, except for that resulting from excessive exogenous insulin administration. If it does occur, it is treated by the intravenous administration of 50% dextrose. Infants, because of their decreased hepatic glycogen stores, are at increased risk for hypoglycemia, particularly with stress. Severe perioperative hypoglycemia may occur in newborns (below 30 mg/dL in full-term infants, below 20 mg/dL in the premature), leading to seizures and the potential for neurologic injury. This is prevented by administering an intravenous maintenance solution with adequate glucose (10% dextrose) and frequent determinations of the baby's blood glucose level.

NUTRITIONAL SUPPORT

Severe nutritional deficiencies can lead to heart failure, and heart failure can result in nutritional deficiencies. The protein-calorie malnutrition syndrome associated with severe chronic congestive heart failure is known as cardiac cachexia. Preoperative malnutrition is a risk factor for postoperative complications and prolonged hospital stay in patients undergoing cardiac surgery. A preoperative albumin level of <3.5 g/dL in elderly patients or <2.5 g/dL in all patients is associated with an increased frequency of postoperative complications (123,124). Preoperative nutritional supplementation, however, is rarely feasible due to the urgency of operation. The realization that preoperative deficiency may exist, however, should lead to early postoperative nutritional assessment and supplementation.

Many infants with congenital heart disease and heart failure are unable to feed normally, and "failure to thrive" frequently enters into the decision to recommend surgical repair for the underlying cardiac lesion. After operation, these patients need early protein and caloric supplementation. Routinely, a nasogastric tube is inserted after operation. Initially, this is used for gastric drainage, but as soon as bowel activity returns, tube feedings may be started. The tube should be fine-bore to prevent obstruction of the nares (infants are nose breathers) and soft to prevent gastric perforation or nasal erosion. Initial feedings in infants consist of a clear fluid such as 5% dextrose at 5 to 10 mL per hour. The residual amount left in the stomach after each hour is determined by aspiration. If low residual amounts are present, tube feedings are advanced both in amount and in substance. For newborns, expressed breast milk may be available; this is preferable to commercially available formulas. The infant may need a pacifier to satisfy the urge to suck. Once on full tube feedings and sucking well (usually after just a few days), the infant is allowed oral intake with the tube in place. Supplements are given by tube until full calories are ingested by mouth.

Likewise, adults who are experiencing postoperative complications (such as difficulty weaning from the ventilator) should receive early postoperative alimentation. In general, adults require about 25 kcal and 1 g of protein/kg of usual body weight per day (125,126). The enteral route is preferred to the intravenous to avoid the problems of maintaining venous access, fluid overload, and infection associated with central venous hyperalimentation. The ileus associated with cardiac surgery usually clears within a few days, and once intestinal activity is present, a small-bore feeding tube is placed through the nose into the stomach or, preferably, advanced into the duodenum. For patients with delayed slow gastric emptying, treatment with metoclopramide (10 mg per the tube once a day) is of value (127). A multitude of commercially available enteral formulas are available, and the type of formula can be tailored to the needs of the patient. Tube feedings are initiated with small volumes of full-strength formula, and the volume is gradually increased until the target volume is reached. Diarrhea is the main side effect, and this may be reduced by the addition of pectin to the formula. Patients should be fed with the head of the bed raised 15 to 30°, and periodic measurement of the gastric residual volume should be made. If the residual exceeds 100 to 150 mL, the feeding rate should be decreased. As the patient's general condition improves, he or she can be converted gradually to a full oral diet with continued tube feeding at a lower rate. Monitoring of the patient's caloric intake ("calorie count") guides the timing of tube feeding discontinuation.

Parenteral ("hyperalimentation") nutrition is required for patients who require nutritional support and are unable to be fed by a feeding tube. This is usually delivered via a central vein, although peripheral vein hyperalimentation is possible. Parenteral feeding solutions typically contain glucose, fat, amino acids, electrolytes, vitamins, and trace minerals. At our hospitals, we use standardized protocols regarding the composition, preparation, and administration of parenteral nutrition. The hospital pharmacists have an active and important role in the formulation of the parenteral nutrition solutions. The patient is monitored closely regarding urine output, serum electrolytes, glucose and blood urea nitrogen, liver enzymes, and blood count. Common complications include hyperglycemia and catheter infection.

Patients with normal preoperative nutritional states and uncomplicated postoperative courses typically have depressed appetites and occasional nausea early after surgery, and this is of little consequence. Generally, they are prescribed a low-salt (2 g of sodium) diet as their total-body sodium is usually elevated, and they are discharged home on a "no-added" salt diet. After about a week, the appetite usually recovers with discharge from the hospital and the return to "home cooking." Patients with coronary artery disease or heart failure undergo dietary counseling by a registered dietitian prior to discharge from the hospital.

CARE OF THE RADIAL ARTERY HARVEST SITE

Complications related to the removal of the radial artery for use as a bypass graft conduit are rare (see Chapter 5), but special measures to closely monitor and document the status of the patient's incision, arm, and hand during the early postoperative period are in order. An unrecognized incisional hematoma could lead to finger ischemia and permanent damage. As a part of the initial assessment of the patient performed upon arrival in the ICU, the hand should be examined for color, capillary refill, temperature, and ulnar artery pulse. The patient's nurse performs this evaluation every hour for the first 4 hours after surgery, and the results are documented in writing. Assessment for fingertip viability and sensation abnormalities is then performed every 4 hours for 24 hours. The arm and hand should be elevated on a pillow to help reduce edema. After 24 hours, the radial artery harvest site incision dressing is removed.

REFERENCES

1. O'Brien WO, Karski JM, Cheng D, et al. Routine chest roentgenography on admission to intensive care unit after heart operations: is it of any value? *J Thorac Cardiovasc Surg* 1197; 113:130–133.
2. Augoustides J, Weiss SJ, Pochettino A. Hemodynamic monitoring of the postoperative adult cardiac surgical patient. *Semin Thorac Cardiovasc Surg* 2000;12:309–315.
3. Flores ED, Lange RA, Hillis RD. Relation of mean pulmonary artery wedge pressure and left ventricular end-diastolic pressure. *Am J Cardiol* 1990;66:1532–1533.
4. Stewart RD, Psyhojos T, Levitsky S, et al. Central venous catheter use in low-risk coronary artery bypass grafting. *Ann Thorac Surg* 1998;66:1306–1311.
5. Pulmonary Artery Catheter Consensus Conference Participants. Pulmonary Artery Catheter Consensus Conference: consensus statement. *Crit Care Med* 1997;25:910–925.
6. Mullerworth MH, Angelopoulos P, Couyant MA, et al. Recognition and management of catheter-induced pulmonary artery rupture. *Ann Thorac Surg* 1998;66:1242–1245.
7. Sirivella S, Gielchinsky I, Parsonnet V. Management of catheter-induced pulmonary artery perforation: a rare complication in cardiovascular operations. *Ann Thorac Surg* 2001;72:2056–2059.
8. Cicenia J, Shapira N, Jones M. Massive hemoptysis after coronary artery bypass grafting. *Chest* 1996;109:267–270.
9. Aral A, Oguz M, Ozberrak H, et al. Hemodynamic advantages of left atrial epinephrine administration in open heart operations. *Ann Thorac Surg* 1997;64:1046–1049.
10. Breisblatt WM, Stein KL, Wolfe CJ, et al. Acute myocardial dysfunction and recovery: a common occurrence after coronary bypass surgery. *J Am Coll Cardiol* 1990;15:1261–1269.
11. Wilkes MM, Navickis RJ, Sibbald WJ. Albumin versus hydroxyethyl starch in cardiopulmonary bypass surgery: a meta-analysis of postoperative bleeding. *Ann Thorac Surg* 2001;72:527–533.
12. Mekontso-Dessap A, Houel R, Soustell EC, et al. Risk factors for post-cardiopulmonary bypass vasoplegia in patients with preserved left ventricular function. *Ann Thorac Surg* 2001;71: 1428–1432.
13. Landry DW, Oliver JA. The pathogenesis of vasodilatory shock. *N Engl J Med* 2001;345:588–595.

14. Morales DLS, Gregg D, Helman DN, et al. Arginine vasopressin in the treatment of 50 patients with postcardiotomy vasodilatory shock. *Ann Thorac Surg* 2000;69:102–106.
15. Rosenzweig EB, Starc TJ, Chen JM, et al. Intravenous arginine-vasopressin in children with vasodilatory shock after cardiac surgery. *Circulation* 1999;100(suppl II):II182–II186.
16. Argenziano M, Chen JM, Cullinanae S, et al. Arginine vasopressin in the management of vasodilatory hypotension after cardiac transplantation. *J Heart Lung Transplant* 1999;18:814–817.
17. Varon J, Marik PE. The diagnosis and management of hypertensive crises. *Chest* 2000;118:214–227.
18. Zabeeda D, Medalion B, Jackobshvilli S, et al. Comparison of systemic vasodilators: effects on flow in internal mammary and radial arteries. *Ann Thorac Surg* 2001;71:138–141.
19. Bojar RM, Rasteger H, Payne DD, et al. Methemoglobinemia from intravenous nitroglycerin: a word of caution. *Ann Thorac Surg* 1987;43:332–334.
20. Kaplan JA, Jones EL. Vasodilator therapy during coronary artery surgery. A comparison of nitroglycerin and nitroprusside. *J Thorac Cardiovasc Surg* 1979;77:301–309.
21. Reves JG, Croughwell ND, Hawkins E, et al. Esmolol for treatment of intraoperative tachycardia and/or hypertension in patients having cardiac operations. *J Thorac Cardiovasc Surg* 1990;100:221–227.
22. Wiest DB. Esmolol: a review of its therapeutic efficacy and pharmacokinetic characteristics. *Clin Pharmacokinet* 1995;28:190–202.
23. Wiest DB, Garner SS, Uber WE, et al. Esmolol for the management of pediatric hypertension after cardiac operations. *J Thorac Cardiovasc Surg* 1998;115:890–897.
24. Sladen RN, Klamerus KJ, Swafford MW, et al. Labetalol for the control of elevated blood pressure following coronary artery bypass grafting. *J Cardiothorac Anesth* 1990;4:210–221.
25. Abernethy DR, Schwartz JB. Calcium-antagonist drugs. *N Engl J Med* 1999;341:1447–1457.
26. Vincent J-L, Berlot G, Preiser J-C, et al. Intravenous nicardipine in the treatment of postoperative hypertension. *J Cardiothorac Vasc Anesth* 1997;11:160–164.
27. Leslie J, Brister N, Levy JH, et al. Treatment of postoperative hypertension after coronary artery bypass surgery. *Circulation* 1994;90:II256–II261.
28. Grossman E, Messerli FH, Grodzicki T, et al. Should a moratorium be placed on sublingual nifedipine capsules given for hypertensive emergencies and pseudoemergencies? *JAMA* 1996;276:1328–1331.
29. McEvoy GK, ed. *American hospital formulary drug information 2002.* Bethesda: American Society of Health-System Pharmacists, 2002:1691.
30. Seitelberger R, Hannes W, Gleichauf, et al. Effects of diltiazem on perioperative ischemia, arrhythmias, and myocardial function in patients undergoing elective coronary bypass grafting. *J Thorac Cardiovasc Surg* 1994;107:811–821.
31. Parolari A, Rubini P, Alamanni F, et al. The radial artery: which place in coronary operation? *Ann Thorac Surg* 2000;69:1288–1294.

32. Acar C, Ramsheyi A, Pagny J-Y, et al. The radial artery for coronary artery bypass grafting: clinical and angiographic results at five years. *J Thorac Cardiovasc Surg* 1998;116:981–989.
33. Brogden RN, Markham A. Fenoldopam. A review of its pharmacodynamic and pharmacokinetic properties and intravenous clinical potential in the management of hypertensive urgencies and emergencies. *Drugs* 1997;54:634–650.
34. Gombotz H, Plkaza J, Mahla E, et al. DA1-receptor stimulation by fenoldopam in the treatment of postcardiac surgical hypertension. *Acta Anaesthesiol Scand* 1998;42:834–840.
35. Hill AJ, Feneck RO, Walesby RK. A comparison of fenoldopam and nitroprusside in the control of hypertension following coronary artery surgery. *J Cardiothorac Vasc Anesth* 1993;7:279–284.
36. Halpenny M, Lakshmi S, O'Donnel A, et al. Fenoldopam: renal and splanchnic effects in patients undergoing coronary artery bypass grafting. *Anaesthesia* 2001;56:953–960.
37. McNaughton PD, Braude S, Hunter D, et al. Changes in lung function and pulmonary capillary permeability after cardiopulmonary bypass. *Crit Care Med* 1992;20:1289–1294.
38. Ranieri VM, Vitale N, Grasso S, et al. Time-course of impairment of respiratory mechanics after cardiac surgery and cardiopulmonary bypass. *Crit Care Med* 1999;27:1454–1460.
39. Mickleborough LL, Maruyama H, Mohamed S, et al. Are patients receiving amiodarone at increased risk for cardiac operations? *Ann Thorac Surg* 1994;58:622–629.
40. Rady MY, Ryan T, Starr NJ. Preoperative therapy with amiodarone and the incidence of acute organ dysfunction after cardiac surgery. *Anesth Analg* 1997;85:489–497.
41. Ferguson GT, Cherniack RM. Management of chronic obstructive pulmonary disease. *N Engl J Med* 1993;328:1017–1022.
42. Higgins TL. Safety issues regarding early extubation after coronary artery bypass surgery. *J Cardiothorac Vasc Anesth* 1995; 9(suppl 1):24–29.
43. Karski JM. Practical aspects of early extubation in cardiac surgery. *J Cardiothorac Vasc Anesth* 1995;9(suppl 1):30–33.
44. Hickey RF, Cason BA. Timing of tracheal extubation in adult cardiac surgery patients. *J Cardiac Surg* 1995;10:340–348.
45. Cheng DCH, Karski J, Peniston C, et al. Morbidity outcome in early versus conventional tracheal extubation after coronary artery bypass grafting: a prospective randomized controlled trial. *J Thorac Cardiovasc Surg* 1996;112:755–764.
46. Cheng DCH, Karski J, Peniston C, et al. Early tracheal extubation after coronary artery bypass graft surgery reduces cost and improves resource use. *Anesthesiology* 1996;85:1300–1310.
47. Ovrum E, Tangen G, Schiott C, et al. Rapid recovery protocol applied to 5658 consecutive "on pump" coronary bypass patients. *Ann Thorac Surg* 2000;70:2008–2012.
48. Heinle S, Diaz K, Fox LS. Early extubation after cardiac operations in neonates and young infants. *J Thorac Cardiovasc Surg* 1997;114:413–418.
49. Price JA, Rizk NW. Postoperative ventilatory management. *Chest* 1999;115:130S–137S.
50. Meade MO, Guyatt G, Butler R, et al. Trials comparing early vs late extubation following cardiovascular surgery. *Chest* 2001;120: 445S–453S.

51. Oikkonen M, Karjalainen K, Kahara V, et al. Comparison of incentive spirometry and intermittent positive pressure breathing after coronary artery bypass graft. *Chest* 1991;99:60–65.
52. Davies LK. Cardiopulmonary bypass in infants and children: how is it different? *J Cardiovasc Vasc Anesth* 1999;13:330–345.
53. Brater DC. Diuretic therapy. *N Engl J Med* 1998;339:387–395.
54. Johnson RG, Shafique T, Sirois C, et al. Potassium concentrations and ventricular ectopy: a prospective observational study in post–cardiac surgery patients. *Crit Care Med* 1999;27:2430–2434.
55. Wait RB, Kahng KU, Dresner LS. Fluids and electrolytes and acid-base balance. In: Greenfield LJ, Mulholland M, Oldham KT, et al., eds. *Surgery: scientific principles and practice,* 2nd ed. Philadelphia: Lippincott–Raven, 1997:254.
56. Gray RJ, Braunstein G, Krutzik S, et al. Calcium homeostasis during coronary bypass surgery. *Circulation* 1980;62:I57–I61.
57. Reiner AP. Massive transfusion. In: Spiess BD, Counts RB, Gould SA, eds. *Perioperative transfusion medicine.* Baltimore: Williams & Wilkins, 1998:360.
58. Meldrum DR, Cleveland JC, Sheridan BC, et al. Cardiac surgical implications of calcium dyshomeostasis in the heart. *Ann Thorac Surg* 1996;61:1273–1280.
59. Chen RH. The scientific basis for hypocalcemic cardioplegia and reperfusion in cardiac surgery. *Ann Thorac Surg* 1996;62: 910–914.
60. Munoz R, Laussen PC, Palacio G, et al. Whole blood ionized magnesium: age-related differences in normal values and clinical implications of ionized hypomagnesemia in patients undergoing surgery for congenital cardiac disease. *J Thorac Cardiovasc Surg* 2000;119:891–898.
61. England MR, Gordon G, Salem M, et al. Magnesium administration and dysrhythmias after cardiac surgery. *JAMA* 1992;268: 2395–2402.
62. Toraman F, Karabulut EH, Alhan HC, et al. Magnesium infusion dramatically decreases the incidence of atrial fibrillation after coronary artery bypass grafting. *Ann Thorac Surg* 2001;72: 1256–1262.
63. Storm W, Zimmerman JJ. Magnesium deficiency and cardiogenic shock after cardiopulmonary bypass. *Ann Thorac Surg* 1997;64: 572–577.
64. Campi J, Radius E, Bar I, et al. Effects of magnesium on myocardial function after coronary artery bypass grafting. *Ann Thorac Surg* 1995;59:942–947.
65. Androgue HJ, Madias NE. Management of life-threatening acid–base disorders: first of two parts. *N Engl J Med* 1998;338: 26–34.
66. Ritter JM, Doktor HS, Benjamin N. Paradoxical effect of bicarbonate on cytoplasmic pH. *Lancet* 1990;336:372–373.
67. Viitanen A, Salmenpera M, Heinonen J, et al. Pulmonary vascular resistance before and after cardiopulmonary bypass: the effect of PaCO2. *Chest* 1989;95:773–778.
68. Fullerton DA, McIntyre RC, Kirson LE, et al. Impact of respiratory acid–base status in patients with pulmonary hypertension. *Ann Thorac Surg* 1996;61:696–701.
69. Androgue HJ, Madias NE. Management of life-threatening acid–base disorders: second of two parts. *N Engl J Med* 1998; 338:107–111.

70. Goodnough LT, Brecher ME, Kanter MH, et al. Transfusion medicine: blood transfusion. *N Engl J Med* 1999;340:438–447.
71. Rebollo MH, Bernal JM, Llorca J, et al. Nosocomial infections in patient having cardiovascular operations: a multivariate analysis of risk factors. *J Thorac Cardiovasc Surg* 1996;112:908–913.
72. Leal-Noval SR, Rincon-Ferrari MD, Garcia-Curiel A, et al. Transfusion of blood components and postoperative infection in patients undergoing cardiac surgery. *Chest* 2001;119:1461–1468.
73. Chelemer SB, Prato BS, Cox PM Jr, et al. Association of bacterial infection and red blood cell transfusion after coronary artery bypass surgery. *Ann Thorac Surg* 2002;73:138–142.
74. Van de Watering LMG, Hermans J, Houbiers JGA, et al. Beneficial effects of leukocyte depletion of transfused blood on postoperative complications in patients undergoing cardiac surgery. *Circulation* 1998;97:562–568.
75. Parolari A, Antona C, Rona P, et al. The effect of multiple blood conservation techniques on donor blood exposures in adult coronary and valve surgery performed with a membrane oxygenator: a multivariate analysis on 1310 patients. *J Cardiac Surg* 1995;10:227–235.
76. Goodnough LT, Brecher ME, Kanter MH, et al. Transfusion medicine: blood conservation. *N Engl J Med* 1999;340:525–533.
77. Hardy J-F, Belisle S, Janview G, et al. Reduction in requirements for allogenic blood products: nonpharmacologic methods. *Ann Thorac Surg* 1996;62:1935–1943.
78. Sowade O, Warnke H, Scigalla P, et al. Avoidance of allogenic blood transfusions by treatment with epoietin (recombinant human erythropoietin) in patients undergoing open-heart surgery. *Blood* 1997;89:411–418.
79. Shimpo H, Mizumoto T, Onoda K, et al. Erythropoietin in pediatric cardiac surgery: clinical efficacy and effective dose. *Chest* 1997;111:1565–1570.
80. D'Ambra MN, Gray RJ, Hillman R, et al. Effect of recombinant human erythropoietin on transfusion risk in coronary bypass patients. *Ann Thorac Surg* 1997;64:1686–1693.
81. Ascione R, Williams S, Lloyd CT, et al. Reduced postoperative blood loss and transfusion requirement after beating-heart coronary operations: a prospective randomized study. *J Thorac Cardiovasc Surg* 2001;121:689–696.
82. Laffey JG, Boylan JF, Cheng DCH. The systemic inflammatory response to cardiac surgery. *Anesthesiology* 2002;97:215–252.
83. Hsu L-C. Biocompatibility in cardiopulmonary bypass. *J Cardioasc Vasc Anesth* 1997;11:376–382.
84. Mahoney CB, Lemole GM. Transfusion after coronary artery bypass surgery: the impact of heparin-bonded circuits. *Eur J Cardiothorac Surg* 1999;16:206–210.
85. Shapira OM, Aldea GS, Zeligher J, et al. Enhanced blood conservation and improved clinical outcome after valve surgery using heparin-bonded cardiopulmonary bypass circuits. *J Cardiac Surg* 1996;11:307–317.
86. Ranucci M, Mazzucco A, Pessotto R, et al. Heparin-coated circuits for high-risk patients: a multicenter, prospective, randomized trial. *Ann Thorac Surg* 1999;67:994–1000.
87. Grossi EA, Kallenbach K, Chau S, et al. Impact of heparin bonding on pediatric cardiopulmonary bypass: a prospective randomized study. *Ann Thorac Surg* 2000;70:191–196.

88. Muehrcke DD, McCarthy PM, Kottke-Marchant K, et al. Biocompatibility of heparin-coated extracorporeal bypass circuits: a randomized, masked clinical trial. *J Thorac Cardiovasc Surg* 1996;112:472–483.
89. Aldea GS, Doursounian M, O'Gara P, et al. Heparin-bonded circuits with a reduced anticoagulation protocol in primary CABG: a prospective randomized study. *Ann Thorac Surg* 1996;62: 410–418.
90. Bannan S, Danby A, Cowan D, et al. Low heparinization with heparin-bonded bypass circuits: is it a safe strategy? *Ann Thorac Surg* 1997;63:663–668.
91. Scott W, Rode R, Castleman B, et al. Efficacy, complications and cost of a comprehensive blood conservation program for cardiac operations. *J Thorac Cardiovasc Surg* 1992;103:1001–1007.
92. Mojcik CF, Levy JH. Aprotinin and the systemic inflammatory response after cardiopulmonary bypass. *Ann Thorac Surg* 2001; 71:745–754.
93. Peters DC, Noble S. Aprotinin: an update of its pharmacology and therapeutic use in open heart surgery and coronary bypass surgery. *Drugs* 1999;57:233–260.
94. Hardy J-F. Pharmacological strategies for blood conservation in cardiac surgery: erythropoietin and antifibrinolytics. *Can J Anaesth* 2001;48:S24–S31.
95. Poullis M, Manning R, Laffan, M, et al. The antithrombotic effect of aprotinin: actions mediated via the protease-activated receptor 1. *J Thorac Cardiovasc Surg* 2000;120:370–378.
96. Levi M, Cromheecke ME, de Jonge E, et al. Pharmacological strategies to decrease excessive blood loss in cardiac surgery: a meta-analysis of clinically relevant endpoints. *Lancet* 1999;354: 1940–1947.
97. Smith PK, Muhlbaier LH. Aprotinin: safe and effective only with the full-dose regimen. *Ann Thorac Surg* 1996;62:1575–1577.
98. Smith CR, Spanier TB. Aprotinin in deep hypothermic circulatory arrest. *Ann Thorac Surg* 1999;68:278–286.
99. Feindt P, Seyfert UT, Volmer I, et al. Celite and kaolin produce differing activated clotting times during cardiopulmonary bypass under aprotinin therapy. *Thorac Cardiovasc Surgeon* 1994; 42:218–221.
100. Dietrich W, Spath P, Zuhlsdorf M, et al. Anaphylactic reactions to aprotinin reexposure in cardiac surgery: relation to antiaprotinin immunoglobulin G and E antibodies. *Anesthesiology* 2001; 95:64–71.
101. Lemmer JH Jr, Stanford W, Bonney SL, et al. Aprotinin for coronary bypass operations: efficacy, safety, and influence on early saphenous vein graft patency: a multicenter, randomized, double-blind, placebo-controlled study. *J Thorac Cardiovasc Surg* 1994; 107:543–553.
102. Alderman EL, Levy JH, Rich JB, et al. Analyses of coronary graft patency after aprotinin use: results from the International Multicenter Aprotinin Graft Patency Experience (IMAGE) trial. *J Thorac Cardiovasc Surg* 1998;116:716–730.
103. Lemmer JH Jr, Stanford W, Bonney SL, et al. Aprotinin for coronary artery bypass grafting: effect on postoperative renal function. *Ann Thorac Surg* 1995;59:132–136.

104. Daily PO, Lamphere JA, Dembitsky WP, et al. Effect of prophylactic epsilon-aminocaproic acid on blood loss and transfusion requirements in patients undergoing first-time coronary artery bypass grafting. *J Thorac Cardiovasc Surg* 1994;108:99–108.
105. Vander Salm TJ, Kaur S, Lancey RA, et al. Reduction in bleeding after heart operations through the prophylactic use of epsilon-aminocaproic acid. *J Thorac Cardiovasc Surg* 1996; 112:1098–1107.
106. Dunn CJ, Goa KL. Tranexamic acid: a review of its use in surgery and other indications. *Drugs* 1999;57:1005–1032.
107. Royston D. Aprotinin versus lysine analogues: the debate continues. *Ann Thorac Surg* 1998;65: S9–S19.
108. Fanashawe MP, Shore-Lesserson L, Reich DL. Two cases of fatal thrombosis after aminocaproic acid therapy and deep hypothermic circulatory arrest. *Anesthesiology* 2001;95:1525–1527.
109. American Regent Laboratories. *Aminocaproic acid product insert.* Shirley, NY: American Regent Laboratories, 1999.
110. McEvoy GK, ed. *American hospital formulary drug information 2002.* Bethesda: American Society of Health-System Pharmacists, 2002:1454–1457.
111. Casati V, Guzzon D, Oppizzi M, et al. Tranexamic acid compared with high-dose aprotinin in primary elective heart operations: effects on perioperative bleeding and allogeneic transfusions. *J Thorac Cardiovasc Surg* 2000;120:520–527.
112. Erstad BL. Antifibrinolytic agents and desmopressin as hemostatic agents in cardiac surgery. *Ann Pharmacother* 2001;35: 1075–1084.
113. Despotis GJ, Levine V, Saleem R, et al. DDAVP reduces blood loss and transfusion in cardiac surgical patients with impaired platelet function identified using a point-of-care test: a double-blind, placebo controlled trial. *Lancet* 1999;254:106–110.
114. Body SC, Birmingham J, Parks R, et al. Safety and efficacy of shed mediastinal blood transfusion after cardiac surgery: multicenter observational study. *J Cardiovasc Vasc Anesth* 1999;13: 410–416.
115. De Varennes B, Nguyen D, Denis F, et al. Reinfusion of mediastinal blood in CABG patients: impact on homologous transfusions and rate of re-exploration. *J Cardiac Surg* 1996;11: 387–395.
116. Martin J, Robitaille D, Perrault LP, et al. Reinfusion of mediastinal blood after heart surgery. *J Thorac Cardiovasc Surg* 2000;120:499–504.
117. Vertrees RA, Conti VR, Lick SD, et al. Adverse effects of postoperative infusion of shed mediastinal blood. *Ann Thorac Surg* 1996;62:717–723.
118. Lin JC, Szwerc MF, Magovern JA. Non-steroidal anti-inflammatory drug-based pain control for minimally invasive direct coronary artery bypass surgery. *Heart Surg Forum* 1999;2: 169–171.
119. Young C, Knudsen N, Hilton A, et al. Sedation in the intensive care unit. *Crit Care Med* 2000;28:854–866.
120. Thourani VH, Weintraub WS, Stein B, et al. Influence of diabetes mellitus on early and late outcome after coronary artery bypass grafting. *Ann Thorac Surg* 1999;67:1045–1052.

121. Van den Berghe G, Wouters P, Weekers F, et al. Intensive insulin therapy in critically ill patients. *N Engl J Med* 2001;345: 1359–1367.
122. Furnary AP, Zerr KJ, Grunkemeier GL, et al. Continuous intravenous insulin infusion reduces the incidence of deep sternal wound infection in diabetic patients after cardiac surgical procedures. *Ann Thorac Surg* 1999;67:352–360.
123. Rich MW. Keller AJ, Schechtman KB, et al. Increased complications and prolonged hospital stay in elderly cardiac surgical patients with low serum albumin. *Am J Cardiol* 1989;63:714–718.
124. Engelman DT, Adams DH, Byrne JG, et al. Impact of body mass index and albumin on morbidity and mortality after cardiac surgery. *J Thorac Cardiovasc Surg* 1999;118:866–873.
125. Cerra FB, Benitez MR, Blackburn GL, et al. Applied nutrition in ICU patients: a consensus statement of the American College of Chest Physicians. *Chest* 1997;111:769–778.
126. Souba WW. Nutritional support. *N Engl J Med* 1997;336:41–48.
127. Genton L, Jolliet P, Pichard C. Feeding the intensive care patient. *Curr Opin Anaesth* 2001;14:131–136.
128. Strong DM, Latz L. Blood-bank testing for infectious diseases: how safe is blood transfusion? *Trends Mol Med* 2002;8:355–358.

Postoperative Complications Involving the Heart and Lungs

Despite advances in cardiac surgery and perioperative care, the prevention and treatment of postoperative complications continue to be an integral part of the care of the cardiac surgery patient. As older, sicker adult patients with more complicated cases undergo surgery with greater frequency, the opportunity for postoperative morbidity and mortality has increased (1). Likewise, infants with congenital heart conditions are undergoing total repair operations at an earlier age than in previous years, with a concomitant increase in the potential difficulties encountered in their early postoperative care. Recognition and treatment of perioperative complications are as important as the performance of the surgery itself. A technically perfect operation can be ruined by poor postoperative care, and a less-than-perfect technical operative result can often be "saved" by appropriate management of postoperative problems.

LOW CARDIAC OUTPUT

A useful definition of the state of significant low cardiac output following heart surgery is the following: the requirement for intra-aortic balloon counterpulsation or significant doses of inotropic drug support for longer than 30 minutes to maintain the systolic blood pressure >90 mm Hg and the cardiac index >2.2 L/min/m^2 (2). Low cardiac output occurs during the early postoperative period in approximately 10% to 20% of patients who undergo cardiac surgery. The incidence of this complication is dependent on the type and severity of the cardiac lesion undergoing repair, preoperative ventricular function, adequacy of myocardial preservation during the procedure, and adequacy of the surgical repair. For example, coronary artery bypass graft (CABG) procedures on patients with normal left ventricular (LV) function have a low incidence of postoperative low cardiac output. In contrast, patients with ischemic mitral valve regurgitation with poor LV function have a notoriously high incidence of low output after mitral valve replacement and coronary bypass surgery.

Although intraoperative technical mishaps or inadequate myocardial protection during surgery can cause damage to a previously normal ventricle, the most important factor determining the incidence of postoperative low output is preoperative ventricular function. Thus, preoperative evaluation of ventricular function is important. Careful review of the patient's cardiac catheterization study—both the hemodynamic measurements (cardiac output, LV end-diastolic pressure, and pulmonary artery pressures) and the left ventriculogram—provides a good indication of the presence or absence of preoperative ventricular dysfunction. Very useful is the preoperative echocardiogram, which provides information about global and segmental myocardial contractility, chamber sizes, and valvular function.

Normal systolic function is associated with an ejection fraction (EF) of 60% to 75%. Moderate LV dysfunction is present when the

EF is 35% to 50%, and severe impairment of contractility is associated with an EF below 35%. The EF is dependent on preload and afterload; therefore, the value should be assessed in the context of the patient's history and other data. The EF, furthermore, reflects only the systolic (ejection) function of the heart. Diastolic dysfunction, reflected as abnormalities in ventricular relaxation and filling, also can result in heart failure and even pulmonary edema, despite the presence of a normal systolic EF (3). Patients with LV hypertrophy are particularly susceptible to diastolic dysfunction.

Preoperative recognition of poor ventricular function leads to alterations in the management of technical aspects of the operative procedure. For example, in patients with poor preoperative LV function, we may place a catheter to vent the left ventricle to prevent ventricular distension, and we frequently use the technique of combined antegrade and retrograde cardioplegia to optimize cardioplegia delivery (see Chapter 2). Likewise, for patients with very poor LV function, a lower perfusion temperature during cardiopulmonary bypass (CPB) (such as 25 to 28°C) may be employed. For the patient with poor preoperative ventricular function, we routinely introduce a femoral artery catheter in the operating room just before beginning surgery to provide access for the expeditious introduction of an intraaortic balloon pump, should one be required in the operating room or during the early postoperative period. Patients with preoperative LVEF of <20% to 25% often have an intraaortic balloon pump placed prior to surgery, either in the catheterization laboratory (under fluoroscopic guidance) or in the operating room prior to making the incision (4).

Management of Low Cardiac Output

When low cardiac output is present early after cardiac surgery, management should follow a logical order of analysis and treatment (Fig. 4-1). First, consideration should be given to the possibility of reversible mechanical factors causing the poor cardiac performance. This is especially true for the patient who had good preoperative ventricular function and who was weaned from CPB without difficulty. Inadequate preload is the most common cause of low cardiac output. The left and right heart filling pressures should be measured and compared with those found to be optimal in the operating room and before surgery. Cardiac tamponade must be ruled out (see Chapter 5). Consideration should be given to the possibility of technical problems related to the operation: occlusion of bypass grafts, embolic obstruction of a coronary artery, prosthetic valve dehiscence or obstruction, residual shunts, or obstruction of a conduit or baffle (5).

The physical examination should be repeated. Patients with severe low cardiac output have cold, poorly perfused extremities and absent peripheral pulses. In infants, an elevated core temperature is often present with a cool periphery. Auscultation should be performed to listen especially for valvular regurgitation murmurs, abnormal prosthetic valve sounds (if a prosthetic valve is present), and muffled heart tones. The arterial blood pressure tracing should be inspected for the presence of an abnormally wide pulse pressure indicative of possible aortic valve regurgitation. The pulmonary artery wedge pressure tracing should be examined for the presence

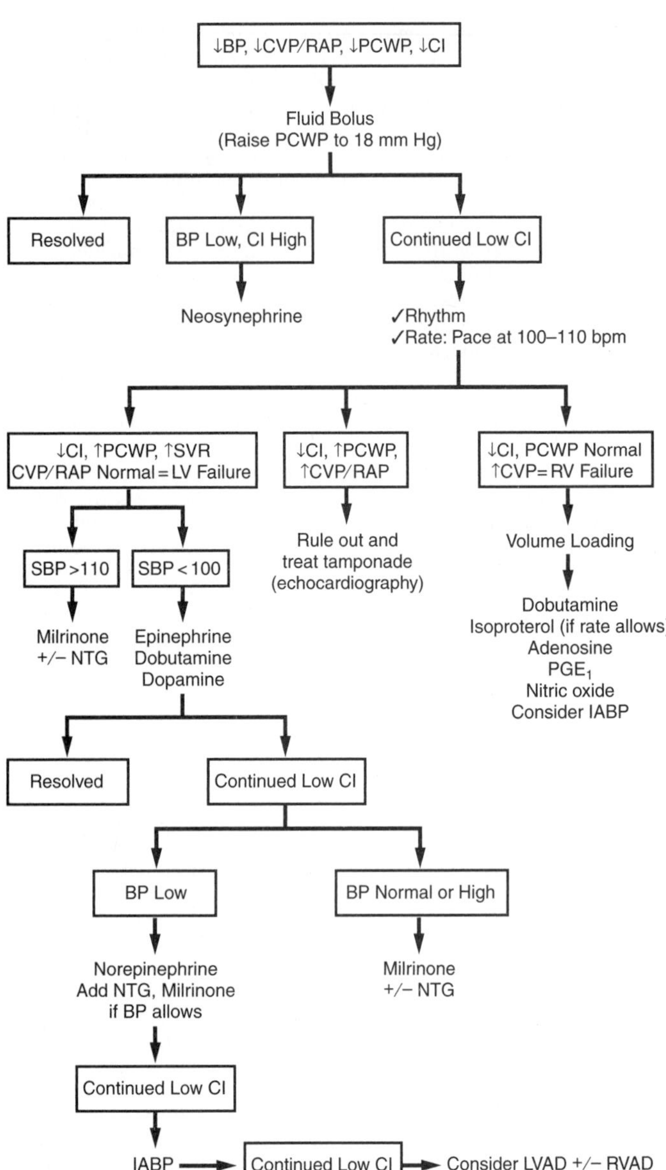

Fig. 4-1. Management algorithm for low cardiac output. BP, blood pressure; CI, cardiac index; CVP, central venous pressure; IABP, intra-aortic balloon pump; LV, left ventricle; LVAD, left ventricular assist device; NPD, nitroprusside; NTG, nitroglycerin; PCWP, pulmonary capillary wedge pressure; PGE_1, prostaglandin E_1; RAP, right atrial pressure; RV, right ventricle; RVAD, right ventricular assist device; SBP, systolic blood pressure; SVR, systemic vascular resistance.

of V waves, suggesting mitral valve regurgitation. The 12-lead electrocardiogram (ECG) should be studied for evidence of ischemia.

Echocardiography provides information about both valvular and ventricular function. In infants, transthoracic echocardiography can be used to visualize the ventricles, assess their contractility, and determine the presence or absence of significant mediastinal blood clots; color flow Doppler can be used to identify residual intracardiac shunts. A bolus of saline injected through a right atrial or central venous catheter will produce a cloud of echocardiographically visible microbubbles ("echo contrast") in the right atrium and ventricle that will appear immediately in the left atrium or ventricle if there is a right-to-left shunt. Likewise, agitated saline injected into the left atrial line will produce echo contrast in the right side if there is a left-to-right shunt.

Early after surgery, transthoracic echocardiography is not as useful in adults as it is in infants. Inability to turn the patient, bandages, mediastinal air, chest tubes, and the adult chest configuration combine to make assessment of the heart by this technique difficult. Transesophageal echocardiography, however, is easily performed by the experienced operator and provides reliable information regarding ventricular filling and function, valvular function, and the presence or absence of tamponade (6).

Occasionally, emergency cardiac catheterization may be indicated to rule out reparable abnormalities. Coronary arteriography may reveal native artery or graft spasm or bypass graft occlusion. If a mechanical cause for the low cardiac output state is identified, immediate surgical repair is usually indicated despite the emotional trauma experienced by both the patient's family and the surgeon in these situations.

While this evaluation is proceeding, efforts to improve the cardiac output and systemic perfusion are begun. The treatment of low cardiac output involves consideration of the heart rhythm, heart rate, status of the ventricular filling pressure (preload), myocardial contractility, and systemic (and pulmonary) vascular resistance (afterload).

Early consideration should be given to the patient's cardiac rhythm and rate. Cardiac output is reduced in the presence of arrhythmias such as heart block, junctional rhythm, atrial fibrillation, and sinus bradycardia. For the severely compromised patient with new-onset atrial fibrillation, synchronized electrical cardioversion is indicated; restoration of normal sinus rhythm or pharmacologic control of a rapid ventricular response to atrial fibrillation will improve the cardiac output. For patients with heart block or junctional rhythm, sequential atrioventricular pacing will restore the atrial contribution to the stroke volume, increasing the patient's cardiac output by 15% to 35% (7). Proper capture of the atrium must be ensured, and for adults, the atrioventricular interval (the time between the pacing impulse to the atrium and the impulse to the ventricle) should be set at 150 to 180 milliseconds; shorter intervals are used for pediatric patients. Even for patients in sinus rhythm, if the heart rate is substantially <100 beats per minute, pacing at the rate of 100 will result in an improvement in the cardiac output (8). For patients with intact atrioventricular conduction, this is accomplished best by pacing only the atrium.

During the first few hours after surgery, patients frequently have a below-normal core temperature, although the importance of this abnormality is not entirely clear. During surgery, the patients are rewarmed to around 36°C (nasopharyngeal) prior to weaning from CPB; excessive or too rapid rewarming is avoided. Patients who undergo surgery without CPB may experience significant cooling, despite measures such as the use of a heated air-warming blanket during surgery. Postoperative hypothermia reduces cardiac output, increases systemic vascular resistance (SVR), and may be associated with increased complications (9). On the other hand, the reduction in oxygen consumption associated with hypothermia may balance the negative hemodynamic effects (10). Shivering occurs in some postoperative patients as a response to hypothermia, although the mechanism is not entirely clear. It does, however, result in increased metabolic rate and oxygen expenditure. For the shivering patient with low cardiac output, treatment with neuromuscular blocking agents or other drugs will decrease oxygen consumption and may improve the patient's hemodynamic status (11,12).

Optimal cardiac output requires adequate preload for LV filling (Fig. 4-2). LV preload may be monitored by measurement of the pulmonary artery diastolic pressure, pulmonary capillary wedge pressure, and, if a catheter was placed intraoperatively, left atrial pressure. Although the normal heart functions well with a pul-

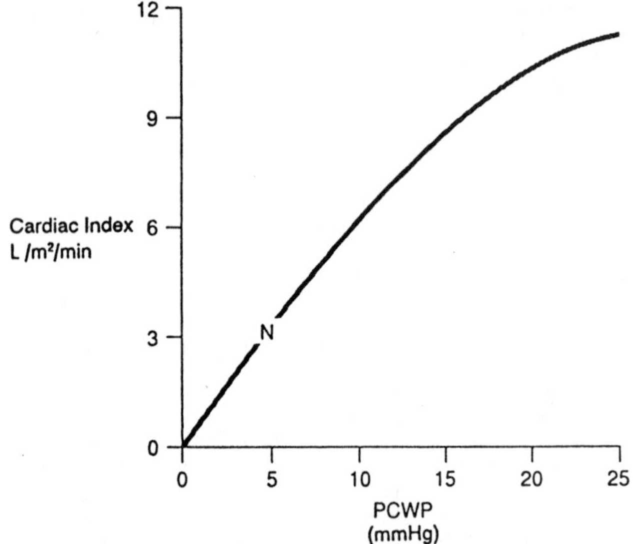

Fig. 4-2. Left ventricular function curve (modified from the Frank–Starling curve). *N* is the normal resting status, and the curve represents normal cardiac output response to changes in filling pressure. PCWP, pulmonary capillary wedge pressure. (From Bartlett RH. *University of Michigan critical care handbook*. 1991, with permission).

monary capillary wedge pressure of 6 to 12 mm Hg, failing hearts require higher filling pressures because of poor compliance of the left ventricle. A trial infusion of 250 to 500 mL of crystalloid or colloid fluid to the adult patient, given over a short period, is an important early maneuver in the management of low output. Raising the LV filling pressure to 15 to 18 mm Hg frequently improves the cardiac output. Patients with LV hypertrophy often have significant diastolic (relaxation) dysfunction and require higher-than-normal filling pressures even though the systolic function is normal. In some patients, very high filling pressures, even up to 25 to 30 mm Hg, are required to optimize LV performance. Knowledge of the preoperative filling pressure is useful. Volume infusion should be administered with care; overfilling of the heart leads to ventricular distention, worsening of the myocardial performance, and pulmonary edema. Either crystalloid (often as 5% dextrose/0.5 N saline) or colloid may be used for volume expansion. Although avoidance of unnecessary blood product transfusion is important, severe anemia in the presence of impaired ventricular function (and loss of ability to compensate for the anemia) results in diminished systemic oxygen delivery. Thus, for patients with low cardiac output after surgery, we often transfuse red blood cells to raise the hematocrit to at least 25% to 27%.

Inotropic Drug Treatment of Low Cardiac Output

Various drugs optimize cardiac output through their effects on myocardial contractility (inotropic effect), their effects on the SVR, or both. Table 4-1 summarizes the commonly used drugs. No one drug is best for all patients with low cardiac output; several drugs may be equally effective in the same hemodynamic setting, and the combined use of several drugs may prove to be most efficacious. Local institutional custom, personal opinion, and, at times, a bit of superstition are often involved in the decision as to which agents are used for which circumstances. Rational selection of drugs to treat low cardiac output requires a basic understanding of the agents available, careful analysis of the hemodynamic abnormalities present, tailoring of the therapy to fit the individual hemodynamic setting, and realization that the patient's state is dynamic, and thus, alterations in the type of drug support administered may be required with the passage of time (13). In general, the drugs used to treat low cardiac output are administered at doses sufficient to achieve a certain end-point (e.g., normalization of blood pressure, cardiac output, and heart rate) rather than a certain specific dose.

All of the available inotropic drugs should be administered via a central vein to ensure delivery into the circulation, to avoid vein irritation, and to prevent extravasation. These agents are usually administered via a catheter in the internal jugular vein or right atrium, but some degree of inactivation of the drug may occur as it traverses the pulmonary circulation. If a left atrial catheter was placed at the time of surgery, it may be used for drug administration that will result in higher coronary and systemic concentrations (14). This route of administration risks the introduction of air emboli into the left heart and should be used only when right heart administration is ineffective and by nursing staff who are experienced in the management of left atrial catheters. Continuous blood pressure monitoring via a radial or femoral artery catheter

Table 4-1. Effects of pharmacologic agents used to treat hypotension and low cardiac output

Drug	Inotropic Effect	Chronotropic Effect	Peripheral Resistance	Cardiac Output	Intravenous Dose Range	Comment
Dobutamine (Dobutrex)	++	+	–	++	2–20 μg/kg/min	May produce more tachycardia than dopamine
Dopamine	++	+	0 or + (dose dependent)	+	2–15 μg/kg/min	Usefulness in renal insufficiency not confirmed
Ephedrine	++	++	0 or +	++	5–25 mg q 10 min (adult dose)	Short-term use only
Epinephrine (Adrenalin)	+++	++	– or 0 or + (dose dependent)	++	0.01–2.0 μg/kg/min (adult: 1–10 μg/min)	β-Receptor agonist at low dose, more α at higher doses; less tachycardia than dobutamine
Isoproterenol (Isuprel)	++	+++	–	++	0.01–2.0 μg/kg/min (adult: 2–10 μg/min)	Usefulness limited by tachycardia

Milrinone (Primacor)	++	0	– –	+	Load 50 µg/kg over 10 min, then 0.375–0.75 µg/kg/min	Reduces PA resistance and pressure; increases flow in arterial grafts; useful for RV failure
Norepinephrine (Levophed)	++	0 or –	+++	++	0.01–0.2 µg/kg/min (adult: 0.5–30 µg/min)	Particularly useful with milrinone or nitroglycerin
Phenylephrine (Neosynephrine)	0	0 or –	+++	0 or –	0.15–0.5 µg/kg/min (adult: 20–180 µg/min)	Used for high–cardiac output/low–blood pressure situation

(+), increase; (–), decrease; 0, no effect; PA, pulmonary artery; RV, right ventricle.

is required for patients receiving significant doses of vasoactive drugs.

Positive inotropic drugs used during the early postoperative period act by increasing the level of intracellular cyclic adenosine monophosphate (cAMP), which has a direct role in the contractile state of the myocardial cells (15). Increased intracellular cAMP results in increased contractility and relaxation, resulting in improved ventricular function. β-Adrenergic agonists (dopamine, dobutamine, epinephrine, norepinephrine, and isoproterenol) stimulate cell surface β1- and β2-receptors, resulting in increased adenylate cyclase activity with increased production of cAMP. β1-Receptors exist predominantly in the myocardium; their activation results in increased speed and force of myocardial contraction, increased rate of automaticity of the sinoatrial node, and faster atrioventricular conduction. The β2-receptors are present predominantly in the smooth muscles of blood vessels and bronchi; their activation results in vasodilation and bronchodilation. α-Adrenergic receptors exist primarily in the peripheral and pulmonary vasculature; α-receptor stimulation causes vasoconstriction.

Dopamine is frequently used for the treatment of reduced cardiac output. A unique feature of this agent is that it has distinctly different hemodynamic effects at different doses. When administered at low doses, 1 to 3 μg/kg per minute, dopamine stimulates the dopamine (DA1) receptors in the renal, mesenteric, coronary, and cerebral circulations, resulting in vasodilation of these vascular beds. Improved renal and mesenteric blood flow results, although the effectiveness of "renal dose" dopamine for the treatment of renal insufficiency is debated (see Chapter 5). At moderate dopamine doses, 3 to 5 μg/kg per minute, dopamine activates β1-receptors, causing increases in myocardial contractility and cardiac output, often without a significant change in the blood pressure. Myocardial oxygen consumption is increased. At high dopamine doses, above 10 to 15 μg/kg per minute, α-adrenergic activation predominates, resulting in vasoconstriction of most vascular beds, tachycardia, increased blood pressure, and increased SVR. In some patients, tachycardia may develop even at moderate doses, thus limiting the effectiveness of dopamine as a positive inotropic agent. Although useful, dopamine is not a strong inotropic agent, probably because part of its action is indirect, through the release of endogenous norepinephrine, which may be depleted in the postoperative heart.

Dobutamine is a popular, effective short-acting agent for treatment of postoperative low cardiac output syndrome. A synthetic sympathomimetic amine, dobutamine acts through stimulation of β1-receptors with no α-receptor effects at any dose (unlike dopamine). It has moderate positive inotropic effects, causes a decrease in peripheral vascular and pulmonary vascular resistances, and increases the heart rate. This combination of increased contractility and decreased afterload can be useful in many patients; thus, dobutamine is often a good first-choice drug for the treatment of mild to moderate low output. Dobutamine may be preferable to moderate- or high-dose dopamine because it increases the cardiac output with a smaller increase in myocardial oxygen consumption (16,17). Frequently, however, the usefulness of dobutamine is limited by the concomitant tachycardia produced. It is administered in a starting dose of 2 to 5 μg/kg per minute, which may be increased to achieve the desired hemodynamic effect (usually up to no more than 12 to 15 μg/kg per minute) or until the heart rate exceeds 100 beats per minute.

Epinephrine is the naturally occurring catecholamine released from the adrenal medulla. Epinephrine acts directly on both α- and β-receptors. At low doses (<0.02 μg/kg per minute), epinephrine activates β1-receptors in the heart and β2-receptors in skeletal muscle blood vessels, causing vasodilation. Myocardial contractility and oxygen consumption, cardiac index, and heart rate all increase, while SVR is often decreased. At low doses, blood may be shunted away from the kidneys and mesentery. At higher doses, the β2 effect is lost, and β1- and α-receptor stimulation predominates. This results in further positive inotropic and chronotropic effects and elevation of the blood pressure but at the cost of increased myocardial oxygen consumption, increased pulmonary artery pressure, and significant increases in vascular resistance that may compromise kidney and other vital organ perfusion. Vasoconstriction, tachycardia, and arrhythmias limit the usefulness of epinephrine at high doses. Epinephrine also reduces tissue glucose uptake and inhibits insulin release in the pancreas, often resulting in hyperglycemia that may require insulin administration. Despite these limitations, epinephrine is a popular agent and is often our first choice for the treatment of moderate low cardiac output syndrome as it compares quite favorably with dobutamine (18). Combined with a vasodilator (such as nitroglycerin), the vasoconstriction caused by higher-dose epinephrine may be lessened with improvement in the overall hemodynamic state.

Norepinephrine, an endogenous neurotransmitter, acts primarily to stimulate β1- and α-receptors with little or no effect on β2-receptors. This results in cardiac stimulation and vasoconstriction. The cardiac effects result in increased cardiac output and increased myocardial oxygen consumption with increased myocardial perfusion as the coronary vessels have a low density of α-receptors. The vasoconstriction effect causes the blood pressure to be increased (often dramatically), and through increased reflex vagal activity, the heart rate usually falls or remains the same. This combination of improved inotropic state, increased blood pressure, improved myocardial blood flow, and reduced heart rate is often quite favorable for the patient suffering severe low cardiac output. The perfusion of different organ systems is variable and depends largely on the relative concentration of α-receptors. Blood flow is redistributed so as to increase heart and brain perfusion, while blood flow to skeletal muscle, skin, and splanchnic beds decreases. Norepinephrine is less arrhythmogenic than epinephrine.

These qualities make norepinephrine particularly useful for treating severe low cardiac output states, especially when associated with hypotension. A starting dose of 0.05 μg/kg per minute is increased as needed to raise the blood pressure and cardiac index. The goal is to return the patient's blood pressure to a level slightly less than his or her usual pressure. For adult patients who were normotensive prior to surgery, this would be a systolic pressure of 80 to 100 mm Hg. Norepinephrine should not be used to raise the blood pressure to supranormal levels. At high doses, the usefulness of norepinephrine is limited by severe peripheral and visceral vasoconstriction that may cause renal insufficiency, intestinal hypoperfusion, and limb ischemia. This is more likely to occur if the patient is hypovolemic; sufficient volume loading should always be accomplished prior to the administration of significant doses of any catecholamine agent.

The concomitant administration of norepinephrine plus a vasodilator such as a phosphodiesterase inhibitor (namely, milrinone) or nitroglycerin is logical, results in further improvement in the cardiac index, and has proven useful for assistance in weaning patients from CPB (19,20). The combination of norepinephrine and milrinone is used frequently in our practices for the treatment of severe postoperative low cardiac output syndrome.

As a rule, norepinephrine should be administered at the lowest effective dose for the shortest necessary period of time. As the patient's cardiac function improves, it is our practice to switch the patient over to a less potent inotropic drug, most commonly dobutamine.

Dopexamine has both β2- and dopamine receptor agonist activity, thus increasing the inotropic state of the heart while also producing a reduction in SVR. Its usefulness, however, is limited by the tendency to cause a significant tachycardia (15).

Isoproterenol stimulates β1-receptors in the heart and β2-receptors in the peripheral vessels, resulting in increases in heart rate, contractility, cardiac output, and myocardial oxygen consumption with a decrease in peripheral vascular resistance. The result is an increase in the cardiac index, due largely to the increased heart rate, with little change in blood pressure. In general, isoproterenol is not recommended for the treatment of postoperative myocardial dysfunction, especially in patients with ischemic heart disease, because it causes a significant increase in myocardial oxygen consumption and is very arrhythmogenic (13). One benefit of isoproterenol is that it lowers pulmonary vascular resistance (PVR), an especially helpful action when reactive pulmonary hypertension and right heart dysfunction are present. This is particularly useful in children with pulmonary hypertension in whom isoproterenol can be infused constantly into a central vein at 0.01 to 0.05 μg/kg per minute if the heart rate is not excessive. It is also used in cardiac transplant patients who may have a slow heart rate and diminished contractility for several days after implantation.

Milrinone increases intracellular cAMP levels by inhibiting the enzyme responsible for cAMP degradation (phosphodiesterase). This results in increased myocardial cell contractility and relaxation plus significant vascular smooth muscle cell relaxation, both favorable effects for the treatment of low cardiac output. Treatment with milrinone causes increased cardiac output and decreased SVR and PVR with minimal effect on myocardial oxygen consumption (15). Milrinone also has the potential for the prevention and treatment of internal mammary artery spasm because of its vasodilatory effect (21). Because of vasodilation, however, arterial blood pressure may fall, and heart rate may increase during treatment. With efficacy comparable with dobutamine, milrinone can be used alone or in conjunction with a catecholamine (22–24). Having a different mechanism of action than the β-adrenergic agonists, the combined administration results in synergistic effects that are often very effective in the treatment of low cardiac output (20). In particular, we have found the simultaneous administration of milrinone and norepinephrine to be very effective. By titrating the relative doses of the two agents, the degree of afterload reduction can be controlled while both agents provide inotropic support via differing mechanisms. For patients with poor preoperative LV function and a significant likelihood of difficulty weaning from CPB and postoperative low cardiac output, we frequently will administer a single dose of milrinone (50 µg/kg) prior to CPB weaning. As CPB support is withdrawn, norepinephrine is infused at a low dose and titrated to offset the milrinone-induced hypotension (if needed) and to provide further inotropic support. If needed, a continuous milrinone infusion of 0.5 µg/kg per minute is instituted (25,26). Milrinone has also been demonstrated to be effective in pediatric cardiac surgery patients and for use in orthotopic heart transplantation (21).

Calcium chloride administered by slow intravenous bolus (10 mg/kg) will raise the patient's blood pressure associated with increases in myocardial contractility and peripheral vascular resistance. This effect, however, is transient, and sustained improvement in the hemodynamic state is not achieved (27). Continuous infusion does not result in sustained improvement in the cardiac index and risks dangerous hypercalcemia. There are multiple potential adverse effects of bolus calcium administration: ventricular irritability, coronary vasospasm, bradycardia, sinus arrest, exacerbation of myocardial reperfusion injury, and possibly pancreatitis. We recommend calcium administration only for documented hypocalcemia.

Digoxin has long been an important part of the treatment of *chronic* congestive heart failure, although its use is largely being replaced by newer drugs (28). For *acute* low cardiac output in adults, however, there is little or no role for digoxin due to its slow onset of action, long half-life, and narrow margin between therapeutic and toxic levels. In children, opinions are mixed regarding the usefulness of digoxin for the treatment of acute myocardial dysfunction (29). Digoxin toxicity occurs at lower serum levels in the presence of hypokalemia, hypomagnesemia, or hypoxia—all conditions that may arise during the early postoperative period. Digoxin has multiple potential interactions with other drugs that are often unpredictable in an individual patient. For these reasons, digoxin is generally not recommended to treat acute low cardiac output in patients following cardiac surgery.

Other inotropic agents have been described for use in cardiac surgical patients with postoperative low cardiac output, although their use is not widespread. Triiodothyronine, administered intra- and postoperatively in CABG patients, may have beneficial hemodynamic effects, may be associated with fewer complications such as atrial fibrillation and myocardial ischemia, and may reduce the need for postoperative mechanical support. These results have not, however, been consistently demonstrated, and widespread use of tri-iodothyronine administration has not been adopted (30,31). The combination of glucose (30% dextrose), insulin (50 U/L), and potassium (80 mEq/L), known as "GIK," infused intravenously at 1.0 mL/kg per hour, improves cardiac output and decreases the need for other inotropic drugs in adult patients undergoing coronary bypass surgery (32). Despite these potential benefits, thyroid hormone and GIK are used infrequently, and, by far, most clinical experience has involved the adrenergic agents and the phosphodiesterase inhibitors as drug treatment for postoperative low cardiac output.

Vasoactive Drugs in the Management of Low Cardiac Output

Management of low cardiac output involves optimization of preload (ventricular filling), contractility (inotropic state), and afterload (SVR and PVR). Drugs that alter the SVR and, thus, the patient's blood pressure are used frequently in the treatment of low cardiac output. Vasodilating drugs decrease the resistance against which the left ventricle ejects (the afterload), thus increasing the cardiac output. If the ventricular preload is adequate, little or no reduction in systemic arterial pressure should result. However, if the blood volume is low, hypotension may occur. This potential complication of vasodilator therapy is, of course, reversible by volume expansion. It is important to remember that blood volume may be low even when central venous or left atrial pressure is normal in the vasoconstricted patient. Afterload reduction results in a decrease in the pulmonary capillary wedge pressure, reflecting decreases in ventricular filling pressure and myocardial wall tension. Afterload-reducing drugs should be used only when ventricular preload is adequate, generally with the pulmonary capillary wedge (or left atrial) pressure being 10 to 15 mm Hg. Continuous blood pressure monitoring is employed when using significant doses of vasodilators.

The agents most commonly used for afterload reduction in the setting of acute low cardiac output are nitroglycerin and nitroprusside. Both are administered by continuous intravenous infusion, have short half-lives, and effectively reduce SVR, although nitroprusside is the more effective (and more toxic) of the two. Chapter 3 provides further discussion of these drugs.

As discussed previously, milrinone has both vasodilatory and inotropic properties, making it particularly useful for the treatment of low cardiac output (21).

Prostaglandin E_1 is a very potent vasodilator used infrequently in adults and occasionally in neonates. For adults or children with pulmonary hypertension (often following cardiac transplantation or mitral valve surgery), it may be infused directly into the pulmonary artery as part of the treatment for right heart failure (33). Due to decreased SVR, norepinephrine infusion may be required to counterbalance systemic hypotension. Similarly, in postoperative patients with pulmonary hypertension, the central venous administration of adenosine (50 μg/kg per minute) has been shown to result in reduced pulmonary artery pressures and increased cardiac output (34).

The use of vasodilators alone in the treatment of low cardiac output is often limited by hypotension; frequently, these drugs are used with an inotropic agent to augment cardiac output and maintain the systemic arterial pressure. Various combinations of an inotropic drug (dopamine, dobutamine, epinephrine, or norepinephrine) plus a vasodilator drug (nitroglycerin, nitroprusside, or milrinone) are used with clinical success. For the patient with hypertension and impaired renal function, fenoldopam may be of value (see Chapter 3).

Drugs that cause peripheral vasoconstriction are sometimes required in the management of patients early after cardiac surgery, usually when the arterial pressure is low, the SVR is low, and the cardiac output is relatively normal or high. Chapter 3 discusses the use of phenylephrine and vasopressin for the treatment of postoperative hypotension. In general, however, pure vasoconstricting drugs are not used for patients with hypotension that occurs in association with low cardiac output. Although the arterial pressure may rise, the cardiac output may fall further due to the increased SVR, which results in decreased organ perfusion. More often, these drugs are indicated to treat "high-output" hypotensive states where the arterial pressure is low, but cardiac output is above normal.

Overall, drug therapy for low cardiac output requires assessment of the hemodynamic situation based on physical examination and invasive measurements. Some patients with postoperative mild to moderate low cardiac output have a depressed cardiac index and normal peripheral vascular resistance. Many of these are successfully treated with moderate-dose dopamine or dobutamine or a low-dose epinephrine infusion. More severe states of low output may require higher-dose epinephrine or norepinephrine with the addition of milrinone and/or a pure vasodilator. For patients with coronary artery disease, nitroglycerin is preferred to nitroprusside as the initial agent for afterload reduction. The simultaneous, but separately controlled, administration of an inotrope/vasopressor drug (such as norepinephrine) and a vasodilator agent allows for separate control of myocardial stimulation and vascular resistance, with the goal being a balance that provides optimal systemic oxygen delivery.

It should be recognized that all patients do not react uniformly to the same inotropic agents and that the patient's hemodynamic status may change over the course of hours. Thus, flexibility, often with some experimentation, is necessary to determine the most suitable agent or combination of agents for a given patient. The recovering patient is weaned from the drugs one by one, with careful monitoring of hemodynamic parameters.

Patients suffering significant low cardiac output despite moderate doses of drug support may require mechanical support of the failing heart. By far, the most common initial form of mechanical support after cardiac surgery is intraaortic balloon counterpulsation (the so-called "balloon pump"). In general, an intraaortic balloon pump is inserted when the patient's cardiac index is <1.8 to 2.0 L/min/m^2 despite moderate doses of inotropic drugs in the absence of hypovolemia or reversible conditions such as tamponade. The topic of mechanical cardiac support is discussed in Chapter 8.

Low Cardiac Output Due to Right Ventricular Failure

Not all instances of postoperative low cardiac output are secondary to failure of the left ventricle. Inadequate output from the right ventricle results in inadequate filling of the left ventricle, decreased LV cardiac output, and poor systemic perfusion. Patients with preexisting pulmonary hypertension (such as those with long-standing mitral valve disease, some transplant patients, or those with chronic left-to-right shunts) or right ventricular (RV) hypertrophy are at particular risk for RV failure. Other causes of RV dysfunction include RV infarction, the performance of a right ventriculotomy necessary for cardiac repair (as in the correction of tetralogy of Fallot), inadequate intraoperative RV protection during aortic cross-clamping, and air embolism into the right coronary artery or bypass graft. Elevation of pulmonary artery pressure, either acute or chronic, produces increased afterload to ejection of the right ventricle with reduced RV output.

The diagnosis of RV failure is based on the demonstration of a low cardiac output with elevated right-sided filling pressures (central venous or right atrial) and relatively normal or decreased left-sided filling pressures (pulmonary capillary wedge or left atrial). If the potential for RV failure is suspected at the time of surgery, placement of a catheter for direct continuous measurement of left atrial pressure is very useful. Increasing right atrial pressure in association with decreasing left atrial pressure is an ominous sign. Echocardiography can be confirmatory by demonstrating poor RV contractility in the presence of relatively normal LV wall motion. Principles in the management of RV failure are to (a) provide adequate preload, (b) reduce RV afterload (PVR), and (c) maintain systemic blood pressure (35). RV output is very dependent on its preload. Volume loading, to a right atrial pressure of 8 to 15 mm Hg (or to 80% of the pulmonary capillary wedge pressure), may be necessary to increase the right heart output. The goal of inotropic drug support is to improve RV contractility and RV myocardial perfusion without increasing PVR. Isoproterenol infusion results in improved contractility and a decrease in PVR. Its usefulness is frequently limited, however, by the tachycardia and systemic vasodilation it causes. Dobutamine is often useful as it frequently does not cause elevation of the pulmonary artery pressure, and if the systemic blood pressure is adequate, nitroprusside may be added to decrease the PVR. Milrinone, by providing inotropic support to the myocardium while simultaneously decreasing PVR, is particularly useful for treating postoperative RV failure. It may, however, cause systemic hypotension, requiring the concomitant use of vasopressor agents. Continuous adenosine administration reduces the PVR and increases cardiac output without reducing the systemic blood pressure and may prove to be very useful for the treatment of RV failure associated with pulmonary hypertension (34). Other, more cumbersome treatments for right heart failure have included prostaglandin E_1 infusion and inhaled nitric oxide (35,36). Finally, even though LV function may be normal, the use of intraaortic balloon counterpulsation may prove helpful, possibly due to beneficial effects on septal wall motion and/or improved coronary blood flow.

When adequately treated, low cardiac output due to right heart failure will frequently be temporary and abate over a period of a few days.

CARDIAC ARREST

Cardiac arrest may occur in the postoperative patient unexpectedly [as in sudden development of ventricular fibrillation (VF)] or as the terminal event after a progressive downhill course (such as refractory low cardiac output syndrome). Patients who suffer unexpected cardiac arrest have the best chance of successful resuscitation, but the complication must be managed quickly and appropriately (37,38). Thus, the ECG and blood pressure are monitored constantly in all patients early after surgery (when the risk of cardiac arrest is the greatest) with alarm systems in place to alert the nursing staff if dangerous abnormalities occur. These alarms are lifesaving and must not be turned off to silence repeated irritating false sensing as this might lead to failure to recognize a potentially reversible, but otherwise fatal, arrhythmia.

Despite the many possible underlying causes of cardiac arrest in the postoperative patient (including arrhythmia, ischemia, pulmonary embolism, abrupt mechanical obstruction of a prosthetic valve, and tamponade), the initial management is the same and follows the basic protocol published by the American Heart Association (39). The technique of cardiopulmonary resuscitation (CPR) involves maintenance of an open airway (with or without mouth-to-mouth breaths) and chest compressions (appropriate to the size of the patient). The universal advanced life support algorithm specifies the following steps for management of cardiac arrest: Perform chest compressions for pulseless patients, defibrillate VF or ventricular tachycardia (VT) until no longer present, gain control of the airway by mask and bag insufflations or endotracheal intubation and provide adequate oxygenation and ventilation, give intravenous boluses of epinephrine (and/or vasopressin), and correct reversible causes (40). Potentially reversible causes include hypovolemia, hypoxia, myocardial ischemia, metabolic abnormalities, drug overdoses, cardiac tamponade, tension pneumothorax, and pulmonary embolism.

Ventricular fibrillation is the most common cause of sudden cardiac arrest. Prompt defibrillation is imperative; delays in defibrillation decrease the chance of successful resuscitation. Even if the patient is not being monitored, a witnessed cardiac arrest can be treated initially with an attempt at "blind" defibrillation, as it is likely that VF is the underlying rhythm. The initial defibrillation shocks should not be delayed for drug administration. The recommended initial adult defibrillation energy dose is 200 J. It is important to place the paddles across the patient's chest in a position that will optimize the amount of energy delivered to the heart (i.e., so that the paddles face each other, as well as possible with the center of the mass of the heart between them). An unsuccessful defibrillation attempt should be followed immediately by a second shock of 200 to 300 J and, if this is unsuccessful, then immediately by a 360-J shock. For children, the initial defibrillation energy dose is 2 J/kg and is increased to 4 J/kg for subsequent shocks (41). Delays in shock delivery, even for administering drugs, should not occur as the sooner defibrillation occurs, the higher the likelihood of resuscitation (42). The use of defibrillators that deliver shocks with a biphasic waveform provide for defibrillation at lower energy levels, thus improving defibrillation efficacy (43).

If defibrillation is not successful after three or more shocks or if >1 or 2 minutes have elapsed, closed chest CPR should begin. A bed board is placed beneath the patient to improve the effectiveness of closed chest cardiac massage. An adequate endotracheal airway is established, ventilation with 100% oxygen is begun, and closed chest massage performed. Moderate hyperventilation is best; frequent measurement of the arterial blood gases is performed if an arterial catheter is present. ECG monitoring is established, if not already in progress. Secure intravenous access is essential, preferably through a central or femoral venous route.

Closed chest cardiac massage restores cardiac output to only about 20% of normal (44). Although a normal systolic blood pressure (70 to 90 mm Hg) may be generated, the mean perfusion pressure is frequently far below normal during CPR. Adequacy of massage may be determined by observing the arterial blood pressure monitor (if an arterial catheter is in place), palpating the peripheral pulses, and examining the patient's pupils, which, if previously dilated, will frequently decrease to normal size. For neonatal patients, CPR employs the "two-thumb-encircling" compression technique (with two thumbs on the sternum and fingers encircling the chest and supporting the back), with the depth of compression being approximately one-third of the anterior–posterior diameter of the chest (45). The usual neonatal compression rate is approximately 90 per minute.

For some postoperative patients, adequate perfusion pressure cannot be generated by closed chest massage because of the instability of the sternum. In others, the presence of a compressing blood clot within the mediastinum may prevent effective CPR. Also, the presence of a prosthetic valve may make closed massage more hazardous because the myocardium can be perforated when compressed against the rigid prosthesis. In these instances, the chest should be reopened for open cardiac massage using the sterile thoracotomy instruments that should be readily available in all properly equipped cardiac surgical intensive care units. Open chest (or "internal") cardiac massage is often more effective than closed chest massage, especially if tamponade is relieved on opening the chest. Care must be taken in reopening the sternotomy incision, particularly if the patient has coronary bypass grafts.

Open massage is performed by placing one hand behind the heart and one hand on the anterior surface of the right atrium and ventricle. The hands should be kept flat while pressing them together at a rate of about 80 to 90 times per minute for adults. Compression begins at the apex and is advanced toward the ventricular outflow tracts. The heart should not be kneaded or squeezed by the fingers as this may cause perforation of the myocardium. Open cardiac massage allows for direct visualization of the heart, safer compressions in the presence of a prosthetic valve, less trauma to mediastinal structures, inspection for causative factors (such as an occluded bypass graft), direct application of pacing wires or internal defibrillation paddles, and direct injection of drugs into the heart or aorta. Fear of infection should not prevent the surgeon from reopening the patient's chest for open resuscitation, as the infection rate among those who survive is low (<10%) (46).

Epinephrine has been the drug of choice for the management of cardiac arrest (47). The combined α- and β-adrenergic agonist properties of epinephrine result in increased SVR, which directs more of the cardiac output to the brain and heart; also, the drug increases myocardial contractility and heart rate. Epinephrine may also facilitate defibrillation. The adult dose is a 1.0-mg intravenous bolus, and this may be repeated every 3 to 5 minutes as needed. In the event that an intravenous catheter is not present, 1.0 to 2.0 mg of epinephrine can be mixed with 10 mL of normal saline (for adults) and injected down the patient's endotracheal tube, although bioavailability may be highly variable. The pediatric dose of intravenous epinephrine for cardiac arrest is 0.01 mg/kg, administered at the same frequency as for adults. If intravenous access is not secure, epinephrine may be administered via the child's endotracheal tube at the dose of 0.1 mg/kg (0.1 mL/kg of 1:1,000 epinephrine solution).

For adults, vasopressin (40 U i.v., one time only) may be administered instead of epinephrine or after one or more epinephrine doses. In this setting, vasopressin may actually be more effective than epinephrine, as it has a longer half-life (10 to 20 minutes) and a lower incidence of adverse effects (48).

Sodium bicarbonate is not recommended for the early treatment of the patient who suffers cardiac arrest and who did not have preexisting metabolic acidosis. Adverse effects of bicarbonate administration in this setting include paradoxical intracellular acidosis and cerebrospinal fluid acidosis, plasma hyperosmolarity, impairment of oxygen delivery by increasing hemoglobin's affinity for oxygen, reduction in coronary perfusion, and alkalemia-induced reduction of cerebral blood flow (44,48). The acidosis that occurs early during cardiac arrest is largely respiratory in etiology, although the arterial blood gases may not accurately reflect this. Actually, it takes 20 to 30 minutes before metabolic acidosis develops during cardiac arrest unless the patient had metabolic acidosis before the arrest. The early administration of sodium bicarbonate in cardiac arrest has not been shown to improve survival, and the drug should be used only to treat a pH of <7.20 that is due to established metabolic causes. The usual dose is 1 mEq/kg; overtreatment (iatrogenic alkalosis) should be avoided.

Although frequently administered, intravenous *lidocaine* is likely not of benefit for the treatment of shock-refractory VF or pulseless VT and may increase the amount of energy required for defibrillation (47). *Amiodarone,* however, may be of benefit in improving the success of subsequent defibrillation attempts and is the *first arrhythmic drug of choice* for ventricular arrhythmias, rather than lidocaine. The initial dose for adults is 300 mg diluted in 20 to 30 mL of normal saline or 5% dextrose in water given by rapid intravenous infusion with repeated doses of 150 mg given if required. Use of magnesium and/or procainamide is not recommended for the treatment of cardiac arrest (48).

After successful resuscitation from cardiac arrest, an arterial catheter should be introduced (if not already present), and the patient should be moved to the intensive care unit (if not already there). A nasogastric tube is often placed, and a pulmonary artery catheter may be useful to aid in the management of the unstable patient. If the arrest rhythm was VF, amiodarone or lidocaine is continued (or started) in an effort to prevent recurrent dysrhythmias. If the cause of the arrest is ischemia and if the ischemia is continuing, then further stabilization can be achieved by the addition of intraaortic balloon pump support. Serial ECGs and measurements of cardiac enzymes to rule out a myocardial infarction (MI) should be ordered. If the patient remains unstable, echocardiography should be performed; if indicated, cardiac catheterization with coronary arteriography may be in order.

Pulseless electrical activity (PEA), previously known as electromechanical dissociation, is a usually fatal cause of cardiac arrest characterized by lack of ejection of blood from the heart despite relatively normal ECG complexes (48). The basic problem is usually the inability of weak ventricular contractions to produce a detectable blood pressure or pulse. Treatment is the institution of CPR, assessment for treatable causes, and administration of epinephrine (adult dose, 1 mg i.v. push, repeat every 3 to 5 minutes). If the PEA rate is quite slow, atropine (adult dose, 1 mg i.v.) may be used following epinephrine. If PEA is due to calcium channel blocker overdose or hyperkalemia, intravenous calcium may be indicated. In the postoperative patient, PEA may due to severe hypovolemia, tamponade, tension pneumothorax, prosthetic valve dysfunction obstruction, severe hypoxia, or pulmonary embolism. When one is confronted with a patient with PEA, these potentially reversible causes must be considered.

Asystole is the total lack of cardiac electrical activity. In the postoperative patient, this is treated by the institution of pacing via the temporary pacing wires that were placed on the heart at the time of surgery. Failure of pacing to initiate ventricular contractions indicates nonfunctional pacing wires (due to lack of contact with the heart or breakage), inappropriate function of the temporary pacemaker, or a globally ischemic or otherwise nonfunctional heart. Transcutaneous pacing may be attempted, but if the heart has irretrievably decompensated, pacing efforts by any method will fail.

POSTOPERATIVE CARDIAC ARRHYTHMIAS

Abnormalities of the heart rhythm occur in more than one-third of patients after open-heart surgery, and thus, the management of these arrhythmias is an almost daily part of the care of the cardiac surgery patients. Although often a benign event, postoperative arrhythmias may be life threatening, may contribute significantly to both short- and long-term morbidity, and often lengthen the patient's duration of hospitalization. The high frequency of postoperative arrhythmias and the potential for serious adverse sequelae make it important to identify them quickly and treat appropriately. Most of the common arrhythmias are successfully managed by routine measures (Table 4-2). The parenterally administered drugs useful in treating postoperative rhythm problems are summarized in Table 4-3.

Postoperative Bradyarrhythmia

A slow heart rate may decrease the cardiac output. The most effective combination of rate and ventricular filling time for adults is approximately 100 to 110 beats per minute. The cardiac output of infants is particularly rate dependent, and bradycardia (<80 beats per minute) should be treated even if the arterial pressure is normal. Sinus bradycardia (heart rate of <70 beats per minute) is frequent in adult patients who are receiving β-adrenergic antagonists in the perioperative period. Other drugs that can cause bradycardia include verapamil, diltiazem, and amiodarone. It is standard practice to attach temporary pacing wires to the right ventricle at the time of operation; most often, atrial wires are also placed. Thus, the simplest treatment of sinus bradycardia is the institution of pacing. Pacing the atrium alone usually suffices as conduction

Table 4-2. Management strategies for postoperative arrhythmias

Arrhythmia	Treatment
Sinus bradycardia, some nodal bradycardias	1. Atrial pacing (DDD mode preferred) 2. Atropine 3. Isoproterenol
Complete heart block, slow nodal rhythm	1. Sequential atrioventricular pacing (DVI mode) 2. Ventricular pacing (VVI mode) 3. Isoproterenol
Nodal rhythm	1. Pacing (atrial if possible) 2. Observe if rate reasonable and blood pressure satisfactory
Premature ventricular contractions	1. Observe if infrequent, chronic, asymptomatic 2. Check blood gases, potassium, magnesium 3. If new or frequent, consider: a. Overdrive pacing b. β-Blocker
Ventricular tachycardia, sustained	1. If hypotensive: electrical cardioversion 2. If stable and LV preserved: procainamide or lidocaine 3. If stable and LV poor: amiodarone
Sinus bradycardia, some nodal bradycardias	1. Atrial pacing 2. Atropine 3. Isoproterenol

Continued

Table 4-2. *Continued*

Arrhythmia	Treatment
Sinus tachycardia	1. Treat underlying cause 2. β-Blocker
Narrow complex paroxysmal supraventricular tachycardia	1. Adenosine to slow and observe etiology
Atrial premature beats	1. Not usually treated 2. β-Blocker
Atrial fibrillation	1. Patient stable and heart rate satisfactory: a. Not always treated; b. Anticoagulation if persists >48 h 2. Unstable and tachycardic: a. Synchronized cardioversion 3. Hemodynamically stable but tachycardic: a. Rate control: i. If LV good: diltiazem or esmolol infusion ii. If LV poor: amiodarone b. Drug conversion: amiodarone or procainamide 4. Persistent or chronic: a. Oral β-blocker and/or digoxin b. Anticoagulation if persists >48 h
Atrial flutter	1. Rapid atrial pacing 2. If ineffective: treat as for atrial fibrillation

LV, left ventricle; see text for description of DDD, DVI, and VVI modes.

Table 4-3. Commonly used parenteral drugs for treating postoperative arrhythmias

Drug	Indications	Adult Dose	Side Effects
Adenosine	Narrow complex paroxysmal supraventricular tachycardia	*i.v. bolus:* 6 mg; may repeat with 12 mg if indicated	Bronchoconstriction, flushing, atrioventricular block; if given for wide complex tachycardia/VT, may cause deterioration
Amiodarone	VF or pulseless VT; wide QRS complex tachycardia	*i.v. bolus:* 150 mg i.v. q 5–10 min (For VF: 300-mg bolus; may repeat 150 mg in 5–10 min)	Hypotension, vasodilation, negative inotropic effect, bradycardia, AV block, hepato- and pulmonary toxicity, nausea, vomiting
	Atrial fibrillation	See Table 4-4	
Digoxin	Atrial fibrillation/flutter (slows ventricular response)	*i.v. load:* 1.0 mg in divided doses over 4–8 h *p.o. load:* 1.0 mg in divided doses over 24 h	Arrhythmias including AV block and bradycardia, anorexia, nausea, vomiting, confusion
Diltiazem	Atrial fibrillation/flutter	*i.v. load:* 0.25 mg/kg over 2 min; may repeat in 15 min *Maintenance:* 5–15 mg/h; titrate for HR 70–120 beats/min with SBP >90 mm Hg	Hypotension, AV block, bradycardia, decreased cardiac output, headache
Esmolol	Atrial fibrillation/flutter; tachycardia	*i.v.:* Begin at 50 μg/kg/min; increase in 50-μg/kg/min increments q 5 min to max 200 μg/kg/min; maintain HR 70–120 beats/min and SBP >90 mm Hg	Bradycardia, hypotension, atrioventricular block reduced cardiac output (transient due to short half-life)

Continued

Table 4-3. *Continued*

Drug	Indications	Adult Dose	Side Effects
Lidocaine	VT, VF	*i.v. bolus:* 1.0–1.5 mg/kg; may repeat with 0.5–1.5 mg/kg in 10 min *Maintenance:* 1–4 mg/min	Confusion, coma, seizures, hypotension, nausea, vomiting
Magnesium sulfate	Torsade de pointes; refractory VF (after lidocaine or amiodarone)	*i.v. bolus:* 1–2 g	May cause hypotension; caution if renal insufficiency present
Procainamide	VT, VF, wide QRS complex tachycardia of uncertain origin, atrial fibrillation/flutter	*i.v. load:* 500–1,000 mg (up to 17 mg/kg); run at 20 mg/min *Maintenance:* 1–4 mg/min; reduce if desired effect seen or hypotension or QRS widening occurs	VT, asystole, hypotension, seizures, thrombocytopenia, lupus-like syndrome
Propranolol	Atrial fibrillation/flutter	*i.v.:* 0.5–1.0 mg q 5 min up to 2–5 mg	Bradycardia, hypotension, reduced cardiac output
Verapamil	Supraventricular tachycardias; atrial fibrillation rate control	*i.v. bolus:* 2.5–10 mg over 2 min; repeat in 10–20 min	AV block, bradycardia, hypotension, reduced cardiac output, constipation

AV, atrioventricular; HR, heart rate; SBP, systolic blood pressure; VF, ventricular fibrillation; VT, ventricular tachycardia.
Note: The listed side effects are not comprehensive, and other adverse reactions to these drugs are known to occur.

through the atrioventricular node is usually preserved. Atrial pacing is more physiologic than sequential atrioventricular pacing or ventricular pacing alone.

If the pacing wires fail to capture and do not provide satisfactory atrial or ventricular pacing, symptomatic bradycardia can be treated acutely with atropine (adult dose, 0.5 to 1.0 mg i.v., may repeat every 3 to 5 minutes to a total dose of 3.0 mg; pediatric dose, 0.02 mg/kg, may repeat every 5 minutes to a total dose of 1.0 mg in a child, 2.0 mg in an adolescent). Longer-term treatment includes continuous intravenous infusion of dopamine (5 to 10 µg per minute), epinephrine (2 to 10 µg per minute), or isoproterenol (adult dose, 2 to 10 µg per minute; pediatric dose, 0.01 to 0.10 µg/kg per minute), external cardiac pacing (which is often painful for the patient), and passage of a temporary transvenous pacing wire.

Various degrees of heart block may develop after surgery, most frequently after valve replacement and congenital procedures that involve manipulations near the atrioventricular conduction system. First-degree block (PR interval >200 milliseconds) is not uncommon, causes no symptoms, usually disappears spontaneously, and requires no treatment. In patients with first-degree heart block, we frequently leave a ventricular demand pacemaker in place as a backup, should the first-degree block worsen. Second-degree block occurs when only some atrial impulses are conducted to the ventricle. If this results in a significant bradycardia, treatment is sequential atrioventricular pacing via the temporary epicardial leads.

Third-degree (complete) heart block is a serious problem as in the postoperative patient, the ventricular escape rate may be only 30 to 40 beats per minute. Complete heart block infrequently occurs in CABG patients (about 4%), is usually self-limiting, and rarely persists after the first postoperative day (49). It is, however, much more common in valve surgery patients, occurring in up to 15% (50,51). Thus, at the time of surgery, secure placement and testing of the pacing wires are important for patients undergoing valve procedures. For complete heart block, sequential atrioventricular pacing is the treatment of choice. Most of these patients will regain normal atrioventricular conduction within hours to days after valve replacement, although a few (presumably due to irreversible injury to the conduction system during surgery) will require placement of a permanent pacemaker prior to discharge from the hospital. No patient with surgically related complete heart block should be discharged from the hospital without pacemaker implantation.

Management of Temporary Cardiac Pacing Systems

Use of temporary pacing for bradyarrhythmia can be lifesaving for the postoperative patient; it is our current standard to attach temporary ventricular (and usually atrial) pacing electrodes to the heart at the time of operation. Optimal placement involves good contact with the myocardium and avoidance of contact with coronary arteries, bypass grafts, and mediastinal drainage tubes (52). The pacing leads exit through the chest wall and are attached to an external pulse generator.

The generator may be one of several types that have the ability to sense native myocardial depolarization and to deliver current to the leads for pacing. Sequential generators provide for both atrial and ventricular pacing and for adjusting the length of time between the atrial and ventricular impulses. The external pulse generator allows for adjusting the amount of current delivered to the heart (in milliamperes) and the sensitivity of sensing. The demand mode of pacing causes the pacemaker to deliver current to the heart only when the sensed rate is below the rate set by the operator. The asynchronous mode provides a pacing current to the heart irrespective of the native heart rate. Most frequently, the demand mode is used with the backup rate setting at 60 beats per minute. The sensitivity of sensing is also adjustable. Failure of pacing (failure to capture) may be due to poor contact between the pacing electrode and the heart, failure to turn on the pulse generator, battery failure, setting the pacer output too low, or poor contact between the pacing leads and the generator. Failure of the device to sense appropriately indicates a loose connection, too low a sensitivity setting, or early battery failure.

Pacing modes are coded by abbreviations. The first letter refers to the chamber being paced (A for atrium, V for ventricle, D for both). The second letter refers to the chamber being sensed (A, V, or D). The third letter denotes the response to the sensed event (I for inhibit, T for trigger, D for triggering of a ventricular complex in response to a sensed atrial complex). Typically, patients with intact conduction early after surgery will have their pacemaker set at the VVI mode with a backup rate of 60 beats per minute. Therefore, if the ventricular rate becomes <60, the ventricle will be paced automatically at 60, irrespective of the status of the atrium or atrioventricular conduction. Patients with bradycardia are often paced using the DDD mode. When intact atrioventricular conduction is present, the DDD mode actually functions as the AAI mode in which the paced atrial complex is conducted naturally to the ventricle. But, if native conduction fails, the ventricle will be paced, thus maintaining the programmed heart rate. This mode is advantageous in patients with variable native sinus node function and/or intermittent atrioventricular block.

Most patients have their epicardial pacing wires removed on the day prior to anticipated discharge from the hospital, preferably in the morning. Although serious bleeding related to wire removal is rare (<1 in 1,000), it may occur and can require emergency sternotomy for control. Thus, instruments for emergency reopening of the patient are available on all well-equipped cardiac surgery units. The wires are extracted by gentle continuous traction while the patient's rhythm is being monitored. If significant resistance to removal is encountered, the wires are pulled taut and cut at the skin level; the retained wire is allowed to retract into the patient. This is also a useful approach for patients that have been anticoagulated with coumadin. After removal, the patient is kept at bed rest for 2 hours, with continuous monitoring for the next 12 to 24 hours. Some patients may experience ventricular arrhythmias during wire removal, although these are generally short lived and do not require treatment (53).

Postoperative Tachyarrhythmias

Approximately one-third of patients who undergo open-heart procedures suffer postoperative tachyarrhythmias. Most of these are supraventricular (atrial fibrillation and flutter) and are easily recognized as such. Occasionally, however, a wide QRS tachycardia occurs, and it may be difficult to determine the exact nature of the arrhythmia.

Wide QRS-Complex Tachycardia

A wide complex tachycardia may be either supraventricular or ventricular in origin; misdiagnosis may lead to improper treatment. If the wide QRS tachycardia is assumed to be supraventricular and is treated with a drug that blocks atrioventricular conduction (such as adenosine, β-blocker, or calcium channel blocker), severe hypotension may result. Thus, in most circumstances, wide complex tachycardia should be considered to be VT and should be treated as such (54).

Thus, electrical cardioversion is often the initial treatment of choice of wide complex tachycardia, particularly if the patient is unstable. If this is not successful or possible, amiodarone is the preferred antiarrhythmic agent for the empiric treatment of wide complex tachycardia of uncertain mechanism, especially if the patient's LV function is poor (EF <40%) (55). If amiodarone does not terminate the arrhythmia, adenosine (6-mg rapid i.v. infusion, followed by 12 mg in 1 to 2 minutes if required) is recommended. Whereas adenosine's action is very short lived, it will frequently terminate broad complex supraventricular tachycardia (SVT) without much effect in VT. Thus, if the tachycardia is supraventricular, adenosine is useful both as a diagnostic and as a therapeutic agent. If these measures are not successful, procainamide should be considered, especially for wide complex tachycardia of unknown type in the patient with good LV function. This type IA antiarrhythmic agent is often effective treatment for VT. Also, although not specifically approved by the Food and Drug Administration for this purpose, it is frequently used for the treatment of supraventricular arrhythmias. Procainamide may convert atrial fibrillation to sinus rhythm and slows conduction in accessory bypass tracts if such are involved in the tachycardia. Procainamide is administered at a rate of 20 mg per minute i.v. up to a total dose of 15 mg/kg. Careful monitoring of the blood pressure and ECG is performed during the loading procedure as it may cause prolongation of the QT interval and act as a negative inotropic agent. It may then be given by continuous infusion at 1 to 4 mg per minute (adult dose) with monitoring of blood levels and the ECG QT interval. Amiodarone remains the drug of choice for the treatment of pulseless VT after electrical cardioversion, but when not effective, refractory wide complex tachycardia may respond to *sotalol* or *bretylium*.

Narrow QRS-Complex Tachycardia

Determining the nature of narrow complex tachycardia may be difficult. Adenosine may be useful in this setting to differentiate SVTs (including atrial dysrhythmias) and junctional tachycardia. SVT is very common during the first few days after open-heart surgery. The most frequently encountered tachycardias are sinus tachycardia (ST), atrial fibrillation, and atrial flutter.

Sinus Tachycardia

ST may be the result of hypovolemia, anemia, fever, agitation, or inadequate pain relief. It may, however, be a compensatory response to compromised cardiac function and may indicate a serious problem such as ongoing myocardial ischemia or tamponade. It is often difficult to differentiate ST from SVT that is due to a re-entrant mechanism (such as in a patient with Wolff–Parkinson–White syndrome). In both arrhythmias, P waves may be difficult to identify. In general, reentrant SVT is faster than ST, with the rate being above 140 in adults, 180 in children, and 220 in infants. Also, SVT is more regular than ST, with no beat-to-beat variability in the R-R interval. When ST is present, evaluation should be undertaken to rule out the presence of a low cardiac output state. This would include physical examination, measurement of arterial pH, an echocardiogram, and, if necessary, placement of a pulmonary artery catheter for thermodilution measurement of the cardiac output.

During the first few hours after surgery, occasional adult patients exhibit ST, often associated with hypertension. This hyperdynamic state is more common in younger male adults and may be related to a greater-than-normal catecholamine response to the stress of operation. ST in the intubated patient early after operation may suggest a patient who is awake and feeling pain, but who cannot move because of continued muscle paralysis.

For patients with uncomplicated ST, the initial treatment is assurance of adequate cardiac filling pressures and adequate pain control. If correction of hypovolemia and pain does not alleviate the tachycardia (and low output is not present), treatment with a β-adrenergic antagonist may be indicated. Esmolol is particularly well suited for this purpose because of its short half-life and rapid reversibility on discontinuation. Caution must be used because hypotension or bradycardia may result, necessitating abrupt discontinuation of the drug.

Atrial Fibrillation and Flutter

In adults, atrial arrhythmias (fibrillation, flutter, and paroxysmal atrial tachycardia) occur in up to 40% of coronary bypass patients and up to 50% of valve surgery patients (56). The incidence is much lower in children. The most common atrial arrhythmia is atrial fibrillation.

Risk factors associated with postoperative atrial fibrillation include older patient age, previous atrial fibrillation, preoperative use of digoxin, history of rheumatic heart disease, chronic obstructive pulmonary disease, and longer aortic cross-clamp (ischemic) time (56,57). It has been suggested that performing coronary bypass surgery without the use of CPB ("off pump") may be associated with a lower incidence of postoperative atrial arrhythmias, although this result has not been consistently demonstrated (58–60). Although the cause of these arrhythmias is unknown, contributing factors may include manipulation and cannulation of the atrium, intraoperative ischemia, and the effects of endogenous and administered catecholamines. It has been hypothesized that some patients may possess inherent electrophysiologic characteristics (involving nonuniform refractoriness of adjacent atrial areas), making them more likely to experience postoperative atrial fibrillation (57,61). Although often considered to be just a "nuisance," postoperative atrial fibrillation contributes to increased lengths of hospital stay, is a cause of patient discomfort, and is associated with an increased incidence of postoperative stroke.

Most commonly, atrial fibrillation develops on the second or third day after surgery, and the reason for this delay is not clear. For most patients, the ventricular rate response to atrial fibrillation is usually 110 to 150 beats per minute, and this rate is generally well tolerated. With the onset of tachycardia, however, the patient frequently feels warm, becomes diaphoretic, and may become anxious. Thus, it is useful to warn patients preoperatively about the possibility (and the generally benign nature) of postoperative atrial fibrillation.

Patients with marginal cardiac function who develop atrial fibrillation may suffer hemodynamic deterioration due to loss of the normal synchronized "atrial kick" that contributes about 10% to 15% to the cardiac output. Rare patients suffer extreme tachycardia (>200 beats per minute) with severe hypotension. Atrial fibrillation is usually recognized by the irregular nature of the ventricular response. Analysis of the patient's arterial blood pressure monitor tracing usually aids in the diagnosis. If the ventricular response is uniform, making the diagnosis more difficult, an atrial electrogram may be obtained by recordings from the atrial pacing wires that were implanted at surgery (Fig. 4-3). This will reveal the atrial complexes that are irregular in rhythm, amplitude, and polarity. Intravenously administered adenosine, which blocks atrioventricular conduction, can be used to cause transient slowing of the ventricular rate, so that atrial activity can be analyzed. Its action is rapid but evanescent; hence, it is useful only for diagnostic, not therapeutic, purposes. It should not be used for wide complex arrhythmias or if the arrhythmia is not certain to be supraventricular in origin as severe deterioration may result.

Atrial flutter is usually characterized by a regular ventricular response with a rate of about 150 beats per minute. This represents an atrial contraction rate of about 300 per minute with 2:1 atrioventricular block allowing for only every other atrial complex to be conducted and to result in ventricular contraction. The degree of block may, however, be variable, resulting in an irregular ventricular response. In atrial flutter, the atrial electrogram will demonstrate regular atrial complexes, usually at 230 to 350 beats per minute, with uniform amplitude and polarity. These atrial "flutter waves" are usually recognizable on the standard ECG tracing and facilitate the diagnosis of atrial flutter. Occasional patients will have faster atrial flutter rates in the range of 340 to 430 beats per minute.

TREATMENT OF ATRIAL FIBRILLATION/FLUTTER. The method of management of atrial fibrillation or flutter depends on the status of the patient. If the patient is hemodynamically compromised, electrical cardioversion is the treatment of choice. This is especially useful for the patient who develops atrial fibrillation or flutter during the first few hours after surgery and is still intubated and under the effect of general anesthesia. Synchronous cardioversion is performed with external paddles, placed a bit more cephalad across the chest wall than for ventricular defibrillation (to place the atria directly in the path of the delivered energy), and begun using 20 to 50 J (0.2 to 1.0 J/kg for infants). It is important to ensure that the *synchronization circuit* of the cardioversion energy source is used to prevent discharge during the T wave of the patient's ECG, as this might result in VF. If the patient is awake, pretreatment with a

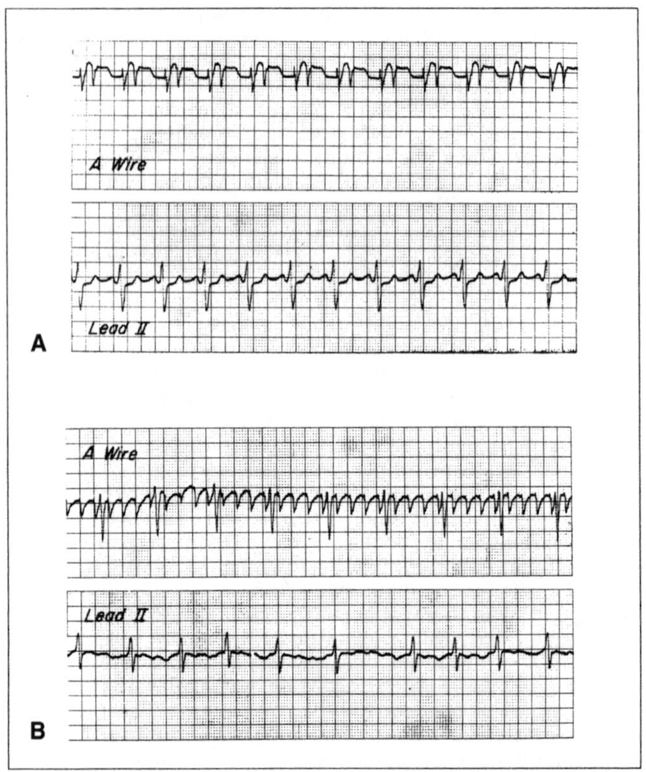

Fig. 4-3. Atrial electrode tracings. Recordings made from atrial electrodes (*A wire*) and corresponding lead II for a patient with normal sinus rhythm (A) and a patient with atrial fibrillation/flutter (B). Atrial activity is much more easily analyzed in the atrial wire tracing than in conventional leads.

short-acting sedative such as midazolam is desirable to prevent pain and memory of the event. If successful conversion is not achieved at the initial energy setting, a higher energy level may be tried, but there is probably no advantage to exceeding 100 J for cardioversion of SVT. Although frequently initially successful, electrical cardioversion of postoperative atrial arrhythmias often provides only temporary restoration of sinus rhythm, probably because the underlying precipitating factors leading to the development of the arrhythmia remain unchanged.

Atrial flutter (but not fibrillation) may be treated by rapid overdrive atrial pacing (62). This is performed by using a pacemaker mode that can deliver up to 800 electrical impulses per minute. The pacemaker is connected to the atrial pacing electrodes (not the ventricular, as this may result in VF), and the atrium is captured by pacing at a rate about 20% faster than the underlying atrial rate (which is usually either two or three times the ventricular rate). When monitoring lead II, evidence of atrial capture is seen when the atrial depolarization wave reverses polarity. Rapid atrial pacing is maintained for 10 to 15 seconds and then abruptly stopped. This often results in conversion of atrial flutter to atrial fibrillation, a rhythm generally more easily controlled by medications.

When atrial fibrillation or flutter occurs several days after surgery, the patient is usually extubated and alert. Drug treatment is usually preferable to electrical cardioversion in this situation. If the patient's average ventricular rate is <110 beats per minute and he or she is comfortable without evidence of hemodynamic compromise, no rate control treatment is necessary.

For patients with atrial tachycardia, but who are hemodynamically relatively stable, treatment of postoperative atrial fibrillation involves *rate control, conversion to sinus rhythm,* and *anticoagulation* if the arrhythmia persists. Rate control may usually be achieved by the administration of a β-adrenergic antagonist, a calcium channel blocking drug, or amiodarone (see Table 4-3). Intravenous diltiazem is a frequently preferred choice for this setting (57,63). Alternatively, continuous esmolol infusion may be used, although this may result in hypotension more often (64). For both drugs, the goal is to reduce the ventricular response to below 110 beats per minute while maintaining the systolic blood pressure above 90 mm Hg. Digoxin can be used to slow the ventricular response to atrial fibrillation, but the effect is slow in onset (up to 6 hours), and we generally prefer diltiazem or esmolol for this purpose.

Amiodarone is effective for the treatment of atrial fibrillation (65). Amiodarone is a complex drug that differs from other available agents and whose exact mechanism of action has not been clarified (55). It has both α- and β-adrenergic inhibitory action in addition to effects on sodium, potassium, and calcium channels. Amiodarone has been used successfully for rate control in atrial fibrillation or flutter that is resistant to other drugs and has become the preferred or one of several preferred antiarrhythmic agents for the treatment of atrial fibrillation or flutter in patients who are hemodynamically stable. It may be administered intravenously or orally. When given intravenously, the major acute side effects are hypotension and bradycardia, both of which are usually manageable with fluid infusion, pressor drug administration, and temporary pacing, if necessary (48). Besides being effective in controlling the heart rate, amiodarone may also cause conversion to sinus rhythm, a beneficial property not shared by diltiazem or the β-blocking drugs. This conversion from atrial fibrillation to sinus rhythm may be associated with thromboembolism in patients who have been in the dysrhythmia for >48 hours. Therefore, it is recommended that amiodarone therapy should be used within 48 hours of atrial fibrillation onset and that if the arrhythmia persists for >48 hours, anticoagulation therapy should be instituted (see following discussion). Amiodarone is a complex, effective, but potentially toxic drug with multiple side effects and drug interactions, particularly with long-term administration (66,67). Side effects associated with chronic amiodarone treatment include pulmonary toxicity (pneumonitis) and abnormalities of liver and thyroid function tests. Additionally, amiodarone potentiates warfarin anticoagulation, and patients receiving maintenance amiodarone doses will usually need a reduction in their warfarin dose (68). In general, the short-term use of amiodarone for postoperative arrhythmia treatment has been found to be safe and effective, but treated patients should be closely observed, keeping the potential for pulmonary and other toxicities in mind (69,70).

For hemodynamically stable patients with new-onset postoperative atrial fibrillation, amiodarone may be administered (initially intravenously and then orally) to slow the heart rate and to encourage conversion to sinus rhythm (Table 4-4) (71). The intravenous route is preferred for converting new-onset atrial fibrillation to sinus rhythm because a prolonged period of oral loading is necessary to achieve a therapeutic effect. For adults, a 150-mg amiodarone intravenous loading dose is administered over 60 minutes followed by 1 mg per minute for 6 hours, then 0.5 mg per minute for 12 to 24 hours, after which the patient may be switched to oral amiodarone. Following conversion to sinus rhythm, oral amiodarone is continued for 2 to 3 weeks and then stopped.

For many years, the mainstay of drug treatment for postoperative atrial tachycardia was digoxin. Because of its slow onset of action, narrow therapeutic–toxic ratio, and various side effects, digoxin has largely been replaced by other drugs for the purpose of acute rhythm management. When administered, serum digoxin levels should be followed. Side effects include dangerous arrhythmias, gastrointestinal complaints, and visual disturbances. Digoxin toxicity is potentiated by hypokalemia; serum digoxin levels are increased in the presence of quinidine, verapamil, and amiodarone. Once begun, digoxin is usually continued for 4 to 6 weeks after operation. In our practices, digoxin is used mostly for the management of chronic atrial fibrillation, particularly when heart failure is also present.

Conversion of atrial fibrillation to sinus rhythm has been reported by the administration of various drugs including amiodarone, procainamide, quinidine, propafenone, and ibutilide. Of

Table 4-4. Amiodarone administration to treat postoperative atrial fibrillation (adult doses)

Loading dose (i.v. infusion)
- 150 mg over 10–20 min (monitor BP), then
- 1 mg/min for 6 h, then
- 0.5 mg/min until taking orally, then
- 200 mg p.o. t.i.d. for 1 wk, then
- 200 mg p.o. b.i.d. for 1 wk, then
- 200 mg p.o. q d for 2 wk, then
- Discontinue amiodarone

BP, blood pressure.
Note: A variety of amiodarone dosing protocols exist. This is one example. The doses should be modified based on patient size. Caution should be used in patients with liver, renal, or pulmonary disease.

these, quinidine is no longer recommended. Propafenone is not currently available in intravenous form in the United States (72,73). Ibutilide is used for the conversion of atrial fibrillation to sinus rhythm, although experience in postoperative patients is limited and it has significant dangerous proarrhythmic effects (57).

When used to produce pharmacologic cardioversion, procainamide is administered as a loading dose followed by a continuous infusion. The procainamide loading dose may be oral (1.0 to 1.5 g) or intravenous (1.0 g). Serious hypotension may result from the rapid intravenous infusion of procainamide; therefore, continuous ECG and blood pressure monitoring are required when the drug is used in this fashion. After conversion, a maintenance dose of 1 to 2 g per day (adult dose, slow-release preparation) may be given. Of note, long-term use of procainamide (for >1 month) is associated with the development of a lupus-like syndrome. In our practices, intravenous or oral amiodarone (although more expensive) has largely replaced procainamide for the purpose of converting recent-onset atrial fibrillation to sinus rhythm.

Patients with postoperative atrial fibrillation are at increased risk for thrombotic stroke. They should therefore be considered for anticoagulation (with heparin and/or warfarin) if the arrhythmia persists for >48 hours, unless contraindications are present (71).

PREVENTION OF ATRIAL FIBRILLATION/FLUTTER. Because atrial arrhythmias are so common after cardiac surgery, a variety of drugs, administered prophylactically, have been investigated to attempt to reduce the incidence of their occurrence. These agents include various β-blockers, sotalol (a β-blocker with additional antiarrhythmic properties), amiodarone, digoxin, procainamide, propafenone, various calcium channel blockers, and magnesium (57,74–76). Many of the studies have significant limitations, and many of the results have been conflicting.

One consistent result of most studies, however, is the demonstration that the prophylactic administration of an oral β-blocker reduces the incidence of postoperative atrial fibrillation by as much as 40% (71,74). For adult patients, we currently favor the use of oral atenolol (adult dose, 12.5 to 25 mg twice per day), which is begun as soon as the patient is taking sips of water. Atenolol is a β1-selective blocker, is generally well tolerated, and at this dose has little effect on bronchial smooth muscle. Contraindications include bradycardia, hypotension, severe ongoing bronchospasm, and uncompensated heart failure. For the patient who was taking a β-blocker prior to surgery, it is important to resume β-blocker therapy soon after the operation to prevent rebound tachycardia and hypertension that may occur upon the abrupt withdrawal.

Prophylactic treatment with amiodarone has been reported to decrease the incidence of postoperative atrial arrhythmias and may be cost-effective (57,77–81). A variety of dosing schedules have been used in these investigations, including beginning oral amiodarone 7 days before operation, a large single oral loading dose on the day before surgery, and the institution of intravenous amiodarone during or early after operation (76). Most of the studies have involved adult coronary artery bypass patients. Overall, prophylactic postoperative β-blockade and amiodarone treatment both reduce postoperative atrial fibrillation. Amiodarone, however, may be more effective (82).

It has been proposed that atrial overdrive pacing (AAI mode) at a rate of about 10 beats per minute above the resting heart rate will reduce the incidence of postoperative atrial fibrillation (83). The results of this practice have, however, been conflicting, and we do not currently use this technique (84,85).

Junctional Ectopic Tachycardia

Postoperative junctional ectopic (nodal) tachycardia is a potentially dangerous arrhythmia that occurs most commonly after congenital heart surgery in neonates and infants, particularly after repair of tetralogy of Fallot (86). When it occurs in an adult, it may be a manifestation of digoxin toxicity. Hypotension, vagolytic drugs, electrolyte abnormalities, and cardiomyopathies are contributing factors for the development and maintenance of this arrhythmia. In this rhythm, the electrical impulse originates in the His–Purkinje system of the ventricles. Atrioventricular dissociation is present, with the atrial rate typically being slower than the ventricular. The diagnosis is based on demonstration of a narrow complex tachycardia with atrioventricular dissociation. Because of the severe tachycardia (200 to 300 beats per minute), ventricular filling time is reduced and severe hemodynamic instability may result. The loss of atrioventricular synchrony reduces the cardiac output even further. Adrenergic stimulation (by exogenous drugs or by patient anxiety and stimulation) frequently increases the heart rate and worsens the situation.

Treatment is directed at optimizing the patient's metabolic state and minimizing adrenergic stimulation with adequate sedation. Cooling of the patient to around 34°C (with cooling blankets and gastric lavage) has been used to reduce the heart rate. Intravenous amiodarone appears to be particularly effective for the treatment of this difficult and dangerous arrhythmia (87,88). Procainamide infusion has also been used with success to control the rapid rate response (89).

Ventricular Tachyarrhythmias

Premature ventricular contractions (PVCs) are impulses that arise in an ectopic ventricular focus. Although common in adult heart disease patients, they are uncommon in children. When present after surgery, PVCs are usually not a problem in themselves, but they may serve as an indicator of less obvious disturbances such as metabolic and electrolyte abnormalities (e.g., hypokalemia, hypoxia, myocardial ischemia, acidosis, alkalosis, or digoxin toxicity). Thus, when new-onset PVCs occur early after surgery, especially at a frequency of >4 to 6 per minute, the patient's blood gases and digoxin (if receiving the drug) and serum potassium levels should be checked. A 12-lead ECG is indicated to rule out ischemia. If this is normal and the patient is otherwise stable, specific treatment is not usually required for unifocal, single PVCs. Due to the potential proarrhythmic side effect of most antiarrhythmic drugs, pharmacologic treatment of asymptomatic PVCs can lead to the development of more dangerous arrhythmias in up to 10% of patients. One safe way to eliminate PVCs is by overdrive pacing, in which the atrium is paced at a rate of 5 to 10 beats per minute faster than the native heart rate. When the heart rate increases in this way, there is less time for ectopic pacemakers to become depolarized to threshold levels and to initiate premature beats.

More serious ventricular tachyarrhythmias occur in about 1% of patients after cardiac surgery. Patients with LV hypertrophy and those undergoing ventricular aneurysm or endocardial resection are at greatest risk for this complication. Prophylactic administration of antiarrhythmic agents (such as lidocaine or procainamide) does not necessarily prevent the development of postoperative ventricular arrhythmias in this group of patients and, because of their proarrhythmic effects (particularly procainamide), may be counterproductive.

Nonsustained VT (NSVT) is defined as three or more ventricular beats occurring at a rate of >100 per minute lasting <30 seconds or without hemodynamic compromise. Occasional episodes of NSVT do not require treatment, although it is prudent to rule out hypokalemia, hypomagnesemia, and hypoxia as contributing factors. Recurrent runs (salvos) of NSVT may be indicative of significant ventricular irritability and the potential for the development of life-threatening VT or VF. Suppression therapy may be instituted, usually in the form of amiodarone, β-blocker drug, or lidocaine infusion. Such treatment may be particularly indicated for patients with poor LV function or who have undergone aortic valve replacement, as these patients are more likely to develop serious arrhythmias. For selected patients, electrophysiologic testing may be indicated (85).

Sustained VT, even if hemodynamically well tolerated, should be treated immediately because deterioration to VF may soon occur. In general, any wide QRS tachycardia should be treated as ventricular in origin until proven otherwise. If the patient is hemodynamically stable, treatment of VT may be begun with amiodarone (preferred), procainamide, or lidocaine. If VT persists, synchronized electrical cardioversion is performed.

If the patient with VT is hypotensive, immediate synchronized cardioversion is indicated. This is accomplished using external paddles applied to the chest wall facing each other to maximize the current flow through the heart. The initial energy dose should be 100 J, and if this is unsuccessful, subsequent attempts are made using 200, 300, and, if required, up to 360 J. The pediatric electrical dose is 2 to 4 J/kg. To help prevent recurrent VT, amiodarone load and infusion are recommended.

VF results in sudden total cessation of the cardiac output and must be treated immediately by electrical defibrillation. See the discussion regarding cardiac arrest earlier in this chapter for further details.

PERIOPERATIVE MYOCARDIAL ISCHEMIA AND INFARCTION

Myocardial ischemia, either transient or irreversible leading to infarction, may occur during and after cardiac surgery. This complication is most frequently associated with coronary artery bypass procedures. In fact, up to 40% of coronary artery bypass surgery patients exhibit some evidence of postoperative ischemia, with the highest incidence occurring within 6 hours of weaning the patient from CPB (90). Early recognition of the presence of myocardial ischemia can lead to treatment to limit the damage that occurs or, in the case of coronary spasm, to effect a complete reversal of the condition.

Perioperative Infarction

When rigorously searched for with frequent ECGs and enzyme determinations, the incidence of definite perioperative MI for first-time (primary) coronary bypass operations is approximately 4%, whereas the incidence in repeat (redo) coronary operations is about 12% (91,92). The incidence in valvular and congenital procedures is lower, but the potential for MI, due to coronary artery injury or embolism, is present with all open-heart operations. Unless extensive ECG, enzymatic, and radionuclide testing is performed, many perioperative MIs go unnoticed. Not surprisingly, the operative mortality in those with perioperative infarcts is increased and the long-term survival is adversely affected (93,94). Efforts to identify preoperative factors predictive of perioperative MI have had conflicting results, although diabetic patients and those undergoing repeat operations consistently have a higher rate of MI.

The diagnosis of perioperative MI may be difficult as there is a continuum of myocardial injury ranging from a small degree of injury to full-blown transmural infarction with the development of classic (new Q-wave) ECG changes. Release of myocardial creatine kinase–myocardial band (CK-MB) isoenzyme is the most studied method to detect perioperative myocardial ischemia and has documented correlation with long-term outcome. The usual pattern of CK-MB isoenzyme release results in a peak of serum enzyme concentrations at 12 to 16 hours after surgery; some release occurs in nearly all patients who undergo cardiac surgery of any type. A significantly greater peak serum level and a more prolonged period of enzyme elevation, however, are observed in those patients who, by other tests, are found to suffer perioperative infarction. In general, for adult coronary bypass surgery patients, peak postoperative CK-MB activity of <20 U/L (with no ECG changes) suggests no significant myocardial injury, whereas CK-MB activity of >50 U/L suggests perioperative infarction (95). Various other CK-MB "cut-off" levels have been suggested to make the diagnosis of perioperative MI. Large infarctions are associated with peak CK-MB values that are >10 times the upper limit of normal. The use of five times the upper limit of normal as the MI "cut-off" increases the sensitivity of the analysis, but reduces specificity by including patients with nonischemic, surgically induced myocardial injury (93).

Troponin I is a cardiac-specific regulatory protein that is released as a result of cardiac, but not skeletal, muscle injury. Following MI, troponin I peaks later (36 hours) and elevated levels persist longer than CK-MB (96). Although useful for making the diagnosis of MI in patients who have not undergone heart surgery, experience using troponin I to diagnose perioperative infarctions is limited and correlation with long-term outcome is not documented (93,97–99).

Significant transmural MI is usually (but not always) associated with ECG changes. The patterns of ECG changes according to the location of the infarct are summarized in Table 4-5. The postoperative ECG is not nearly as sensitive as cardiac enzyme analysis for the diagnosis of perioperative infarction, but the presence of new Q waves is essentially 100% diagnostic. A significant number of patients will have "diagnostic" elevations of CK-MB, but will not

Table 4-5. Electrocardiographic (ECG) identification of acute myocardial infarction (MI) location

ECG changes associated with transmural MI
1. Hyperacute or inverted T waves
2. ST-segment elevation
3. New Q wave (longer than 0.04 second duration or >1/3 height of QRS complex)

ECG changes associated with non-Q wave (subendocardial) MI
1. ST-segment depression
2. Inverted T waves

Location of Infarction	ECG Leads Demonstrating ECG Changes Listed Above
Anteroseptal	V_1, V_2
Anteroapical	V_2, V_3
Anterolateral	V_4–V_6, aVL
Large anterior	V_1–V_6
Lateral	I, aVL, V_5, V_6
Inferior	II, III, aVF
Posterior[a]	V_1, V_2, V_3

[a]The changes in a posterior MI are mirror images of those in anterior infarctions, i.e., inverted hyperacute T waves and ST-segment depression.

demonstrate new Q waves. Nearly all patients with new Q waves, however, will have high CK-MB levels. Patients with new left bundle branch block and elevated CK-MB levels are also considered to have experienced an MI.

Perioperative MI may occur during surgery (due to injury to a coronary artery or intracoronary embolism) or may occur early after the operation (due to closure of a bypass graft). In fact, nearly 10% of all vein grafts are closed at 1 week after surgery (91). Grafts that suffer early closure are often grafts that have been placed to small, diffusely diseased arteries (100). The amount of myocardium at risk may be limited and graft closure not clinically recognized. On the other hand, closure of a graft to a major artery that is perfusing a large amount of myocardium may be quite serious. In general, however, early postoperative graft patency cannot be predicted on the basis of elevated postoperative cardiac enzymes alone. ECG correlation improves the ability to make the diagnosis of closure of a graft.

Patients suspected to have suffered an uncomplicated perioperative MI are treated essentially the same as those who experience a normal, uncomplicated postoperative course, although nitroglycerin is administered intravenously for 24 to 48 hours if the patient's blood pressure will allow. Complications such as low cardiac output and arrhythmias are managed as described elsewhere in this chapter. Prophylactic lidocaine administration is not indicated. After recovery, it is often useful to obtain some measure of the patient's EF (by nuclear angiography or echocardiography) to allow for determination of the extent of damage incurred. It often is determined that no significant decrease in the EF has occurred, a finding that can be reassuring for the patient and the surgeon alike. Patients with demonstrable damage may benefit long term from cardioactive drug treatment (β-blocker and/or angiotensin enzyme inhibitor), which should be managed by the patient's cardiologist.

Coronary Artery Spasm

Coronary artery spasm during the early postoperative period after coronary artery bypass surgery can be an unrecognized cause of sudden, severe cardiovascular collapse that may be fatal (101,102). This complication often presents as acute hypotension with the ECG demonstrating ST-segment elevation, although VT, VF, or atrioventricular block also may occur as initial manifestations. When this happens in the operating room, nitroglycerin may be injected directly into vein grafts for relief of the spasm. When it occurs in the postoperative patient, calcium channel blocking agents are administered (intravenous diltiazem at 5 to 10 mg per minute or nifedipine sublingually in 10-mg increments). Whereas peripheral intravenously administered nitroglycerin is usually not solely effective for the coronary spasm, it should be given if the patient's blood pressure allows. Emergency coronary arteriography to confirm the diagnosis of coronary spasm and for direct injection of vasodilator drugs into the affected coronary artery or vein graft is likely the most effective management strategy. If the patient is severely hypotensive or suffers cardiac arrest, emergency sternotomy should be performed for open cardiac massage and direct injection of vasodilator drugs (e.g., nitroglycerin in 0.2-mg increments).

PULMONARY COMPLICATIONS

Abnormalities of gas exchange or ventilation are not unusual after cardiac surgery. In fact, nearly all patients develop atelectasis to various degrees. Preoperative identification of patients at risk for pulmonary complications and proper attention to postoperative pulmonary care will help minimize the incidence and severity of these complications. Adults with acquired heart disease may have been heavy cigarette smokers and may suffer significant chronic obstructive lung disease. Despite the preoperative presence of significantly abnormal pulmonary function test results, however, successful surgery may usually be achieved in these patients (103,104). Thus, even severe preoperative pulmonary dysfunction is not usually a contraindication to cardiac surgery when the benefits of the planned operation are judged to outweigh the risk. Preoperative pulmonary (spirometric) function testing and blood gas determination will aid in determining the patient's risk of postoperative pulmonary complications and will provide baseline information for postoperative comparison (105).

Atelectasis

Radiographic evidence of atelectasis is present during the early postoperative period in most patients who have undergone heart surgery. Most commonly, the left lower lobe is affected, the degree of atelectasis is subsegmental, and the radiographic appearance is exacerbated after the patient is extubated. Examination of the patient usually reveals crackles, even though congestive heart failure is not present.

Although the sternotomy incision is less painful and less debilitating than lateral thoracotomy incisions, a significant decrease in pulmonary function still occurs after cardiac surgery via this approach. CPB increases lung water content, thus resulting in further abnormalities of ventilation and gas exchange early after surgery. In adults undergoing coronary bypass procedures, there is a reduction of at least 25% to 50% in forced vital capacity and forced expiratory volume in 1 second postoperatively. This decrease may be larger in patients who have undergone mobilization of the internal mammary artery than those who have not (106,107). Vigorous pulmonary toilet, with frequent use of the incentive spirometer and early ambulation, is generally effective treatment for postoperative atelectasis. As the patient becomes more active, the atelectasis clears, although some may remain radiographically evident on the predischarge chest radiograph. Bronchoscopy is rarely necessary.

Bronchospasm

Bronchospasm is occasionally encountered either intra- or postoperatively. Patients at increased risk are those with preexisting asthma and those who suffer chronic obstructive lung disease with a reactive component. When present during closure of the sternum, hyperinflation of the lungs may cause hypotension due to compression of the heart as the sternal halves are being brought together. If present during the early postoperative period in the ventilated patient, severe bronchospasm may result in hypoxemia and high ventilatory pressures.

Acute bronchospasm is treated by the administration of β-adrenergic bronchodilators by either the intravenous or the inhalation route. For the patient suffering acute bronchospasm with hemodynamic compromise due to lung hyperinflation, intravenous low-dose epinephrine (0.25 to 0.50 μg per minute for adults) provides both bronchodilation and inotropic support. Inhalation administration of epinephrine may also be performed and is effective. Drugs with more selective β2 action, such as albuterol and metaproterenol, will have fewer cardiovascular effects (predominantly tachycardia) and a longer duration of action. These may be administered via the endotracheal tube from a nebulizer or, for extubated patients, from a metered-dose inhaler (108). Corticosteroids, although slower to act, are also effective and do not result in wound-healing problems when used as a short course during the perioperative period (109). For patients with known severe reactive airway disease, we frequently administer steroids several hours preoperatively and for a few days postoperatively. Chronic bronchospasm may be treated with inhaled corticosteroids, the nonsteroidal antiinflammatory agent cromolyn sodium, and/or theophylline. These agents are not, however, generally used for acute management of bronchospasm following cardiac surgery.

Asthmatic patients having elective or even urgent surgery can be managed effectively by pretreatment with a leukotriene inhibitor such as montelukast (10 mg by mouth at night) or zafirlukast (20 mg by mouth twice a day). These are initiated, if possible, approximately 1 week before surgery.

It should be remembered that bronchospasm might be a manifestation of pulmonary edema. Thus, for the postoperative patient with new-onset dyspnea and wheezing, a chest x-ray film is indicated. If pulmonary edema is present, diuresis is the mainstay of the treatment, although bronchodilator therapy may still be of use.

Phrenic Nerve Injury

Temporary or permanent injury to one or both phrenic nerves may occur during cardiac surgery. In some patients, this happens as the result of direct trauma such as during mobilization of the internal mammary artery or during a difficult dissection in a patient undergoing reoperation. In others, it may be the result of cold thermal injury if ice–saline slush is placed within the pericardial sac during aortic cross-clamping for the purpose of myocardial protection.

In adults undergoing surgery using topical ice slush, radiographic evidence of phrenic nerve dysfunction may occur in up to 25% of patients. This is associated with an increased incidence of postoperative atelectasis and the appearance of an elevated (usually left) hemidiaphragm on postoperative chest radiographs (110). Although many adult patients with unilateral phrenic nerve dysfunction may not be severely compromised, if both phrenic nerves are injured, severe morbidity may result (111). Use of a foam pad placed between the ice and the pericardium to insulate the left phrenic nerve from the slush can effectively lower the incidence of this complication. Thus, some use an insulating pad routinely and others use cold saline irrigation instead of slush. In most adults, postoperative phrenic nerve dysfunction does not result in serious consequences, and diaphragmatic function returns with time, although up to 25% of those affected do not fully recover diaphragmatic function, which may be particularly debilitating for patients who suffered preoperative chronic obstructive pulmonary disease (112).

In children, phrenic nerve paralysis occurs in approximately 1.5% of patients and can be a serious problem (113). Infants do not tolerate loss of hemidiaphragmatic function as well as adults and may not be able to be weaned from mechanical ventilation as the result of the injury. Definitive diagnosis is based on the demonstration of paradoxical movement of the diaphragm during fluoroscopic or ultrasound examination. In the patient who is receiving positive-pressure ventilation, the paralyzed diaphragm may appear normal on the chest radiograph; thus, one of these tests is necessary to confirm the diagnosis of phrenic nerve paralysis. Diaphragmatic paralysis should be suspected in the pediatric patient who cannot be weaned from the ventilator as expected. In some patients, diaphragmatic function will return, but if ventilatory dependency lasts >2 weeks, consideration should be given to performing a diaphragmatic plication procedure, especially for children <2 years old. This procedure will often allow extubation of the previously ventilator-dependent patient (114).

Phrenic nerve dysfunction following heart–lung and lung transplantation is an important clinical problem that results in prolonged need for ventilator support and intensive care unit stay (115).

Prolonged Respiratory Insufficiency

Most patients are extubated within 6 hours of surgery. Some patients, particularly elderly ones or those who have had long operations, may be too somnolent for early extubation. Factors associated with the need for prolonged ventilator support after coronary artery surgery are increased age, preoperative heart failure, intraoperative fluid retention, postoperative intraaortic balloon requirement, perioperative stroke, and the need for more blood transfusions (116). In these patients, ventilator support is continued and repeated efforts to wean are made; extubation is usually achieved within 24 hours. After this time period, failure to wean is usually due to either oxygenation failure (characterized by low Po_2 levels) or ventilatory failure (with high CO_2 levels) or both. When weaning failure occurs, efforts are directed at optimization of the patient's cardiac performance and volume status, correction of ongoing metabolic abnormalities, reduction in narcotic and sedative drug administration, and provision of sufficient nutrition. Bronchoscopy may be indicated, particularly if bronchial mucous plugging is suspected to be present. After 10 to 14 days of ventilator dependency and intubation, tracheostomy is often performed. This provides for better patient comfort, lower airway resistance, and reduced bacterial contamination of the lower airway, but does increase the risk of mediastinitis.

Patients who need prolonged positive-pressure ventilation require careful management. No patient dependent on a respirator for his or her life should be left unattended. Ventilator alarm systems must remain activated at all times. Periods off the respirator (required for tracheal care, x-ray films, etc.) must be limited to 1 or 2 minutes at a time, and the monitor should be watched for the appearance of ventricular irritability or bradycardia indicative of hypoxia. A self-inflating bag (Ambu bag) connected to an oxygen supply must be at each bedside. Whenever a patient appears to be ventilated improperly or if there is any question of machine malfunction, the nurse, respiratory therapist, or physician in attendance should immediately begin hand ventilation while the problem is being resolved.

Determining the adequacy of mechanical ventilation is based on physical examination, pulse oximetric measurement of the arterial oxygen saturation, and arterial blood gas analysis. The patient who "looks comfortable" may be surprisingly hypoxic; thus, the use of pulse oximetry to continuously measure the patient's arterial oxygen saturation is standard. The pulse oximeter, however, does not provide information regarding Pco_2 and acid–base status and should not be relied on as the sole method of monitoring the ventilator-dependent patient. Periodic blood gas determinations are essential.

A useful method of quantitating the lung's ability to transfer oxygen to the blood is to determine the alveolar–arterial (A-a) gradient:

$$\text{A-a gradient} = [713\,(F_io_2) - (P_aco_2/0.8)] - P_ao_2$$

The A-a gradient is an estimate of the degree of intrapulmonary shunting. The normal value for a young patient is approximately 10, rising to 25 for the elderly patient.

The A-a gradient can be measured daily to provide a valuable objective index of progress in patients who cannot undergo extubation early after surgery. When the gradient is <350 mm Hg and if the patient's hemodynamic condition is stable, steps toward extubation (such as a trial of breathing on pressure support or a T-tube setup) are made.

An early goal of prolonged ventilatory management is to reduce the patient's inspired oxygen concentration (F_iO_2) to below 50%. Prolonged exposure to concentrations above this level is associated with detrimental changes in the lungs. Thus, we use the lowest F_iO_2 that will yield an arterial oxygen saturation of 92% to 94%. The addition of positive end-expiratory pressure (PEEP) will frequently allow for improved oxygenation at lower F_iO_2. Patients who are fluid overloaded (as are many cardiac surgery patients early after operation) should undergo vigorous diuresis as long as adequate cardiac function is maintained. For some patients, especially those with concomitant renal insufficiency, hemofiltration can be useful. This technique provides for the removal of excess fluid in addition to the elimination of cardiopulmonary toxic substances that may be contributing to the respiratory failure.

The patient undergoing prolonged ventilatory support must not be allowed to starve. Failure to maintain nutrition may impair respiratory muscle function and further hamper efforts at weaning the patient from the ventilator. If it is anticipated that extubation and normal feeding are more than a few days away (or if a few days have already passed), then nutrition must begin. If bowel activity is present, a soft small-bore nasogastric tube may be used for enteral feedings; if not, central venous hyperalimentation is begun.

Preferences for the route of endotracheal intubation differ among institutions. In general, the oral route is preferred when the period of intubation is expected to be short. This route of intubation is often easier to perform, but can cause trauma to the mouth and is uncomfortable for the awake patient. The nasal route is more comfortable, but is associated with sinusitis and pressure necrosis of the skin of the nares (contributed to, in some patients, by low cardiac output).

Prolonged endotracheal intubation is uncomfortable and has the potential for local complications such as vocal cord ulceration and posterior commissure stenosis. This has led some surgeons to recommend performance of a tracheostomy in ventilator-dependent patients after a set period (such as 10 or 14 days). On the other hand, early tracheostomy following cardiac operation is a risk factor for developing mediastinitis (117,118). Thus, a policy of performing a tracheostomy after a specified period of intubation may not be applicable to all cardiac surgery patients. Likewise, complications of a tracheostomy include tracheal ulceration, bleeding, tracheoinnominate fistula, and late tracheal stenosis. Generally, we wait at least 10 days (and often longer) after the original cardiac procedure before proceeding with a tracheostomy. Use of the percutaneous dilatational tracheostomy technique may be preferable for surgeons who have experience with this method (119,120).

Despite the increased risk of mediastinitis, for those patients who have been ventilator dependent for some time and clearly are not going to be weaned in the near future, a tracheostomy is recommended. The tracheostomy tube is more comfortable for the patient, allows for more convenient management of pulmonary secretions, and is useful during a slow weaning protocol. This latter feature is particularly valuable as the patient may be disconnected from the ventilator (or placed on a positive-pressure support system) for increasingly longer periods of time as the ability to breathe on his or her own improves. This avoids the trials of extubation and, sometimes, reintubation, which are traumatic and dangerous for the patient and may be required to wean the patient from prolonged endotracheal intubation.

Acute Respiratory Distress Syndrome

Acute respiratory distress syndrome (ARDS) is a form of severe respiratory insufficiency that may occur in the presence of relatively normal cardiac function. It is characterized by injury to both the alveolar vascular endothelial and the alveolar epithelial cells, resulting in increased capillary permeability, alveolar flooding, impaired removal of edema fluid from the alveolar space, and reduced surfactant production (121). This results in extravasation of protein-containing fluid in the alveolar space, hypoxemia, decreased lung compliance, increased work of breathing, diffuse pulmonary infiltrates on chest radiograph, and pulmonary hypertension (122). Although the cause is not known, ARDS appears to result from, at least in part, a florid inflammatory process that has been termed *systemic inflammatory response syndrome,* which may be contributed to by the use of CPB (123). ARDS after cardiac surgery is rare, occurring in <1% of patients, but has a high mortality rate (124,125).

Treatment of postoperative ARDS is largely supportive. Prevention and treatment of infections and nutritional supplementation (preferably by the enteral route) are important. Diuresis to reduce preload while maintaining adequate cardiac output may be helpful in reducing lung water. The optimal method of ventilator management for patients with ARDS is not clear. However, the use of smaller tidal volumes (6 mL/kg of body weight) and maintaining plateau pressure (airway pressure after a 0.5-second pause at the end of inspiration) below 30 cm H_2O has been associated with lower ARDS mortality (126). A moderate level of PEEP (5 to 8 cm H_2O) is used to lower the F_iO_2 to below 60% while maintaining the arterial saturation above 90%, if possible. A relatively high ventilatory rate may be needed to prevent severe hypercarbia. There are no medications currently used for the specific early treatment of ARDS; routine use of glucocorticoids is not recommended (121).

Pneumothorax

Pneumothorax may occur in patients after open-heart surgery, especially when they are receiving positive-pressure ventilation. It is more common in those with preexisting obstructive or bullous disease and those requiring significant levels of PEEP. Tension pneumothorax may develop quickly in the mechanically ventilated patient; this possibility should be kept in mind during the evaluation of a patient who has suddenly decompensated. Although breath sounds may be diminished on the affected side, the noise produced by the ventilator and other noise in the intensive care unit may cause the breath sounds to appear equal despite the presence of a large pneumothorax. Other clues to the presence of tension pneumothorax include distended neck veins and tracheal deviation away from the involved hemithorax. If the patient is severely hypotensive and a pneumothorax is strongly suspected, treatment is begun by inserting a 16-gauge intravenous catheter (cannula-over-needle type) into the pleural space. A rush of air exiting from the chest through the cannula, associated with hemodynamic improvement of the patient, confirms the diagnosis. If the patient is sufficiently stable, then a chest x-ray film may be obtained before definitive therapy. This will reveal collapse of the lung and, if tension is present, shifting of the mediastinal structures away from the affected side.

Definitive therapy is the placement of a chest tube (Fig. 4-4). The insertion site is usually at the fourth or fifth interspace in the anterior axillary line. For pneumothorax, the tube is directed superiorly. For adequate drainage of blood or fluid, the tube should be directed either posteriorly or along the diaphragm. The anterior axillary line is preferred because more posteriorly located tubes are more uncomfortable. The diaphragm rises as high as the sixth intercostal space laterally; therefore, the insertion site should not be lower than this interspace.

Pleural Effusions

Postoperative pleural effusions are very common in cardiac surgery patients, occurring in 40% to 90% of patients, depending on the modality used to make the diagnosis (127). Typically, the effusions become evident after the second postoperative day, are usually small in size, and are most often on the left side. They may be more common in patients who have had the internal mammary artery mobilized for use as coronary artery bypass conduit. The use of ice slush for cooling of the heart may also be a contributing factor. Patients with chronic congestive heart failure frequently have pleural effusions before surgery, and although these may be drained during surgery, it is not unusual for the effusions to recur. Most of the effusions, particularly smaller ones, will resolve with diuresis and time. Larger effusions, particularly in patients with impaired lung function, will result in dyspnea and will require drainage. Most often, in our practices, drainage is achieved by ultrasound-guided thoracentesis performed by the radiologist (128). In a few patients, significant effusions will recur and require repeat thoracentesis or chest tube placement. Rarely, the effusion is difficult to drain (often due to loculations) and causes compression and entrapment of the lung. For these patients, decortication may be indicated.

For many patients, especially those undergoing coronary artery bypass, we frequently place a flexible small diameter silastic drainage tube into the left pleural space. The exterior end of the tube is attached to a collection bulb. This tube remains in place after the larger chest tubes are removed and is removed when the daily drainage falls below 100 mL. This usually occurs by the third or fourth postoperative day. Use of this supplemental drain is associated with a decreased incidence of symptomatic left pleural effusions (129).

Chylothorax, due to injury to the thoracic duct, is a rare complication that may occur especially in children who undergo surgery for congenital lesions. Continued drainage of the protein-

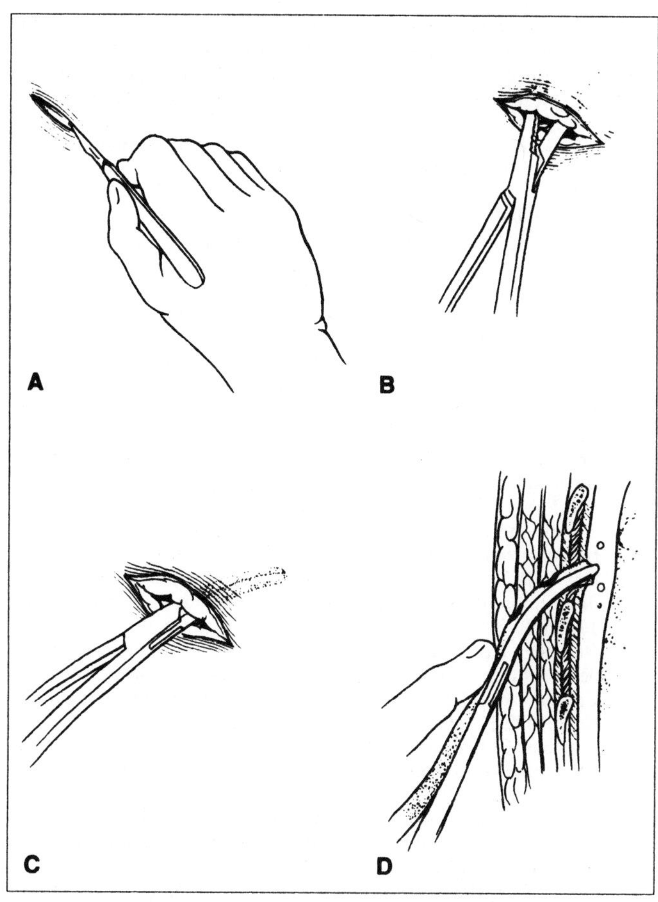

Fig. 4-4. Insertion of a chest tube. A chest tube may be inserted safely, even in patients with coagulopathy who are on ventilators, if proper technique is used. Under local anesthesia, a small incision is made and a tunnel dissected bluntly through the subcutaneous tissues to the rib (A). A tract through the intercostal muscles is created bluntly *over* the superior surface of the rib selected to avoid trauma to the intercostal vessels that follow the inferior edge (B and C). A gloved finger may be inserted into the pleural space to verify that the lung is not adherent, if in doubt. A pleural tube of adequate caliber (*not* a Foley catheter) is guided into the pleural space with a clamp (D), attached to a water seal drainage system, and sutured securely.

rich fluid may result in malnutrition. Conservative management includes closed drainage, total parenteral nutrition, and a diet of medium-chain triglycerides. In some patients, chylothorax is a major problem and may require treatment by thoracic duct ligation, application of fibrin glue, talc pleurodesis, and/or pleuroperitoneal shunt (130). For adults with chylothorax, the use of video-assisted thoracoscopy has been advocated (131).

REFERENCES

1. Ferguson TB, Hammill BG, Peterson ED, et al. A decade of change–risk profiles and outcomes for isolated coronary artery bypass grafting procedures, 1990–1999: a report from the STS National Database Committee and the Duke Clinical Research Institute. *Ann Thorac Surg* 2002;73:480–490.
2. Rao V, Ivanov J, Weisel RD, et al. Predictors of low cardiac output syndrome after coronary artery bypass. *J Thorac Cardiovasc Surg* 1996;112:38–51.
3. Beattie S. Heart failure with preserved LV function: pathophysiology, clinical presentation, treatment, and nursing implications. *J Cardiovasc Nurs* 2000;14:24–37.
4. Dietl CA, Berkheimer MD, Woods EL, et al. Efficacy and cost-effectiveness of preoperative IABP in patients with ejection fraction of 0.25 or less. *Ann Thorac Surg* 1996;62:401–409.
5. Doty DB. The surgeon's response to a low-output state after cardiopulmonary bypass: etiologies and remedies. *J Cardiac Surg* 1990;5:256–262.
6. Reichert SL, Visser CA, Koolen JJ, et al. Transesophageal echocardiography in hypotensive patients after cardiac surgery. Comparison with hemodynamic parameters. *J Thorac Cardiovasc Surg* 1992;104:321–326.
7. Hartzler GO, Maloney JD, Curtis JJ, et al. Hemodynamic benefits of atrioventricular sequential pacing after cardiac surgery. *Am J Cardiol* 1977;40:232–236.
8. Eichorn EJ, Diehl JT, Konstam, MA, et al. Left ventricular inotropic effect of atrial pacing after coronary artery bypass grafting. *Am J Cardiol* 1989;632:687–692.
9. Insler SR, O'Connor MS, Leventhal MJ, et al. Association between postoperative hypothermia and adverse outcome after coronary artery bypass surgery. *Ann Thorac Surg* 2000;70:175–181.
10. Kim YD, Katz NM, Ng L, et al. Effects of hypothermia and hemodilution on oxygen metabolism and hemodynamics in patients recovering from coronary artery bypass operations. *J Thorac Cardiovasc Surg* 1989;97:36–42.
11. Kranke P, Eberhart LH, Roewer N, et al. Pharmacological treatment of postoperative shivering: a quantitative systematic review of randomized controlled trials. *Anesth Analg* 2002;94:453–460.
12. Zwischenberger JB, Dechert RE, Kirsh MM, et al. Suppression of shivering decreases oxygen consumption and improves hemodynamic stability during postoperative rewarming following cardiopulmonary bypass. *Surg Forum* 1985;36:11–13.
13. DiSesa VJ. The rational selection of inotropic drugs in cardiac surgery. *J Cardiac Surg* 1987;2:385–391.
14. Aral A, Oguz M, Ozberrak H, et al. Hemodynamic advantages of left atrial epinephrine administration in open heart operations. *Ann Thorac Surg* 1997;64:1046–1049.

15. Doyle AR, Dhir AK, Moors AH, et al. Treatment of perioperative low cardiac output syndrome. *Ann Thorac Surg* 1995;59:S3–S11.
16. Fowler MB, Alderman EL, Oesterle SN, et al. Dobutamine and dopamine after cardiac surgery: greater augmentation of myocardial blood flow with dobutamine. *Circulation* 1984;70:1103–1111.
17. Disesa VJ, Brown E, Mudge GH, et al. Hemodynamic comparison of dopamine and dobutamine in the postoperative volume-loaded, pressure-loaded and normal ventricle. *J Thorac Cardiovasc Surg* 1982;83:256–263.
18. Butterworth JF IV, Prielipp RC, Royster RL, et al. Dobutamine increases heart rate more than epinephrine in patients recovering from aortocoronary bypass surgery. *J Cardiothorac Vasc Anesth* 1992;6:535–541.
19. Lathi KG, Shulman MS, Diehl JT, et al. The use of amrinone and norepinephrine for inotropic support during emergence from cardiopulmonary bypass. *J Cardiothorac Vasc Anesth* 1991;5:250–254.
20. Hardy JF, Searle N, Roy M, et al. Amrinone, in combination with norepinephrine, is an effective first-line drug for difficult separation from cardiopulmonary bypass. *Can J Anaesth* 1993; 40:495–501.
21. Levy JH, Bailey JM, Deeb GM. Intravenous milrinone in cardiac surgery. *Ann Thorac Surg* 2002;73:325–330.
22. Kikura M, Levy JH, Michelsen LG, et al. The effect of milrinone on hemodynamics and left ventricular function after emergence from cardiopulmonary bypass. *Anesth Analg* 1997;85:16–22.
23. Yamada T, Takeda J, Katori N, et al. Hemodynamic effects of milrinone during weaning from cardiopulmonary bypass: comparison of patients with a low and high prebypass cardiac index. *J Cardiothorac Vasc Anesth* 2000;14:367–373.
24. Feneck RO, Sherry KM, Withington PS, et al. Comparison of the hemodynamic effects of milrinone with dobutamine in patients after cardiac surgery. *J Cardiothorac Vasc Anesth* 2001;15: 306–315.
25. Lobato EB, Florete O Jr, Bingham HL. A single dose of milrinone facilitates separation from cardiopulmonary bypass in patients with pre-existing left ventricular dysfunction. *Br J Anaesth* 1998;81:782–784.
26. Prielipp RC, MacGregor DA, Butterworth JF IV, et al. Pharmacodynamics and pharmacokinetics of milrinone administration to increase oxygen delivery in critically ill patients. *Chest* 1996; 109:1291–1301.
27. Tinker J. Potent inotropes are the drugs of choice after cardiopulmonary bypass. *J Cardiothorac Vasc Anesth* 1987;1:256–259.
28. Hauptman PJ, Kelly RA. Digitalis. *Circulation* 1999;99:1265–1270.
29. Latifi S, Lidsky K, Blumer JL. Pharmacology of inotropic agents in infants and children. *Prog Pediatr Cardiol* 2000;12:57–79.
30. Mullis-Jansson SL, Argenziano M, Corwin S, et al. A randomized double-blind study of the effect of triiodothyronine on cardiac function and morbidity after coronary bypass surgery. *J Thorac Cardiovasc Surg* 1999;117:1128–1135.
31. Klemperer JD, Klein I, Gomez M, et al. Thyroid hormone treatment after coronary-artery bypass surgery. *N Engl J Med* 1995; 333:1522–1527.

32. Lazar HL, Philippides G, Fitgerald C, et al. Glucose–insulin–potassium solutions enhance recovery after urgent coronary artery bypass grafting. *J Thorac Cardiovasc Surg* 1997;113:354–362.
33. D'Ambra MN, LaRaia PJ, Watkins WD, et al. Prostaglandin E-1: a new therapy for refractory right heart failure and pulmonary hypertension after mitral valve replacement. *J Thorac Cardiovasc Surg* 1985;89:567–572.
34. Fullerton DA, Jones SD, Grover FL, et al. Adenosine effectively controls pulmonary hypertension after cardiac operations. *Ann Thorac Surg* 1996;61:1118–1123.
35. Vlahakes GJ. Management of pulmonary hypertension and right ventricular failure: another step forward. *Ann Thorac Surg* 1996;61:1051–1052.
36. Fullerton DA, Jaggers J, Wollmering MM, et al. Variable response to inhaled nitric oxide after cardiac surgery. *Ann Thorac Surg* 1997;63:1251–1256.
37. El-Banayosy A, Brehm C, Kizner L, et al. Cardiopulmonary resuscitation after cardiac surgery: a two-year study. *J Cardiothorac Vasc Anesth* 1998;12:390–392.
38. Suominen P, Palo R, Sairanen H, et al. Perioperative determinants and outcome of cardiopulmonary arrest in children after heart surgery. *Eur J Cardiothorac Surg* 2001;19:127–134.
39. American Heart Association. Guidelines 2000 for cardiopulmonary resuscitation and emergency cardiovascular care: International Consensus on Science. *Circulation* 2000;102(suppl I):I1–I384.
40. Kloeck W, Cummins RO, Chamberlain D, et al. The universal advances life support algorithm: an advisory statement from the Advanced Life Support Working Group of the International Liaison Committee on Resuscitation. *Circulation* 1997;95:2180–2182.
41. Nadkarni V, Hazinski MF, Zideman D, et al. Pediatric resuscitation: an advisory statement from the Pediatric Working Group of the International Liaison Committee on Resuscitation. *Circulation* 1997;95:2185–2195.
42. Eisenberg MS, Mengert TJ. Cardiac resuscitation. *N Engl J Med* 2001;344:1304–1313.
43. Bardy GH, Marchlinski FE, Sharma AD, et al. Multicenter comparison of truncated biphasic shocks and standard damped sine wave monophasic shocks for transthoracic ventricular defibrillation. *Circulation* 1996;94:2507–2514.
44. Torres NE, White RD. Current concepts in cardiopulmonary resuscitation. *J Cardiothorac Vasc Anesth* 1997;11:391–407.
45. American Heart Association. Pediatric advanced life support. *Circulation* 2000;102(suppl I):I291–I357.
46. Fiser SM, Tribble CG, Kern JA, et al. Cardiac reoperation in the intensive care unit. *Ann Thorac Surg* 2001;71:1888–1893.
47. Kern KB, Paraskos JA. Task force 1: cardiac arrest. *J Am Coll Cardiol* 2000;35:832–846.
48. Guidelines 2000 Conference on CPR and ECC. Sections 5,6 and 7: Pharmacology I and II; a guide to the international ACLS algorithms. *Circulation* 2000;102(suppl I):I112–I165.
49. Baerman JM, Kirsh MM, deBuitler M, et al. Natural history and determinants of conduction defects following coronary bypass surgery. *Ann Thorac Surg* 1987;44:150–153.

50. Keefe DL, Griffin JC, Harrison DC, et al. Atrioventricular conduction abnormalities in patients undergoing isolated aortic or mitral valve replacement. *Pacing Clin Electrophysiol* 1985;8:393–398.
51. Gordon RS, Ivanov J, Cohen G, et al. Permanent cardiac pacing after a cardiac operation: predicting the use of permanent pacemakers. *Ann Thorac Surg* 1998:66:1698–1704.
52. Del Nido P, Goldman BS. Temporary epicardial pacing in the cardiac surgical patient. *J Cardiac Surg* 1989;4:99–103.
53. Carroll KC, Reeves LM, Anderson G, et al. Risks associated with removal of ventricular epicardial pacing wires after cardiac surgery. *Am J Crit Care* 1998;7:444–449.
54. American Heart Association. Advanced cardiovascular life support. *Circulation* 2000;102(suppl I):I158–I165.
55. American Society of Health-System Pharmacists. Amiodarone. In: McEvoy GK, ed. *AHFS drug information 2001.* Bethesda: American Society of Health-System Pharmacists, 2001:1514–1531.
56. Creswell LL. Postoperative atrial arrhythmias: risk factors and associated adverse outcomes. *Semin Thorac Cardiovasc Surg* 1999;11:303–307.
57. Hogue CW, Hyder ML. Atrial fibrillation after cardiac operation: risks, mechanisms, and treatment. *Ann Thorac Surg* 2000;69:300–306.
58. Hravnak M, Hoffman LA, Saul MI, et al. Atrial fibrillation: prevalence after minimally invasive direct and standard coronary artery bypass. *Ann Thorac Surg* 2001;71:1491–1495.
59. Tamis-Holland JE, Homel P, Durani M, et al. Atrial fibrillation after minimally invasive direct coronary artery bypass surgery. *J Am Coll Cardiol* 2000;36:1884–1888.
60. van Dijk D, Nierich AP, Jansen EWL, et al. Early outcome after off-pump versus on-pump coronary bypass surgery: results from a randomized study. *Circulation* 2001;104:1761–1766.
61. Cox JL. A perspective on postoperative atrial fibrillation. *Semin Thorac Cardiovasc Surg* 1999;11:299–302.
62. Peters RW, Weiss DN, Carliner NH, et al. Overdrive pacing for atrial flutter. *Am J Cardiol* 1994;74:1021–1023.
63. Tisdale JE, Padhi ID, Goldberg AD, et al. A randomized, double-blind comparison of intravenous diltiazem and digoxin for atrial fibrillation after coronary artery bypass surgery. *Am Heart J* 1998;135:739–747.
64. Schwartz M, Michaelson EL, Sawin HS, et al. Esmolol: safety and efficacy in postoperative cardiothoracic patients with supraventricular tachyarrhythmias. *Chest* 1988;93:705–711.
65. Vardos PE, Kochiadakis GE, Igoumenidis NE, et al. Amiodarone as a first-choice drug for restoring sinus rhythm in patients with atrial fibrillation. *Chest* 2000;117:1538–1545.
66. Connolly SJ. Evidence-based analysis of amiodarone efficacy and safety. *Circulation* 1999;100:2025–2034.
67. Goldschlager N, Epstein AE, Naccarelli G, et al. Practical guidelines for clinicians who treat patients with amiodarone. *Arch Intern Med* 2000;160:1741–1748.
68. Sanoski CA, Bauman JL. Clinical observations with the amiodarone/warfarin interaction. *Chest* 2002;121:19–23.

69. Ashrafian H, Davey P. Is amiodarone an underrecognized cause of acute respiratory failure in the ICU? *Chest* 2001;120:275–282.
70. Dimopoulou I, Marathias K, Daganou M, et al. Low-dose amiodarone-related complications after cardiac operations. *J Thorac Cardiovasc Surg* 1997;114:31–37.
71. Fuster V, Ryden LE, Asinger RW, et al. ACC/AHA/ESC Guidelines for the Management of Patients with Atrial Fibrillation: executive summary. *J Am Coll Cardiol* 2001;38:1231–1265.
72. Grace AA, Camm AJ. Quinidine. *N Engl J Med* 1998;338:35–43.
73. Falk RH. Atrial fibrillation. *N Engl J Med* 2001;344:1067–1078.
74. Crystal E, Connolly SJ, Sleik K, et al. Interventions on prevention of postoperative atrial fibrillation in patients undergoing open heart surgery. *Circulation* 2002;106:75–80.
75. Wurdeman RL, Mooss AN, Mohiuddin SM, et al. Amiodarone vs sotalol as prophylaxis against atrial fibrillation/flutter after heart surgery: a meta-analysis. *Chest* 2002;121:1203–1210.
76. Haan CK, Geraci SA. Role of amiodarone in reducing atrial fibrillation after cardiac surgery in adults. *Ann Thorac Surg* 2002; 73:1665–1669.
77. Daoud EG, Strickberger SA, Man KC, et al. Preoperative amiodarone as prophylaxis against atrial fibrillation after heart surgery. *N Engl J Med* 1997;33:1785–1790.
78. Guarnieri T, Nolan S, Gottlieb SO, et al. Intravenous amiodarone for the prevention of atrial fibrillation after open heart surgery: the Amiodarone Reduction in Coronary Heart (ARCH) trial. *J Am Coll Cardiol* 1999;34:343–347.
79. Maras D, Boskovic SD, Popovic Z, et al. Single-day loading dose of amiodarone for the prevention of new-onset atrial fibrillation after coronary artery bypass surgery. *Am Heart J* 2001;141:E8.
80. White CM, Giri S, Tsikouris JP, et al. A comparison of two individual amiodarone regimens to placebo in open heart surgery patients. *Ann Thorac Surg* 2002;74:69–74.
81. Mahoney EM, Thompson TD, Veledar E, et al. Cost-effectiveness of targeting patients undergoing cardiac surgery for therapy with intravenous amiodarone to prevent atrial fibrillation. *J Am Coll Cardiol* 2002;40:737–745.
82. Solomon AJ, Greenberg MD, Kilborn MJ, et al. Amiodarone versus a beta-blocker to prevent atrial fibrillation after cardiovascular surgery. *Am Heart J* 2001;142:811–815.
83. Rho RW, Bridges CR, Kocovic D. Management of postoperative arrhythmias. *Semin Thorac Cardiovasc Surg* 2000;12:349–361.
84. Blommaert D, Gonzalez M, Mucumbitsi J, et al. Effective prevention of atrial fibrillation by continuous atrial overdrive pacing after coronary artery bypass surgery. *J Am Coll Cardiol* 2000;35:1411–1415.
85. Cheng MK, Augostini RS, Asher CR, et al. Ineffectiveness and potential proarrhythmia of atrial pacing for atrial fibrillation prevention after coronary artery bypass grafting. *Ann Thorac Surg* 2000;69:1057–1063.
86. Dodge-Khatami A, Miller OI, Anderson RH, et al. Impact of junctional ectopic tachycardia on postoperative morbidity following repair of congenital heart defects. *Eur J Cardiothorac Surg* 2002; 21:255–259.
87. Michael JG, Wilson WR Jr, Tobias JD. Amiodarone in the treatment of junctional ectopic tachycardia after cardiac surgery

in children: report of two cases and review of the literature. *Am J Ther* 1999;6:223–227.
88. Shah MJ, Rhodes LA. Management of postoperative arrhythmias and junctional ectopic tachycardia. *Pediatr Cardiac Surg Ann* 1998;1:91–102.
89. Mandapati R, Byrum CJ, Kavey RE, et al. Procainamide for rate control of postsurgical junctional tachycardia. *Pediatr Cardiol* 2000;21:123–128.
90. Mangano DT, Study of Perioperative Ischemia (SPI) Research Group. Myocardial ischemia following cardiac surgery: preliminary findings. *J Cardiac Surg* 1990;5:288–293.
91. Alderman EL, Levy JH, Rich JB, et al. Analyses of coronary graft patency after aprotinin use: results from the International Multicenter Aprotinin Graft Patency Experience (IMAGE) trial. *J Thorac Cardiovasc Surg* 1998;116:716–730.
92. Levy JH, Pifarre R, Schaff HV, et al. A multicenter, double-blind, placebo-controlled trial of aprotinin for reducing blood loss and the requirement for donor-blood transfusion in patients undergoing repeat coronary artery bypass grafting. *Circulation* 1995;92:2236–2244.
93. Klatte K, Chaitman BR, Theroux P, et al. Increased mortality after coronary artery bypass graft surgery is associated with increased levels of postoperative creatinine kinase–myocardial band isoenzyme release. *J Am Coll Cardiol* 2001;38:1070–1077.
94. Yokoyama Y, Chaitman BR, Hardison RM, et al. Association between new ECG abnormalities after coronary revascularization and five-year cardiac mortality in BARI randomized and registry patients. *Am J Cardiol* 2000;86:819–824.
95. Birdi I, Angelini GD, Bryan AJ. Biochemical markers of myocardial injury during cardiac operations. *Ann Thorac Surg* 1997;63:879–884.
96. Joint European Society of Cardiology/American College of Cardiology Committee. Myocardial infarction redefined—a consensus document of the Joint European Society for Cardiology/American College of Cardiology Committee for the redefinition of myocardial infarction. *J Am Coll Cardiol* 2000;36:959–969.
97. Vermes E, Mesguich M, Houel R, et al. Cardiac troponin I release after open heart surgery: a marker of myocardial protection? *Ann Thorac Surg* 2000;70:2087–2090.
98. Kost GJ, Kirk JD, Omand K. A strategy for the use of cardiac injury markers (troponin I and T, creatine kinase-MB mass and isoforms, and myoglobin) in the diagnosis of acute myocardial infarction. *Arch Pathol Lab Med* 1998;122:245–251.
99. Greenson N, Macoviak J, Krishnasway P, et al. Usefulness of cardiac troponin I in patients undergoing open heart surgery. *Am Heart J* 2001;141:447–455.
100. Paz MA, Lupon J, Bosch X, et al. Predictors of early saphenous vein aortocoronary bypass graft occlusion. *Ann Thorac Surg* 1993;56:1101–1106.
101. Paterson HS, Jones MW, Baird DK, et al., Lethal postoperative coronary artery spasm. *Ann Thorac Surg* 1998;65:1571–1573.
102. Lemmer JH Jr, Kirsh MM. Coronary artery spasm following coronary artery surgery. *Ann Thorac Surg* 1988;46:108–115.
103. Samuels LE, Kaufman MS, Morris RJ, et al. Coronary artery bypass grafting in patients with COPD. *Chest* 1998;113:878–882.

104. Bando K, Sun K, Binford RS, et al. Determinant of longer duration of endotracheal intubation after adult cardiac operations. *Ann Thorac Surg* 1997;63:1026–1033.
105. Crapo RO. Pulmonary-function testing. *N Engl J Med* 1994; 331:25–30.
106. Shapira N, Zabatino SM, Ahmed S, et al. Determinants of pulmonary function in patients undergoing coronary bypass operations. *Ann Thorac Surg* 1990;50:268–273.
107. Wahl GW, Swinburne AJ, Fedullo AJ, et al. Effect of age and preoperative airway obstruction on lung function after coronary artery bypass grafting. *Ann Thorac Surg* 1993;56:104–107.
108. Nelson HS. β-Adrenergic bronchodilators. *N Engl J Med* 1995; 333:499–506.
109. Matthay MA, Wiener-Kronish JP. Respiratory management after cardiac surgery. *Chest* 1989;95:424–434.
110. Curtis JJ, Nawarawong W, Walls JT, et al. Elevated hemidiaphragm after cardiac operations: incidence, prognosis, and relationship to the use of topical ice slush. *Ann Thorac Surg* 1989; 48: 764–768.
111. Chandler KW, Rozas CJ, Kory RC, et al. Bilateral diaphragmatic paralysis complicating local cardiac hypothermia during open heart surgery. *Am J Med* 1984:77:243–249.
112. Katz MG, Katz R, Schachner A, et al. Phrenic nerve injury after coronary artery bypass grafting: will it go away? *Ann Thorac Surg* 1998;65:32–35.
113. De Leeuw M, Williams JM, Freedom RM, et al. Impact of diaphragmatic paralysis after cardiothoracic surgery in children. *J Thorac Cardiothorac Surg* 1999;118:510–517.
114. Watanabe T, Trusler GA, Williams WG, et al. Phrenic nerve paralysis after pediatric cardiac surgery. *J Thorac Cardiovasc Surg* 1987;94:383–388.
115. Ferdinande PG, Bruyninck F, Van Raemdonck D, et al. Phrenic nerve dysfunction after heart–lung and lung transplantation. *J Heart Lung Transplant* 2002;21:142–145.
116. Habib RH, Zacharias A, Engoren M. Determinants of prolonged mechanical ventilation after coronary artery bypass grafting. *Ann Thorac Surg* 1996;62:1164–1171.
117. Curtis JJ, McKenney CA, Walls JT, et al. Tracheostomy: a risk factor for mediastinitis after cardiac operation. *Ann Thorac Surg* 2001;72:731–734.
118. Stamenkovic SA, Morgan IS, Pontefract DR, et al. Is early tracheostomy safe in cardiac patients with median sternotomy incisions? *Ann Thorac Surg* 2000;69:1152–1154.
119. Byhahn C, Rinne T, Halbig S, et al. Early percutaneous tracheostomy after median sternotomy. *J Thorac Cardiovasc Surg* 2000;120:329–334.
120. Melloni G, Muttini S, Gallioli G, et al. Surgical tracheostomy versus percutaneous dilatational tracheostomy. A prospective-randomized study with long-term follow-up. *J Cardiovasc Surg (Torino)* 2002;43:113–121.
121. Ware LB, Matthay MA. The acute respiratory distress syndrome. *N Engl J Med* 2000;342:1334–1349.
122. Peruzzi WT, Franklin ML, Shapiro BA. New concepts and therapies of adult respiratory distress syndrome. *J Cardiothorac Vasc Anesth* 1997;11:771–786.

123. Asimakiopoulos G, Smith PLC, Ratnatunga CP, et al. Lung injury and acute respiratory distress syndrome after cardiopulmonary bypass. *Ann Thorac Surg* 1999;68:1107–1115.
124. Milot J, Perron J, Lacasse Y, et al. Incidence and predictors of ARDS after cardiac surgery. *Chest* 2001;119:884–888.
125. Christenson JT, Aeberhardt J-M, Badel P, et al. Adult respiratory distress syndrome after cardiac surgery. *Cardiovasc Surg* 1995;4:15–21.
126. Acute Respiratory Distress Syndrome Network. Ventilation with lower tidal volumes as compared with traditional tidal volumes for acute lung injury and the acute respiratory distress syndrome. *N Engl J Med* 2000;342:1301–1308.
127. Cohen M, Sahn SA. Resolution of pleural effusions. *Chest* 2001;119:1547–1562.
128. Qureshi N, Momin ZA, Brandstetter RD. Thoracentesis in clinical practice. Heart Lung 1994;23:376–383.
129. Payne M, Magovern GJ, Benckart DH, et al. Left pleural effusion after coronary artery bypass decreases with a supplemental pleural drain. *Ann Thorac Surg* 2002;73:149–152.
130. Bond SJ, Guzzetta PC, Snyder ML, et al. Management of pediatric postoperative chylothorax. *Ann Thorac Surg* 1993;56:469–472.
131. Fahimi H, Casselman FP, Mariani MA, et al. Current management of postoperative chylothorax. *Ann Thorac Surg* 2001;71: 448–451.

Postoperative Complications Involving Other Organ Systems

BLEEDING AFTER HEART SURGERY

Management of early postoperative bleeding is a familiar task for those who care for cardiac surgery patients. Some bleeding occurs after all cardiac operations, and it is significant enough to require early reexploration to control hemorrhage in 2% to 4% of patients (1,2). In adults, excessive postoperative bleeding occurs in association with repeat operations, emergency procedures, preoperative cardiogenic shock, combined procedures, female gender, small body mass index, older age, peripheral vascular disease, renal insufficiency (creatinine >1.8 g/dL), poor nutrition (albumin <4 g/dL) and in patients who have experienced prolonged cardiopulmonary bypass (CPB) durations (3,4).

Extensive preoperative laboratory testing of hemostasis parameters is not necessary; careful medical history of bleeding tendencies usually suffices, with further testing performed in patients with a history of bleeding problems. A simple screening question is to ask the patient if he or she has previously had tooth extractions and, if so, if excessive bleeding occurred with the procedure; patients who have had teeth pulled without difficulty are unlikely to have a serious congenital bleeding abnormality. Certainly, the history taking should include a careful review of the patient's medications, with particular emphasis on recent ingestion of aspirin, clopidogrel, and nonsteroidal antiinflammatory agents. For patients without a history of bleeding or easy bruising, we routinely measure only the platelet count prior to surgery. If the patient does have bleeding tendencies or has been on warfarin, the preoperative prothrombin time (PT), international normalized ratio, and activated partial thromboplastin time (aPTT) are also determined. Patients who are receiving warfarin prior to surgery may not, however, have increased bleeding. Thus, needed surgery should not be postponed, and it is not required to reverse the warfarin effect prior to operation (5,6).

In children, the determinants of excessive postoperative bleeding are not well defined, but preoperative cyanosis is a risk factor. Due to their smaller blood volume, children are more affected by hemodilution from the bypass circuit volume, with a larger reduction in platelets and soluble coagulation factors occurring as a result. Furthermore, neonates may be relatively deficient in various coagulation factors (such as factors XII and II) and coagulation inhibitors (such as antithrombin III) (7). Prostaglandin E_1 inhibits platelet function, and preoperative treatment with this agent may result in more bleeding. Polycythemic cyanotic children have lower levels of fibrinogen and other clotting factors with increased fibrin split products that contribute to postoperative bleeding.

Excessive bleeding after open heart surgery may be due to one or several of many factors including inadequate surgical hemostasis (surgical bleeding), platelet depletion, platelet dysfunction, plasma clotting factor deficiency, residual heparin effect (incomplete reversal by protamine), excessive protamine administration, hypothermia, increased fibrinolytic activity, and consumption coagulopathy (8). For the patient suffering excessive bleeding early after heart surgery, the major problem is determining whether the bleeding is secondary to a reversible coagulation abnormality or whether it is due to a surgical cause such as a leaking suture line.

Mediastinal drainage tubes are routinely placed at the completion of the operation and are attached to suction collection receptacles. These allow for frequent measurements of the rate of bleeding. Although there is no strict definition of "excessive" postoperative bleeding, concern is raised when the mediastinal tube output exceeds 4 to 5 mL/kg per hour during the first few hours after operation. Typically, postoperative bleeding decreases significantly during the first 3 to 4 hours after surgery and becomes relatively minimal (<0.5 to 1.0 mL/kg per hour) by 6 hours. When the bleeding exceeds these general guidelines, efforts must be made to determine the presence or absence of treatable conditions (e.g., coagulopathy) and whether to return the patient to the operating room for surgical exploration. When the rate of bleeding is massive (i.e., >8 to 10 mL/kg per hour), the prompt return of the patient to the operating room for exploration is nearly always indicated. Clues to the presence of surgical bleeding include the continuous excessive chest tube output in a patient with relatively normal coagulation studies and the sudden development of significant drainage in the patient who was previously not bleeding, especially in conjunction with hemodynamic instability.

Nonsurgical (microvascular) bleeding after cardiac surgery using CPB is a multifactorial problem. Contributors include reduced platelet number and function, hemodilution from the extracorporeal circuit solution, activation of the hemostatic system caused by the interaction of blood with the bypass circuit surfaces (which are not covered by endothelium), activation of the extrinsic clotting system due to tissue trauma, and fibrinolysis. The central mediator in the process of clot formation is the generation of thrombin, which acts to convert fibrinogen to fibrin, the basic building block of clot. To prevent thrombosis during CPB, heparin, acting to catalyze endogenous antithrombin III, is administered, although some degree of thrombin formation and subclinical clot formation does occur, even in the presence of "adequate" heparinization. This subclinical thrombin production and clot formation result in consumption of clotting factors during CPB. Other effects of thrombin include the release of tissue plasminogen factor (with subsequent plasmin generation and fibrinolysis), activation of protein C, and release of tissue factor inhibitor. CPB also induces a complex series of reactions involving both enzyme cascades and cellular elements collectively termed the "systemic inflammatory response." This phenomenon is the result of the activation of complement, kallikrein, bradykinin, leukocytes, platelets, endothelium, and other mediators of inflammation and is due to contact of the blood elements with the nonendothelialized surface of the bypass tubing and oxygenator, surgical trauma, and reperfusion of transiently ischemic tissue (especially lung) (9,10).

Coronary artery bypass graft (CABG) procedures performed without the use of CPB result in less activation of the inflammatory responses and are generally associated with less postoperative bleeding and fewer transfusions (11,12). While such "off-pump" operations are not practical for valve procedures or all coronary bypass operations, they have an important role in the management of coronary disease patients.

Platelets and Bleeding in Cardiac Surgery Patients

Platelet abnormalities, either in quantity or in quality, are the most common cause of nonsurgical postoperative bleeding following procedures using CPB (13).

Thrombocytopenia

Postoperative thrombocytopenia may result from hemodilution due to the priming volume of the CPB circuit. In patients with a normal preoperative platelet count, this usually does not, however, result in a platelet count below 100,000 platelets/mm^3. Long CPB durations will result in a greater decrease in the platelet count due to consumption. Postoperative thrombocytopenia is likely to be more frequent in patients who required intraaortic balloon pump or ventricular assist device placement before surgery.

Patients treated with heparin may develop *heparin-induced thrombocytopenia* (HIT). This acquired syndrome of thrombocytopenia, with or without thrombosis, is an antibody-mediated drug reaction that occurs in about 2.5% of heparin-treated patients, usually after 7 to 8 days of therapy (14). Laboratory detection of the heparin-dependent IgG antibody confirms the diagnosis of HIT. This condition is less common following treatment with low molecular weight heparin (LMWH) as compared with the unfractionated type and appears to be more common following the administration of bovine heparin as compared with porcine heparin (15). Severe thrombocytopenia may result, and thrombotic events (such as deep venous thrombosis and limb arterial occlusion) occur in up to 30% of affected patients. Although not a common cause of early postoperative thrombocytopenia and bleeding in heart surgery patients, HIT should be kept in mind for the postoperative patient who is experiencing an unexplained decline in the platelet count. Treatment of HIT is removal of all sources of heparin (including catheter flush solutions). Platelet transfusions are *not* recommended as both bleeding and thrombotic complications may result. Following discontinuation of all heparin administration, the patient's platelet count usually begins to rise in 1 to 2 days. If anticoagulation is required, synthetic direct inhibitors of thrombin that do not cross-react with the HIT antibody, such as argatroban or lepirudin (recombinant hirudin), may be used in the treatment of patients with HIT (16–18).

Platelet Dysfunction

An important cause of postoperative microvascular bleeding is the variable and temporary decrease in platelet function that accompanies surgery using extracorporeal circulation. Post-bypass platelet dysfunction is likely related to platelet activation and degranulation (depletion of active intracellular mediators) during bypass as the result of contact with the nonendothelialized surfaces of the bypass circuit (tubing and oxygenator) and/or to direct trauma to the platelet glycoprotein (GP) membrane receptors, in particular, the GP Ib receptor. In addition, heparin itself activates platelets to some degree. As a result, prolongation of the patient's bleeding time early after cardiac surgery is common; this abnormality usually disappears within 2 to 4 hours after the procedure. CABG procedures performed without CPB may have less bleeding, at least in part, because the platelets are not subjected to the effects of the extracorporeal circulation circuit.

Drugs That Cause Platelet Dysfunction

Drug-induced platelet dysfunction is a major concern for cardiac surgeons. The use of various antiplatelet agents by cardiologists to treat acute coronary syndromes (unstable angina and myocardial infarction) or as adjuncts to percutaneous coronary interventions (angioplasty and stent placement) has become routine (19,20). Table 5-1 lists the commonly administered platelet inhibitors.

ASPIRIN. Aspirin is administered routinely for acute coronary syndromes and percutaneous interventions. Aspirin permanently inhibits platelet cyclooxygenase activity within 1 hour of ingestion of a single dose. This induces a defect in thromboxane A_2-dependent function, thereby inhibiting platelet activation, leading to impaired platelet aggregation and clot formation. Efficacy of aspirin treatment, in a variety of cardiovascular settings, has been well demonstrated (21). After a single aspirin dose is ingested, all platelets that are present in the patient become inhibited and the free aspirin is rapidly cleared from the plasma. The anucleate platelets cannot manufacture more cyclooxygenase, and therefore, the platelets are affected for the remainder of their existence. Platelets have a lifespan of about 10 days; so after about 5 days, <50% of the platelets present in the patient are aspirin inhibited, assuming no further aspirin ingestion. Generally, aspirin-treated patients who undergo cardiac surgery bleed more and require more transfusions (especially of platelets) than patients who have not received aspirin within several days of operation, although there is some conflicting evidence in this regard (4,22–25). In general, patients who receive aspirin prior to CABG do not suffer excessive complication rates and appear, in fact, to have improved short-term outcomes, including lower mortality (26,27). The drug aprotinin has been shown to reduce postoperative bleeding and transfusions when administered during CABG surgery in aspirin-treated patients (28,29).

Aspirin treatment improves CABG patency. When used for this purpose, aspirin should be given early postoperatively (within 6 hours of surgery); this avoids the increased bleeding effects while maintaining the beneficial effects on early graft patency (30). It is our custom to administer aspirin (325 mg) by rectal suppository to coronary bypass patients within 6 hours after arrival in the intensive care unit as long as excessive bleeding is not present.

CLOPIDOGREL AND TICLOPIDINE. Clopidogrel (Plavix) and ticlopidine (Ticlid) are thienopyridines with platelet inhibitory properties and demonstrated effectiveness when used to treat patients with coronary and vascular disease. Both inhibit, via a liver-transformed metabolite, adenosine diphosphate–induced platelet aggregation (21,31). Because of associated toxicity, primarily hema-

Table 5-1. Commonly used platelet-inhibiting drugs

	Aspirin	Clopidogrel	Abciximab	Eptifibatide	Tirofiban
Mechanism of action	Cyclooxygenase inhibitor	Inhibits ADP-mediated aggregation	Inhibits platelet membrane IIb/IIIa receptor	Inhibits platelet membrane IIb/IIIa receptor	Inhibits platelet membrane IIb/IIIa receptor
Onset of action	<1 h	<2 h (with loading dose)	<1 h	<1 h	<1 h
Effective duration of action	Irreversible (lasts for life of platelet); 7–10 d	Irreversible (lasts for life of platelet); 7–10 d	Biological effect for 12–24 h	4–6 h	4–6 h
Implications for surgery	Not clear; may be desirable to discontinue if possible, but not necessary; may cause more bleeding, but may have advantageous effects	If elective, discontinue drug for 5–7 d before operation	May cause more bleeding, but effect is reversible with platelet transfusion; not a contraindication to emergency surgery	Effect wears off relatively quickly; emergency surgery not associated with bleeding problems	Effect wears off relatively quickly; emergency surgery not associated with bleeding problems

tologic, ticlopidine has been replaced by the safer drug clopidogrel. Given orally only, clopidogrel is frequently administered at 75 mg per day, and with this dose, it requires several days before a steady state of approximately 50% inhibition of adenosine diphosphate–induced platelet aggregation is achieved. Large loading doses, commonly 300 mg, are frequently administered to patients prior to undergoing percutaneous coronary interventions such as stent placement. Following this dose, significant platelet inhibition and prolongation of the bleeding time are achieved within hours (32). Like aspirin, the clopidogrel platelet inhibitory effect is permanent for the affected platelets, and it requires 5 to 7 days for the effect to wear off. When given for these purposes, clopidogrel is usually administered in conjunction with aspirin, resulting in an additive effect. Clopidogrel-treated patients who require cardiac surgery have increased rates of bleeding, blood product transfusion, and need for early reoperation for bleeding (as high as 7%) (33). When a patient taking clopidogrel is considered for surgery, the increased risk of bleeding must be weighed against the risk of postponing the procedure. For totally elective patients, we discontinue the patient's clopidogrel for 4 to 7 days before operation. If the operation is urgent or emergency in nature, we proceed with the procedure but expect to transfuse platelets.

PLATELET GLYCOPROTEIN IIB/IIIA RECEPTOR INHIBITORS. Platelet aggregation, essential for clot formation, is mediated by the platelet membrane GP receptor denoted GP IIb/IIIa. Inhibition of this receptor results in powerful interference with platelet function and thrombosis and reduces complications in patients with acute coronary syndromes or who are undergoing percutaneous coronary intervention procedures. Drugs that specifically inhibit the GP IIb/IIIa receptor include abciximab, eptifibatide, and tirofiban. All three are administered by the intravenous route only. These drugs are used in patients with myocardial infarction or unstable angina and those undergoing percutaneous coronary angioplasty and stent placement. Occasionally, patients treated with IIb/IIIa inhibitors require coronary bypass procedures while under the effect of the IIb/IIIa inhibitor in addition to other antiplatelet drugs such as aspirin and clopidogrel. Because of the increased risk of bleeding complications, an understanding of the IIb/IIIa inhibitors is important for those who participate in the care of patients treated with these agents.

Abciximab (ReoPro) is an antibody directed against the GP IIb/IIIa receptor that improves the results of percutaneous coronary interventions and is efficacious in the treatment of acute coronary syndromes. Abciximab has a very strong affinity for the platelet GP IIb/IIIa receptor. After administration of a bolus dose of abciximab, the GP IIb/IIIa receptors are quickly bound by the antibody and inhibited while free drug is rapidly cleared. As no free drug remains in the patient's plasma, subsequent platelet transfusions effectively reverse the abciximab effect by diluting the abciximab that has become platelet bound. When a patient recently treated with abciximab needs surgery, the drug should be immediately discontinued, but protamine and platelets should not be administered prior to operation unless serious ongoing bleeding is present. Postponing surgery for 12 to 48 hours, often while maintaining the patient on heparin, will result in improved platelet aggregation and may be practical for stable patients. If necessary for ongoing ischemia, however, abciximab-treated patients should not be denied emergency surgery that is otherwise indicated, although they are likely to require platelet transfusions (34–37). Unless required for uncontrollable bleeding, platelets should not be given preoperatively as this might precipitate closure of a critically stenotic major coronary artery and will subject the transfused platelets to the adverse effects of CPB.

Eptifibatide (Integrilin) and *tirofiban* (Aggrastat) are molecules smaller than abciximab that have lesser degrees of affinity for the platelet GP IIb/IIIa receptor and shorter durations of action. They are generally not associated with increased bleeding in patients who require urgent coronary bypass surgery soon after discontinuation of the drug (38–40).

The use of potent platelet-inhibiting drugs has improved the care of coronary artery disease patients but, at times, has complicated the life of surgeons. Most often, patients requiring emergency bypass surgery for failed coronary interventions have received multiple antiplatelet agents, and these drugs have additive effects. These patients can, however, be successfully operated upon without an increased incidence of serious complications. Surgery, if otherwise indicated due to ongoing ischemia or critical anatomy, should *not* be withheld because of the drug-induced platelet defect that is present.

Clotting Factors and Fibrinogen

CPB, because of hemodilution and consumption, results in decreases in plasma clotting factor concentrations, especially factors V and VIII (41). Generally, however, the postoperative levels usually remain well above the level (25% to 30% of normal) required for normal hemostatic function. Thus, clotting factor deficiency is not a frequent cause of postoperative bleeding. It may, however, play a role in patients who have received massive transfusions of packed red blood cells, due to further dilution of the clotting factors, and in very polycythemic patients whose plasma volume is reduced. Assessment of plasma clotting factor function is by measurement of the PT. This test of the extrinsic portion of the clotting system has a normal upper-limit value of 13 seconds, although values of up to 16 seconds indicate sufficient clotting factor concentration to effect relatively normal clotting under most circumstances. For the bleeding patient with prolongation of the PT, treatment of clotting factor deficiency consists of the administration of a sufficient quantity of fresh frozen plasma. Thus, 15 mL/kg of fresh frozen plasma (3 to 4 U for the average-size adult) is administered while the patient's filling pressures (central venous and pulmonary artery diastolic or wedge pressure) are monitored to avoid fluid overload. If the PT is prolonged but the patient is not bleeding, plasma transfusion is not indicated, and the patient is closely observed.

Fibrinogen is necessary for clot formation, but hypofibrinogenemia is not a frequent contributor to postoperative bleeding. Although reductions in fibrinogen levels occur following CPB, a significant deficiency is not present unless the level falls below 70 mg/dL. Causes of hypofibrinogenemia in postoperative patients include consumptive coagulopathy, major hemorrhage, fibrinolytic therapy, excessive fibrinolysis, and uncommon hereditary disorders. If the patient is bleeding and a low fibrinogen level is confirmed, treatment with cryoprecipitate is indicated. In general, however, hypofibrinogenemia is an uncommon cause of postoperative bleeding and usually occurs in conjunction with other indicators of an ongoing coagulopathy. If the patient is not bleeding significantly, transfusion of cryoprecipitate is not indicated.

Heparin

In order to prevent thrombosis within the CPB circuit during surgery, large doses of heparin are administered to the patient. Heparin, a negatively charged polysaccharide, catalyzes the naturally occurring coagulation inhibitor antithrombin III, and its action is dependent upon adequate antithrombin III levels (42,43). Heparin sensitivity is variable among individuals and is lower in pediatric patients. At the end of the CPB period, heparin is reversed by the administration of protamine. Protamine, a positively charged polypeptide, binds with heparin, removing it from antithrombin III, and the ability of the blood to coagulate is restored. During CPB, the adequacy of heparinization is most commonly measured by the activated clotting time (ACT). Quantification of the heparin concentration based on protamine neutralization may also be used, but should be employed in conjunction with a test of the heparin effect such as the ACT. The ACT test tubes utilize an activator (either celite or kaolin) to cause coagulation of the blood placed into the tube. Duration of the clotting time is a measure of the heparin effect. Various protocols for maintenance of adequate intraoperative anticoagulation are utilized (44). After completion of bypass and the administration of protamine, the reappearance of circulating heparin in the blood with resultant bleeding (so-called "heparin rebound") has been described (41). This is attributed to the return of administered heparin from the extravascular to the intravascular space and to the shorter half-life of protamine as compared with heparin. The incidence of heparin rebound and its contribution to postoperative bleeding are uncertain. In any event, incomplete reversal of heparin by protamine is suggested by a prolongation of the ACT or the aPTT, although these tests are not specific for heparin. Determination of the thrombin time using blood drawn directly from the patient's vein (to avoid contamination by heparin flush solution) will confirm the presence or absence of residual heparin. Treatment of demonstrated residual heparin effect is by the administration of protamine, which should be given slowly to avoid hypotension. The empiric administration of protamine to the patient with normalized ACT and/or aPTT is not advised; protamine excess can result in greater perioperative blood losses (41).

Low molecular weight heparin (LMWH) preparations, derived by depolymerization of unfractionated heparin, are effective for the treatment of acute coronary syndromes and deep venous thrombosis. Due to ease of administration by subcutaneous injection and the lack of need for laboratory monitoring, LMWH is frequently used in heart disease patients. Occasionally, surgeons are called upon to operate on patients who have recently received LMWH, and the presence of recently administered LMWH is associated with increased postoperative bleeding and transfusions (45,46).

LMWH activity, in contrast to that of unfractionated heparin, is not accurately measurable by tests such as the ACT or aPTT and is not effectively reversed by protamine (47). We therefore suggest that patients who are scheduled to undergo cardiac surgery that are being treated with LMWH be switched over to continuous unfractionated heparin infusions 24 hours prior to the surgical procedure to allow time for the LMWH activity to wear off.

Fibrinolysis

The tissue trauma of surgery, particularly in conjunction with the use of extracorporeal circulation, causes increased release of tissue plasminogen activator, with a resultant increase in the breakdown of fibrin, namely, the process of fibrinolysis. Fibrinolysis occurs to some degree in all patients after cardiac surgery, probably to a greater degree in those who underwent procedures using CPB and likely more in those with cyanotic heart disease. Excessive fibrinolysis is associated with increased postoperative bleeding, and drugs that inhibit fibrinolysis are administered to reduce bleeding. Laboratory studies suggestive of fibrinolysis include a shortened euglobulin clot lysis time, decreased fibrinogen level, and elevated levels of D-dimers and fibrinogen degradation products. A positive D-dimer result is indicative of fibrinolysis although not necessarily to a pathologic extent. Elevation of both the D-dimers and the fibrinogen degradation products may indicate the presence of disseminated intravascular coagulation (41). The relative contribution of fibrinolysis to postoperative bleeding is unclear, although drugs with antifibrinolytic activity (aprotinin, aminocaproic acid, and tranexamic acid) are associated with reduced postoperative bleeding when administered during cardiac surgery (see Chapter 3). Aprotinin is the most extensively studied and effective of the currently available drugs that have antifibrinolytic action (48–50).

Disseminated Intravascular Coagulation

Serious consumption coagulopathy (or disseminated intravascular coagulation) is an unlikely cause of early postoperative bleeding. Decreases in fibrinogen and plasminogen levels occur with open-heart surgery, but these return to normal after 12 to 24 hours. Sufficient plasma levels of fibrinogen are, however, required for normal hemostasis. Hemodilution and prolonged bypass time (with subclinical consumption of fibrinogen occurring in the oxygenator) may lead to insufficient levels of plasma fibrinogen in the absence of pathologic consumption, and administration of cryoprecipitate may be indicated.

MANAGEMENT OF THE BLEEDING PATIENT

When excessive bleeding is present, replacement of the blood loss at a rate sufficient to maintain the patient's red cell volume and intravascular volume at desired levels is required. Although blood conservation and avoidance of blood product transfusion are important, overzealous application of these principles may result in dangerous anemia or hypovolemia, particularly if the rate of blood loss suddenly increases. Whereas lower hematocrit levels may be acceptable for the nonbleeding patient, if the patient is bleeding excessively, it is wise to provide a margin of safety and transfuse blood so as to maintain the hematocrit in the 23% to 26% range. Control of hypertension, if present, will help reduce the rate of bleeding. For this purpose, an intravenous infusion of a short-acting agent such as nitroglycerin, nitroprusside, or esmolol is administered (Chapter 3).

Massive bleeding mandates prompt reoperation. There are no definite criteria to assist in the recognition of patients with surgically correctable causes of excessive mediastinal bleeding. Surgical bleeding is, however, more likely to be present if the patient has high mediastinal tube output with relatively normal coagulation test parameters or if the patient, who was not bleeding initially, develops sudden excessive output. If the patient is sufficiently stable for transport, reentry may be performed in the operating room. This is preferable, as recannulation and CPB support may be required to correct a difficult-to-reach bleeding site. If the patient is very unstable, however, reexploration may be performed in the intensive care unit. It is important for every cardiac surgical intensive care unit to have a sterile set of instruments (including wire cutters and sternal retractor) and a good light source ready at all times for this purpose. Often, the bleeding site can be repaired in the intensive care unit. If not, it is usually possible to control the bleeding with digital pressure and transfuse the patient until he or she is sufficiently stable for transfer to the operating room for definitive repair. Open resuscitation in the intensive care unit results in surprisingly few infections if sterile technique is used and antibiotics are administered (51).

When the rate of bleeding is excessive but not massive, the decision whether to reoperate may be a difficult one. The approach to this situation is to correct the hemostatic abnormalities as best as possible and, if bleeding continues, then proceed with exploration. A useful algorithm for the management of the bleeding patient is shown in Fig. 5-1.

Examination of the patient may provide clues to the nature of the patient's bleeding. Diffuse oozing from the skin incision and intravenous catheter sites suggests a platelet abnormality, failure of blood within the mediastinal tubes to clot suggests a platelet or coagulation factor abnormality or both, and the presence of clotted blood in the patient's tubes suggests relatively normal hemostatic function and the presence of surgical bleeding.

Laboratory studies regarding the patient's clotting status are essential. When the patient is bleeding excessively, the following studies should be drawn, preferably by a new venipuncture: platelet count, PT, aPTT, and fibrinogen level.

Platelet dysfunction is the most common cause of microvascular (nonsurgical) postoperative bleeding following CPB, particularly in patients who have been treated with platelet inhibitors prior to surgery. Therefore, for the actively bleeding patient, transfusion of platelets is indicated, even if the platelet count has not been determined or if it is in the relatively normal range. Although the patient's platelet count may be relatively normal, the platelets may be dysfunctional and not provide for adequate clot formation. At our institutions, for patients requiring platelet transfusions, apheresis platelet units are used; these provide the approximate platelet volume of six random donors but are obtained from a single volunteer, thus limiting the exposure to the recipient. Children

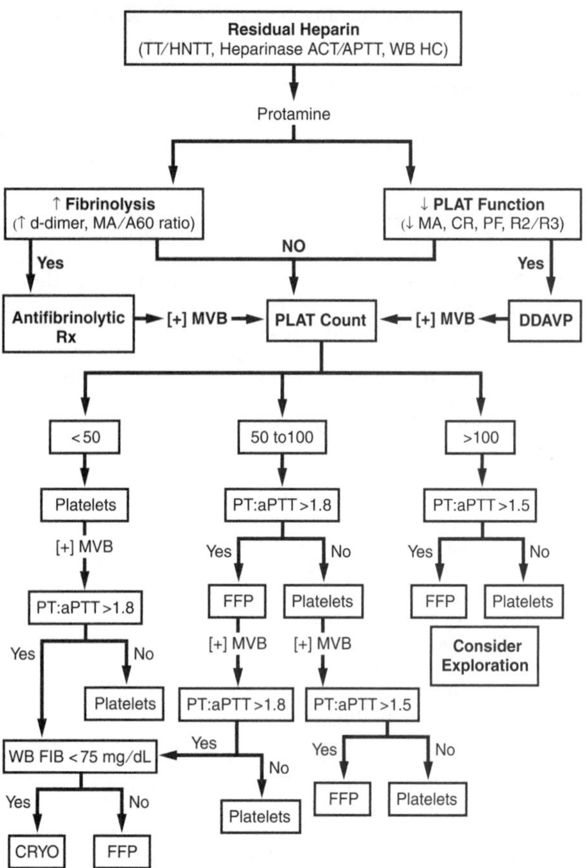

Fig. 5-1. Treatment algorithm for patients with excessive post–cardiopulmonary bypass microvascular bleeding. TT/HNTT, whole-blood thrombin time/heparin-neutralized thrombin time test (Hemochron); heparinase ACT, heparinase kaolin-activated clotting time test (ACT); heparinase aPTT, heparinase-activated partial thromboplastin time test (CoaguCheck Plus); WB HC, whole-blood heparin concentration cartridge (Hepcon instrument); D-dimers, whole-blood D-dimer assay (SimpleRED test); MA, maximum amplitude (thromboelastograph); MA/A60 ratio, maximum amplitude/amplitude at 60 minutes (thromboelastograph); CR, clot ratio values (hemoSTATUS cartridge; Hepcon); PF, platelet force measurements (Hemodyne); R2/R3, R2 and R3 slope values (Sonoclot); WB FIB, whole-blood fibrinogen test (Hemochron); platelets, platelet transfusion (6 U of random donor or apheresis unit equivalent); DDAVP, desmopressin acetate; antifibrinolytic Rx, antifibrinolytic therapy (e.g., ϵ-aminocaproic acid, tranexamic acid, aprotinin); FFP, plasma therapy (2 U of fresh frozen plasma); (+) MVB, continued microvascular bleeding; PT:aPTT, prothrombin time and activated partial thromboplastin time control values (values/mean values from a normal reference population); PLAT Count, platelet count (1,000/µL). (From Despotis GJ, Levine V, Saleem R, et al. DDAVP reduces blood loss and transfusion in cardiac surgical patients with impaired platelet function identified using a point-of-care test: a double-blind, placebo-controlled trial. *Lancet* 1999;354:106–110, with permission).

receive 5 to 10 mL/kg of platelet concentrate, whereas adults receive 1 apheresis platelet unit (equal in volume to about 6 random donor platelet units).

After transfusion, the platelet count should be repeated. If bleeding continues and the count is <75,000/mm^3, a repeat platelet transfusion should be performed.

If the patient's PT is >17 to 18 seconds (or 1.5 times the laboratory control), then a plasma clotting factor deficiency is likely present and treatment with fresh frozen plasma (2 to 3 U for an adult, or 15 mL/kg) is indicated. Plasma is not indicated for a PT of <16 seconds, and other causes for the ongoing bleeding should be sought. If the PT is abnormal but the patient is not bleeding, plasma is not indicated.

For the bleeding patient, if the PT is normal but the aPTT is significantly prolonged (1.5 times control value), consideration should be given to the possibility of a continued heparin effect and to the administration of more protamine. The presence of unneutralized heparin may also be confirmed by use of the ACT, thrombin time, or heparin concentration measurement (Hepcon). Treatment is the administration of more protamine (usually 25 to 50 mg, slowly, for an adult). It should be noted that the aPTT is prolonged by the presence of aprotinin, and this prolongation does not necessarily indicate the presence of coagulopathy or heparin effect. If the patient is not bleeding, transfusion of plasma or cryoprecipitate is not necessary, despite a longer-than-normal aPTT.

If the patient is bleeding and the fibrinogen level is <100 mg/dL, transfusion of cryoprecipitate is indicated. Each unit of cryoprecipitate contains about 250 mg of fibrinogen, and this will raise the adult plasma fibrinogen level by about 10 mg/dL. The usual adult dose is 10 U. The pediatric dose is 1 U of cryoprecipitate/5 kg of body weight.

Excessive postoperative bleeding results in the need for red cell transfusion, sometimes in large volumes. This can be reduced by the use of autotransfusion blood collection systems, but this blood is devoid of platelets and plasma coagulation factors, and if the bleeding persists, plasma and/or cryoprecipitate may be required as indicated by the appropriate laboratory studies.

Cardiac Tamponade

The most serious acute result of excessive postoperative mediastinal bleeding is the development of cardiac tamponade, which is a potentially fatal complication that may develop slowly or rapidly and may be difficult to diagnose (52). Often, this develops in the patient who initially has rapid bleeding, which then suddenly slows as coagulation defects have been corrected. Blood within the chest tubes begins to clot, and the tubes no longer drain well; blood collects within the mediastinum, putting pressure on the heart, resulting in tamponade. The classic physical examination signs of tamponade (muffled heart sounds, jugular venous distention, Kussmaul's sign, and pulsus paradoxus) may be difficult to discern or may be absent in the intubated patient in the noisy intensive care unit environment. Hypotension, narrowed pulse pressure, tachycardia, low mixed venous oxygen saturation, and elevated venous pressures are nonspecific and may be present as the result of either tamponade or ventricular dysfunction. Hemodynamic measurements will demonstrate elevation of the central venous pressure to the level of the left heart filling pressure (left atrial, pulmonary artery capillary wedge, or pulmonary artery diastolic pressure), referred to as "equalization of filling pressures." In many patients, the chest radiograph may reveal a widened mediastinal shadow, although this is also common in postoperative patients without tamponade.

Echocardiography is a generally accurate method to determine the presence of cardiac tamponade. The finding of compression (diastolic collapse) of the right atrium is a sign of increased intrapericardial pressure, although diastolic collapse of the right ventricle is more specific for tamponade (53). Occasional patients, especially with regional tamponade with a loculated blood collection located posterior or lateral to the heart, may not be easily diagnosed by transthoracic echocardiography. In this instance, transesophageal echocardiography is superior to transthoracic echocardiography for making the diagnosis.

Even if echocardiography does not demonstrate tamponade, a high index of suspicion still must be maintained; immediate decompression may be lifesaving for the patient who has acutely decompensated for uncertain reasons. Frequently, if urgent decompression is needed, it may be accomplished by opening the inferior portion of the patient's wound and introducing a gloved finger into the mediastinal space. If the diagnosis of tamponade is correct, the surgeon (and patient) will be rewarded by an outpouring of bloody fluid and rapid improvement in the patient's hemodynamic status. If this does not produce relief, the surgeon should proceed with sternotomy in the intensive care unit; this may be accomplished with considerable success (51). Patients with tamponade who are stable may be transferred to the operating room for a reentry sternotomy and clot removal, generally with minimal complications and little or no increase in the length of hospital stay. *The greatest danger is that cardiac tamponade may go unrecognized and untreated.* Thus, a high level of suspicion should be maintained, and there should be little hesitancy to reexplore the patient who may be suffering postoperative tamponade.

Tamponade may also develop later in the patient's postoperative course, even after discharge from the hospital (54,55). In this setting, the presentation is usually not obvious, and the patient may appear to be suffering from congestive heart failure or myocardial insufficiency. Frequently, patients with delayed cardiac tamponade have been treated with warfarin. General malaise, lack of appetite, exertional dyspnea, and rising creatinine levels are clues to the diagnosis; echocardiography will confirm or rule out the condition. Treatment is drainage, either by percutaneous catheter placed by echocardiographic guidance or by limited sternotomy and placement of pericardial tubes (56).

RENAL FAILURE

Postoperative renal insufficiency of some degree develops in 5% to 10% of patients undergoing cardiac surgery, with approximately 1% requiring postoperative dialysis (57–59). Preoperative factors associated with postoperative renal failure are those associated with poor cardiac performance (such as cardiomegaly), advanced atherosclerotic disease (such as prior heart surgery), recent administration of intravenous contrast agent, reduced baseline kidney function (elevated creatinine level), and advanced age (56,58). In general, valve procedures have a higher rate of this complication. Intraoperative variables associated with postoperative renal failure include the length of time on CPB and the insertion of an intraaortic balloon pump (58). The use of aprotinin during coronary bypass surgery may occasionally be associated with a mild, reversible increase in the postoperative serum creatinine level but not with an increased incidence of serious renal toxicity or the need for postoperative dialysis (60,61). Performance of CABG on the beating heart, not using CPB ("off pump"), may result in less postoperative renal impairment as compared with that from conventional "on-pump" procedures (62).

Renal failure after cardiac surgery is usually secondary to acute tubular necrosis as the result of impaired kidney perfusion, with drug toxicity and cholesterol emboli being other potential causes. Acute tubular necrosis is a reversible process, although proper management is required to prevent secondary complications (hyperkalemia, fluid overload, and uremia) until renal function returns.

In the early postoperative period, the presence of renal insufficiency should be suspected in the patient with reduced urinary output (<0.5 mL/kg per hour for 2 to 3 consecutive hours) and rising creatinine levels. To be sure that the patient's bladder catheter is not obstructed, it is irrigated with a small of volume of sterile saline (30 to 60 mL for adults). Renal ultrasound is performed to exclude ureteral obstruction and evaluate kidney size. (Small kidneys suggest chronic renal insufficiency.) Any medications that may contribute to renal insufficiency, including nonsteroidal antiinflammatory drugs (such as ketorolac and ibuprofen) or angiotensin-converting enzyme inhibitors (such as lisinopril and captopril), should be discontinued.

Next, it must be ensured that the patient has adequate intravascular volume and cardiac output as hypovolemia and low cardiac output will further contribute to kidney injury. If filling pressures are low or normal (central venous or pulmonary capillary wedge pressure <15 to 18 mm Hg), a fluid challenge should be given. If the hematocrit is low (<23% to 26%), the red blood cell volume should be increased with packed red blood cell transfusion. Otherwise, a bolus infusion of 500 to 1,000 mL of crystalloid solution or 5% albumin may be administered over 30 to 60 minutes (10 mL/kg for pediatric patients).

If there is little or no response to the fluid challenge, a large dose of furosemide (100 to 200 mg i.v. for adults, 2 to 4 mg/kg i.v. for infants) with or without a concomitant dose of chlorothiazide (0.5 to 1.0 g i.v.) is sometimes successful in initiating urine flow. Alternatively, a continuous infusion of furosemide may be effective in maintaining satisfactory urine output in the patient who has sufficient preload (63,64). For infants, the continuous furosemide dose is 0.1 to 0.4 mg/kg per hour; the adult dose is 5 to 40 mg per hour. Low-dose dopamine (2 to 3 mg/kg per minute i.v.) has been used to improve urine flow, although the evidence for this practice is not conclusive, and side effects such as tachyarrhythmias and pulmonary shunting may occur. Therefore, the routine use of dopamine to treat acute renal failure is no longer recommended (65–69).

Despite these measures, oliguric renal failure may develop, and even very high doses of diuretics will not be effective in maintaining urine output. Should this occur, efforts are directed to preventing complications of the oliguric state. Fluid intake should be limited to daily output plus about 500 mL in adults. Frequent physical examination will help to follow the state of hydration of the patient. Potassium should not be administered unless the serum level falls below 3.5 mEq/L. Even then, replacement should be done cautiously, in small amounts, and frequent determinations of the serum potassium level are required to recognize hyperkalemia early. Magnesium-containing antacids should be discontinued and replaced with aluminum or calcium antacids to prevent hypermagnesemia and to decrease intestinal absorption of phosphate. Patients on drugs eliminated by renal excretion must be monitored carefully, and dosages should be changed as indicated. Examples would include cimetidine and cefazolin. Aspirin should be discontinued. Serum levels of aminoglycoside antibiotics, digoxin, antiarrhythmic agents, and other drugs should be followed closely, and doses should be decreased as indicated. Consultation with the hospital-based pharmacist is of considerable value in this situation.

For most oliguric patients, intervention will be required at some point to treat hyperkalemia, acidemia, fluid overload, or complications of uremia such as lethargy and pericarditis. Peritoneal dialysis can be performed conveniently at the bedside and is particularly useful for infants with renal failure (70). Conventional hemodialysis may not be well tolerated by patients with recent cardiac surgery because of the possibility of hypotension and cardiovascular collapse. For adult patients, continuous renal replacement (venovenous hemofiltration) therapies have proven to be very successful for the management of acute renal failure (71). In this technique, gradual filtration of the blood is accomplished at a rate slower than hemodialysis, and filtrate removal is by hydrostatic pressure. Solutes (such as potassium, urea, and creatinine) accompany the fluid, and the removed fluid is replaced with physiologic (potassium-free) solution as needed. Larger molecules such as heparin, insulin, and vancomycin are also removed by hemofiltration. Up to 500 mL per hour of fluid may be removed. Continuous renal replacement therapies allow for better control of fluid and metabolic parameters, particularly in hemodynamically unstable patients. Venovenous hemofiltration employs a pump to remove venous blood (from a femoral or subclavian vein), does not rely on arterial pressure, provides good control of the blood flow and filtration rate, and has become the technique of choice in most intensive care units.

Nonoliguric renal failure after cardiac surgery is generally much easier to manage. When the patient urinates in satisfactory or even excessive amounts, it is important to accurately monitor urine output, daily weight, and serum electrolyte concentrations. Replacement should be provided as indicated to prevent hypovolemia and electrolyte abnormalities, usually by matching the urine output with administration of 0.5 N-normal saline.

Acute renal failure requiring dialysis after cardiac surgery is a complication associated with high mortality, but most of the patients who die also suffer complications of other organ systems. Contemporary management, however, is improving the prognosis of patients with this postoperative complication (72,73).

INFECTIOUS COMPLICATIONS

Although less common in pediatric patients, serious infectious problems complicate cardiac operations in a significant proportion of adult patients. Pneumonia and wound infections are the most common sites. Infectious complications of cardiac surgery can lead to considerable morbidity, increased length of hospital stay, increased hospitalization cost, and greater risk of death (74,75).

Pneumonia

Postoperative pneumonia occurs in 1% to 5% of cardiac surgery patients. The frequent cause is aspiration of contaminated oropharyngeal secretions, with gram-positive bacteria being the most common organism (76). Postoperative pneumonia is associated with preoperative smoking and chronic obstructive pulmonary disease, the need for reintubation or mechanical ventilation for >48 hours, the transfusion of >4 U of blood, the presence of a nasogastric tube, and prolonged intensive care unit stay (77,78). The diagnosis of pneumonia is based on the presence of fever, elevated white blood count, the development of an infiltrate on chest x-ray film, and a sputum culture that grows a predominant organism. Prolonged prophylactic antibiotic treatment does not provide protection from pneumonia, and the suspicion of the presence of pneumonia should be confirmed by microbiological examinations of the sputum. For patients with hospital-acquired pneumonia, initial treatment with an aminoglycoside such as gentamicin plus cefotaxime, ceftriaxone, or imipenem is a reasonable first choice pending results of culture, antibiotic susceptibility testing, and clinical response (79). Treatment of confirmed pneumonia is by administration of specific antibiotics, aggressive pulmonary toilet, and ventilator support as required.

Wound Infections and Mediastinitis

Wound infections after a sternotomy incision may be superficial, involving only the skin and subcutaneous fat, or they may be deep, involving the sternum and underlying mediastinal structures. They are clearly an important contributor to postoperative morbidity and mortality in patients undergoing cardiac surgery (80).

Superficial infections are characterized by drainage from the wound and local inflammation while the underlying sternum remains stable. In this instance, removal of the overlying skin sutures, culture of the drainage, administration of antibiotics, and local dressings are often successful treatment.

Bacterial mediastinitis occurs in about 1.25% of patients undergoing open-heart surgery and is associated with increased short- and long-term mortality rates (81,82). In our experience, the incidence in children is lower. The reported incidence in heart transplantation patients is, however, higher (83). In various published reports, the risk factors identified for the development of serious postoperative sternal wound complications include obesity, presence of emphysema, repeat operations, prolonged operative time, early chest reexploration for postoperative bleeding, need for blood transfusion of >5 U, prolonged postoperative mechanical ventilation, and prolonged postoperative low cardiac output (84,85). The use of both the left and the right mammary (internal thoracic) arteries for coronary bypass conduits is associated with an increased incidence of sternal wound complications, particularly in diabetic patients (86,87). The decision to use bilateral internal mammary arteries must therefore weigh both the benefit of increased long-term graft patency and the potential risk of sternal wound problems. Such decisions are individualized based on the age of the patient and the presence of other medical problems.

Patients with tracheostomies are at increased risk for sternal incision infections because of the close proximity of the incision to the tracheal stoma, which is colonized by bacteria. If the tracheostomy is present before the sternotomy, all efforts should be made to isolate the stoma from the incision during the procedure and to avoid connecting the mediastinal dissection with the plane of the pretracheal fascia. If the tracheostomy is required postoperatively, the skin incision should be placed as high as possible, taking care to limit the dissection so that it does not communicate with the previous substernal dissection. The sternal wound should be protected from the tracheostomy by dressings. Despite such precautions, patients who require tracheostomy after cardiac operation have a higher incidence of mediastinitis and mortality than those who do not require tracheostomy (88). The use of electric clippers to remove chest hair, rather than manual shaving, is associated with a lower incidence of mediastinitis and is standard at our hospitals (89).

Prophylactic antibiotic administration is associated with decreased incidences of infection in cardiac surgery patients (90,91). The most common organism associated with sternal wound infections is *Staphylococcus,* with coagulase-negative *Staphylococcus* having a high incidence of methicillin resistance representing a significant proportion (92). The prophylactic antibiotic of choice is cefazolin or cefuroxime, with vancomycin being used at institutions where methicillin-resistant *Staphylococcus* is an important pathogen (93). Vancomycin should not, however, be used routinely as it promotes the emergence of vancomycin-resistant organisms (94). The intravenous antibiotic infusion is begun in the operating room during preparations for surgery but before making the incision. The adult cefazolin dose is 1 to 2 g, and the pediatric dose is 15.0 mg/kg of body weight. Often, a second 1-g cefazolin dose (for adults) is given to the patient after weaning from CPB. Postoperatively, the patient receives the same dose of cefazolin every 8 hours for 24 to 48 hours. Patients who are allergic to cefazolin and those with serious penicillin allergies (due to the real but low incidence of cross-reactivity) receive vancomycin instead of cephalosporin.

Generally, diabetes mellitus is associated with an increased incidence of infection (95). For diabetic patients, careful intra- and postoperative control of the blood glucose level using continuous intravenous insulin infusion appears to reduce the incidence of deep sternal wound infection, and this technique is used routinely by our groups (96).

The early diagnosis of sternal infection and mediastinitis after cardiac surgery can be difficult. Many infections are not evident until after the patient has been discharged from the hospital. In particular, infections due to coagulase-negative staphylococci may be difficult to recognize as they often present late and have less apparent signs and symptoms (97). The standard chest radiograph is of little value in predicting infection or sternal dehiscence. A vertical sternal lucency (the so-called "sternal stripe") is frequently seen on early postoperative chest x-ray film, but is not a sensitive indicator of infection or dehiscence in the absence of other findings. In some patients, fever, leukocytosis, and a positive blood culture will be the first manifestations of a hidden infection that only later becomes obvious. The most common early sign is fluid drainage from the wound; sternal instability usually develops subsequently. Sterile sternal dehiscence with instability but no drainage sometimes occurs, requiring rewiring, but this is not an infectious complication. In some patients, the diagnosis of sternal infection and mediastinitis may not be clear-cut, and in this situation, chest CT may be of value (98). If infection is present, there is often a mediastinal soft tissue mass with bilateral pleural effusions, excessive mediastinal fluid with air-fluid levels, bone destruction, and separation of the sternum. Needle aspiration of the mediastinum under CT scan guidance for gram stain and culture of the fluid obtained may also be performed to aid in the diagnosis of mediastinitis.

Treatment of serious sternotomy wound infections depends on the stage of the process at the time of diagnosis (75,99). If early, when the sternum is not destroyed, success may be achieved by prompt reoperation, debridement of the sternal edges, copious irrigation of the mediastinum, placement of retrosternal irrigation and drainage catheters, rewiring of the sternum, and closure of the fascia and skin. Appropriate intravenous antibiotics are administered for at least 7 days. A dilute antibiotic solution, chosen according to gram stain results, is infused slowly through the irrigating catheters, with the fluid exiting via the drainage catheters. The irrigations are continued until the drainage fluid is sterile by culture (usually 3 to 5 days). Although frequently successful, this method has potential serious complications such as erosion of the catheters into mediastinal structures and systemic toxicity from absorption of the irrigating antibiotic. For these reasons, this technique is usually reserved for particular patients and is not commonly used in our practices (100).

Our most frequent approach to treating serious mediastinitis is a single-stage procedure in which radical debridement of the sternum and cartilage is performed with advancement of muscle flaps, using the pectoralis major and/or rectus muscles. Depending on the degree of sternal resection required, the remaining bone may or may not be reapproximated. Soft Silastic drains are placed beneath the muscle flaps and laced to gentle suction. This technique, often performed in conjunction with a plastic surgeon, is associated with low mortality and morbidity and reduces the length of hospital stay as the patient may be discharged with the drains in place, with planned removal in the office when the daily drainage volume becomes sufficiently small. Our experience with the early aggressive use of muscle flap closure of the seriously infected mediastinum has been excellent, and considerable success, both in adults and in children, has been reported in the literature (101–105).

More long-standing, advanced infections are associated with large amounts of suppurative fluid in the mediastinum, loss of integrity of the sternum, and diffuse cellulitis of the skin and subcutaneous tissues. These patients may require opening the sternum, exposing and draining the mediastinum, and packing the wound with moist gauze, which is changed at frequent intervals. After control of the infection and formation of a healthy-appearing bed of granulation tissue, secondary closure with or without muscle flap advancement is performed. This method, however, requires a very extended hospitalization and risks hemorrhage from the heart (usually the right ventricle) or other mediastinal structures secondary to the dressing changes (106).

In all instances, attention to the patient's nutritional state is of prime importance. Consultation with the hospital-based dietitian, daily calorie counts, and vitamin supplementation are necessary for patients with wound infection. If oral intake is insufficient, early tube or parenteral feeding should be administered to avoid malnutrition and to augment healing.

Infections at the site of saphenous vein harvest site are not rare and are more likely to occur in obese patients. Drainage of noninfected serosanguinous fluid from leg incisions is common, and application of dry dressings and leg elevation usually results in resolution. Often, this drainage is the result of an underlying hematoma that has liquefied, and the fluid drains out the neighboring skin incision. True infections are manifested by erythema, induration, and undue tenderness to palpation. If underlying fluctuance is present, incision and drainage, followed by open packing and secondary healing, in addition to treatment with appropriate antibiotics are indicated. Major infections can lead to the need for skin grafts, vascular procedures, and even amputations (107).

Catheter Sepsis

Most frequently, central venous catheters for monitoring and fluid administration purposes are placed in the patient's internal jugular vein. The rate of infection for this access site is low, whereas use of the femoral and/or the subclavian vein is associated with a higher rate of infectious complications (108). Infection of an intravenous catheter can lead to fever, bacteremia, toxicity, shock, endocarditis, and bacterial seeding of the patient's fresh sternotomy incision. Patients who have been hospitalized for a period of time before surgery or who have been transferred from an outside institution should be closely inspected to rule out the presence of phlebitis. Catheters or sheaths placed via the groin into the femoral artery or vein at the time of cardiac catheterization should be removed preoperatively if other access sites are possible, the patient is not heparinized, and surgery will not be performed for 12 to 24 hours. If surgery is imminent, we remove these groin cannulas postoperatively as soon as hemostatic function has returned, usually within 12 to 24 hours. In particular, femoral vein catheters are associated with an increased incidence of venous thrombosis and infection (109). If an infected peripheral intravenous catheter site is found preoperatively and the patient is stable, it is best to postpone the surgery and treat the patient with antibiotics (and vein excision, if required) for several days. Sterile technique is mandatory when monitoring and access catheters are placed by the anesthesiologist or surgeon in the operating room.

When a postoperative patient develops a fever early after surgery, atelectasis is the most likely cause. Catheter infection, however, can also occur very early after surgery, and this must be kept in mind as it can lead to severe sepsis. Infected central lines are usually not associated with redness or drainage at the insertion site. Thus, if the fever persists, blood cultures should be drawn, the catheter should be removed, and its tip should be cultured. In general, if central venous access is still needed for the care of the patient, this should be achieved through a new site rather than by exchanging the suspect catheter with a new one over a guidewire.

GASTROINTESTINAL COMPLICATIONS

Gastrointestinal (GI) complications occur in about 2% of patients who undergo cardiac surgery. They are often insidious in onset, difficult to diagnose, and severe in their consequences. The most likely cause of these complications is visceral hypoperfusion during or in the early postoperative period following cardiac surgery (110). Risk factors for postoperative GI complications include older age, peripheral vascular disease, congestive heart failure, triple-vessel coronary disease, long periods of CPB, blood transfusions, use of an intraaortic balloon pump, vasopressor support, and reexploration for postoperative bleeding (111,112). Severe digestive tract complications are more common following cardiac transplantation and acute aortic dissection procedures as compared with coronary or valve operations and are more common after combined or valve operations as compared with isolated coronary procedures (113). Overall, the serious GI complications have a high mortality rate, up to 50%. Clinical manifestations of these problems may be subtle in the patient who has recently undergone open-heart surgery, and a high index of suspicion is required to make the diagnosis. The most common complications encountered are ileus, bleeding, intestinal ischemia, cholecystitis, pancreatitis, and colonic pseudoobstruction.

Intestinal Ileus

Failure of the intestinal contents to progress normally is not uncommon following major surgery and narcotic administration. To some degree, intestinal ileus is present in all patients following cardiac surgery, but when prolonged, it will lengthen the time of hospital stay and may lead to the need for parenteral alimentation. Severe ileus occurs in <1% of patients. Clinically, the patient may be nauseated, but severe abdominal pain is absent. The abdomen is usually distended and bowel sounds absent. Signs of peritoneal irritation are not generally present. An abdominal radiograph reveals mildly dilated bowel loops but without signs of bowel obstruction such as severe dilatation of the proximal small bowel and absence of air in the colon and rectum. Treatment of paralytic ileus is conservative, with avoidance of narcotics as much as possible, placement of a nasogastric suction tube, and support with intravenous fluids and calories as indicated. A trial of metoclopramide (10 mg i.v. every 6 to 8 hours) may be of value, especially in diabetic patients. The patient should be followed closely as differentiation between ileus and bowel obstruction may sometimes be difficult. With time, resolution of ileus occurs.

Gastrointestinal Tract Bleeding

Significant GI tract bleeding occurs in 0.5% to 1% of cardiac surgery patients, most commonly adults. Despite the seriousness of this problem when it does occur, for routine patients with no known predisposition to GI bleeding, prophylactic drug treatment may not be warranted (114,115). For patients with known duodenal or gastric ulcer disease, continuation of their usual treatment up until the time of surgery with early resumption after surgery should be performed. Critically ill patients do benefit from stress ulcer prophylaxis (116). Cardiac surgery patients who develop severe postoperative complications (such as cardiogenic shock, respiratory failure, sepsis, and/or renal failure) are at increased risk of stress-related mucosal damage and are therefore candidates for prophylactic therapy. For this situation, antisecretory therapy with a histamine-2 blocker such as famotidine or a proton pump inhibitor such as pantoprazole is indicated. Our current favored regimen for the prophylactic treatment of stress-related mucosal damage is famotidine, which may be given by mouth as a tablet, by nasogastric tube as a suspension, or by intravenous infusion.

GI bleeding will be manifest by the appearance of blood in the nasogastric tube drainage or by the development of melanotic stools (or both). When a significant amount of bleeding has occurred, the patient may become hypovolemic and hemodynamically unstable. Management involves placement of secure intravenous access, determination of the patient's hematocrit and coagulation status, gastric lavage, and consultation with a gastroenterologist. For the unstable patient, a central venous catheter should be placed for volume and blood administration, and central venous pressure should be measured to guide fluid therapy. Blood should be typed and cross-matched for transfusion as indicated, and other preparations for a possible emergency laparotomy should be made. Endoscopy is performed to determine the source of GI bleeding. In many patients, localized upper GI tract bleeding sites (duodenal or ulcer ulcers) may be treated endoscopically by electrocoagulation or epinephrine injection at the site of the bleeding vessel. Following such treatments, medical treatment is continued, and bleeding recurrence rates are generally low. If rebleeding does occur, then surgical treatment may be indicated.

Medical management is often successful as the treatment of diffuse gastritis and is important in the management of duodenal and gastric ulcer disease. For this purpose, options include oral antacids and antisecretory drugs. A histamine-2 inhibitor such as ranitidine and famotidine or one of the proton pump inhibitor agents such as pantoprazole or omeprazole is frequently used. For this purpose, pantoprazole may be administered as a continuous intravenous infusion (adult dose, 80-mg load followed by 8 mg per hour). For patients with documented *Helicobacter pylori* infection and duodenal ulcer disease, omeprazole (or lansoprazole) is administered in conjunction with antibiotics (often clarithromycin and amoxicillin) for a 2-week course.

If the patient has experienced melena or bloody diarrhea but upper endoscopy is negative, lower GI tract bleeding is present and colonoscopy should be performed. Etiologies include mesenteric ischemia, bleeding from a polyp or diverticulum, or antibiotic-associated colitis secondary to *Clostridium difficile.* Treatment is specific to the cause.

Perforation of a duodenal (or gastric) ulcer is now a rare occurrence after cardiac operations. The patient, if awake, experiences sudden and severe abdominal pain that often radiates to the shoulder. No bowel sounds are heard on examination, and there is rigidity with signs of peritoneal irritation. An upright portable chest or cross-table lateral abdominal radiograph usually shows free air underneath the diaphragm, although this finding is not always present. Management of GI perforation requires gastric tube suction, fluid resuscitation as indicated, and antibiotic coverage. General surgical consultation should be obtained promptly, as surgical closure of the perforation (with or without a definitive peptic ulcer disease procedure) is often required (117).

Intestinal Ischemia

Mesenteric ischemia may be occlusive (due to an embolus) or nonocclusive due to impaired perfusion as may occur during cardiac surgery, especially in patients with mesenteric arterial stenoses or diffuse atherosclerosis. It may also occur after repair of aortic dissections in which successful perfusion of the mesenteric circulation is not achieved. Diagnosis of intestinal ischemia may be difficult, and it may not become evident until several days after surgery. Some patients may have a preoperative history of postprandial abdominal pain, anorexia, and weight loss indicative of chronic mesenteric arterial obstruction. Most often, however, the affected postoperative patient complains of diffuse abdominal pain and may have peritoneal signs on examination. Fluid resuscitation and nasogastric suction should be implemented, and the patient should be frequently examined. If deterioration occurs (increasing pain, tachycardia, fever), laparotomy should be performed to rule out or treat intestinal infarction. In this situation, a preoperative mesenteric arteriogram may be in order. The mortality rate of intestinal ischemia requiring surgical exploration is high. Cholesterol emboli can cause multisystem complications, including renal or GI complications. Although frank bowel ischemia leading to an acute picture can occur, lesser degrees of involvement can produce delayed perforation or late intestinal stenosis.

Acute Cholecystitis

Acute cholecystitis (most frequently acalculous) occurs in <1% of cardiac surgery patients, but is often associated with multiorgan failure and therefore a high mortality rate (118). The patient often complains of right upper quadrant pain, may be febrile, and commonly has leukocytosis. A variable degree of hyperbilirubinemia and abnormal liver enzyme levels may be present. A septic hemodynamic pattern may develop, characterized by hypotension, low vascular resistance, and relatively high cardiac output. Physical examination is often difficult because the patient will frequently guard when palpated because of the nearby sternotomy incision. Abdominal ultrasonography is the first diagnostic test and is very helpful if an enlarged gallbladder with a thickened wall is demonstrated. Hepatobiliary scans are also useful, but they have a significant incidence of false-positive results in patients who have recently undergone major surgery. The diagnosis, however, should be pursued because untreated cholecystitis can result in gangrene of the gallbladder. In some cases, the condition may be treated endoscopically (by papillotomy), but most often cholecystectomy is performed, usually by the laparoscopic approach. In critically ill patients, a percutaneous cholecystostomy tube can palliate this condition. When the patient has recovered, if cholelithiasis and duct obstruction are ruled out by contrast cholecystography, the percutaneously placed tube may be removed 4 to 6 weeks following insertion. Of note is the observation that ongoing bile drainage can cause marked sensitivity to warfarin.

Acute Pancreatitis

Asymptomatic elevation of both the serum pancreatic and the nonpancreatic isoamylase levels occurs in about one-third of patients after CPB (119). It is speculated that the relative hypoperfusion of the pancreas during the period of CPB, calcium administration, high-dose narcotic anesthesia, and vasoconstriction secondary to vasopressors may contribute to pancreatic injury. Clinically evident pancreatitis in the postoperative patient often becomes apparent on the fourth or fifth postoperative day when the patient complains of abdominal pain and nausea, vomiting, or anorexia. An elevated serum amylase level may confirm the diagnosis. Treatment consists of withholding oral feedings and, if an ileus is present, placement of a nasogastric tube for suction drainage of the stomach. Postoperative pancreatitis is usually self-limiting, and most patients are able to restart a clear liquid diet within a few days. Severe hemorrhagic pancreatitis necessitating surgical drainage is very rare.

Acute Hepatic Failure

Acute hepatic failure most often accompanies prolonged low cardiac output in adult patients receiving maximum supportive therapy such as catecholamines, intraaortic balloon pumping, and dialysis. It occurs rarely in children. Along with profound jaundice, hypoglycemia and coagulopathy may develop. Management consists mainly in general measures to support the circulation and provide nutrition and close monitoring of blood chemical constituents. Vitamin K and fresh frozen plasma should be administered if bleeding occurs. The mortality rate of fulminant hepatic failure following open-heart surgery is very high.

Nausea, Dysphagia, and Hiccups

Some degree of postoperative nausea, occasionally with vomiting, is not unusual in cardiac surgery patients, likely the result of reduced GI motility and narcotic administration (120). In most patients, this may be successfully treated with prochlorperazine given by rectal suppository (25 mg) or intramuscular injection (5 to 10 mg) or by intravenous ondansetron (2 to 4 mg). For some patients, metoclopramide is successful in improving GI motility and relieving nausea.

Difficulty swallowing may occur after cardiac operations, especially in older patients in association with neurologic complications, although in some affected patients, no cause for the swallowing difficulty is identified (121). Treatment is maintenance of nutrition with enteral or parenteral feeding, precautions to avoid aspiration, and consultation with a speech/swallowing therapist for modification of eating behavior and swallowing technique. Recovery of swallowing may be protracted, but usually occurs.

Painful swallowing after cardiac surgery is not uncommon. Irritation from previously placed endotracheal and nasogastric tubes may be causative, but in some patients, the odynophagia may be due to overgrowth of *Candida albicans* in the oropharynx or esophagus (122). Simple oropharyngeal *Candida* (thrush) is treated with oral nystatin. All antibiotics are discontinued unless absolutely needed to treat a documented infection. This is nearly always successful. Serious esophageal infections are diagnosed by barium swallow and/or endoscopy and may require intravenous antifungal treatment for control.

Postoperative hiccups are a troublesome problem for some patients. Often thought to be due to diaphragmatic irritation that occurred during the procedure, the cause of hiccups is not really known and may be related to drugs (especially benzodiazepines and corticosteroids), esophageal distension, or gastroesophageal reflux, or it may be of central nervous system origin (123). Suggested treatments are many and varied, although chlorpromazine is the only drug approved for the disorder (124). The starting adult dose is 25 to 50 mg by mouth three or four times per day. The course of treatment should be short as side effects may develop with prolonged treatment.

NEUROLOGIC COMPLICATIONS

Cerebral dysfunction after cardiac surgery is an increasingly common and difficult problem in cardiac surgery as the patient population becomes older and patients have more complicating medical problems and undergo increasingly complex operations. For adults, the incidence of adverse cerebral outcomes may be as high as 6%, with about 2% to 3% suffering severe injuries (focal deficit or coma) and 3% suffering less severe but important derangements (deterioration in intellectual function, memory deficit, or seizures) (125–127). Not surprisingly, postoperative cerebral dysfunction is associated with increases in mortality, length of hospital stay and the need for long-term care facilities.

Commonly recognized clinical risk factors for postoperative neurologic dysfunction are advanced age (older than 70 years), hypertension, diabetes mellitus, smoking, and previous stroke. Other factors associated with postoperative strokes in adults include carotid artery bruit or known obstruction, atherosclerosis of the ascending aorta, poor left ventricular function, peripheral vascular disease, prolonged CPB time, and perioperative myocardial infarction (128–131). Procedures requiring hypothermic circulatory arrest are more likely to be associated with adverse cerebral outcomes, especially for elderly patients (132).

Efforts to prevent neurologic injury in cardiac surgery patients center largely on modifications of intraoperative technique. For CABG procedures, performing the operation without the use of CPB ("off pump") may be associated with less early postoperative cognitive impairment, although the long-term benefit may be limited (133–136). The administration of the serine protease inhibitor aprotinin during coronary bypass surgery is associated with a reduced incidence of stroke (49,137). Avoidance of perioperative cerebral hyperthermia may also help reduce the magnitude of neurologic dysfunction following CPB (138,139). Postoperative atrial fibrillation that persists for >48 hours is associated with an increased incidence of stroke and is an indication for anticoagulation of the affected patient to prevent thromboembolism (140).

Stroke

A perioperative stroke is the result of irreversible ischemic death of brain matter, resulting in a gross neurologic deficit such as hemiparesis. Although often considered a "postoperative" complication, most strokes begin during the operative procedure. It is not until several hours after surgery, when the patient's anesthetic has worn off, that the deficit can be appreciated. Ischemia of the brain may occur secondary to global hypoperfusion due to inadequate blood flow and perfusion pressure during surgery, and this may be exacerbated by the presence of occlusive lesions in the patient's cerebral vessels. More commonly, however, strokes are the result of emboli to the cerebral circulation (141,142). Emboli to the brain during surgery may be composed of atherosclerotic debris, thrombus, fat, or air. Generally recognized risk factors for stroke occurring with CABG include advanced age (over 70 years), previous stroke, hypertension, diabetes, cigarette smoking, and carotid bruit.

Patients with carotid artery occlusive disease have an increased risk of perioperative stroke, and routine carotid artery scanning in older patients is advocated by some authorities (143,144). In our practices, preoperative scanning is performed in patients with bruits or heart murmurs that could mask the auscultation of bruits, patients with previous strokes, and patients with known peripheral vascular disease. Patients in need of coronary bypass surgery who have asymptomatic carotid stenosis usually undergo coronary bypass surgery alone unless critically stenotic carotid disease is present (such as severe bilateral carotid stenoses). For patients with critically stenotic or symptomatic carotid disease, combined carotid endarterectomy and coronary bypass procedure or coronary surgery plus carotid artery stent placement may be indicated (145,146).

Patients with atherosclerosis of the ascending aorta have an increased risk of adverse cerebral outcomes with cardiac surgery. Intraoperative examination by transesophageal echocardiography may be useful in identifying patients at increased risk for embolic stroke by revealing the presence of atherosclerotic plaque in the thoracic aorta (ascending, arch or descending) (147). Ultrasound examination of the ascending aorta using a hand-held (epiaortic) transducer is also a useful technique (148) (see Fig. 2-10). When plaque is found to be present, it is usually possible to modify the locations of aortic cannulation and cross-clamp application so as to avoid the plaque and thereby, it is hoped, reduce the chance of plaque material embolism. In some patients, the degree of calcification present may require significant alterations in the operative plan. For CABG procedures, this could mean performing the grafts with the patient on bypass but without cross-clamping the diseased aorta, the use of arterial grafts only so as to avoid the manipulation associated with sewing vein grafts to the ascending aorta, or avoiding CPB altogether and performing the procedure "off pump" (beating heart technique) (149). For the very severely diseased aorta, replacement may be indicated. In our practices, intraoperative epiaortic ultrasound has been found to be quick and simple to perform and is generally used in patients over 70 years of age.

Small lipid emboli may be associated with cerebral dysfunction following the use of CPB. The source of the fat appears to be from the reinfusion of blood suctioned from the pericardial sac during the procedure, and the microemboli may be detected in the brain as lipid deposits that create small capillary and arteriolar dilatations that are associated with ischemic injury and neuronal dysfunction. Reducing the volume of blood returned directly to the patient through the arterial circuit (through the use of a cell-saving device) may be associated with a lower burden of lipid microembolization (150).

Large thrombus emboli are less common than microemboli. Patients with chronic atrial fibrillation, left atrial enlargement, left ventricular aneurysms, or large recent left ventricular infarctions may have mural thrombi attached to the affected chamber. In these patients, manipulation of the heart during surgery can lead to thrombus embolism and stroke. Thus, patients with left-side intracardiac thrombi identified by preoperative or intraoperative echocardiography are at increased risk for perioperative stroke.

Smaller air emboli can damage the brain; thus, careful de-airing of the heart is required whenever procedures on the left side of the heart are performed. Use of intraoperative transesophageal echocardiography allows the surgeon to visualize air in the heart and to pursue de-airing maneuvers prior to weaning the patient from CPB. Massive air embolism can occur from a variety of intraoperative mishaps. It may be prevented to some degree by bubble sensor devices, arterial line filters, and careful de-airing of the heart before resumption of contractions. If a massive air embolism does occur during CPB, immediate treatment by Trendelenburg positioning of the patient, placement of a stab wound in the ascending aorta for air escape, and retrograde perfusion through the superior vena cava is recommended (151). One form of therapy specific for the treatment of air embolism to the brain is the hyperbaric oxygen chamber. If available, hyperbaric oxygen therapy should be employed without delay after completion of the operation as there is a clear relationship between outcome and treatment delay (152). This form of therapy can result in dramatic reversal of neurologic deficits that have occurred in some patients who have suffered large air emboli.

Symptomatic visual abnormalities occur occasionally after open-heart surgery (153). Potential etiologies include retinal emboli, anterior ischemic optic neuropathy, and occipital lobe infarction (cortical blindness). Embolism and hypoperfusion are causes; severe anemia during the operation and preexisting glaucoma contribute (154).

Treatment of the patient who has suffered a perioperative stroke is largely supportive and expectant. Maintenance of adequate oxygenation, oxygen-carrying capacity, and acid–base status is of prime importance. Metabolic causes of encephalopathy (such as medications, narcotic or alcohol withdrawal, endocrinologic disorders, and renal or hepatic failure) and psychiatric etiologies should be considered and treated as well as possible (155). As soon as it is realized that the patient is definitely not awakening from anesthesia normally or that there is a focal neurologic deficit present, discussion with the family should be undertaken so as to alert them to the presence of the complication. When the patient is sufficiently stable to be transported, a computed tomographic (CT) scan of the head should be obtained. Although CT scans are often normal early in the course of a stroke, the scan will rule out large intracerebral hemorrhages and cerebral edema. With intracerebral hemorrhage ruled out, anticoagulation of the patient may be in order, especially if the stroke is thought to be due to thrombotic embolus. Consultation by a qualified and empathetic neurologist will assist both in management of the patient and in helping to address the questions raised by the naturally concerned family members.

Neurobehavioral Disturbances

Alterations in mental function not associated with focal neurologic deficits are relatively common in patients after open-heart surgery utilizing CPB. Such changes may include various degrees of confusion and disorientation, memory deficits, problem-solving deficits, coordination problems, or even psychosis. Clinically obvious neurobehavioral alterations (encephalopathy) occur in approximately 7% of postoperative patients (156). The recognized incidence of cognitive decline after coronary bypass surgery is higher when standardized preoperative and postoperative testing is performed, although there is considerable variation in the incidence depending on the criteria used to make the diagnosis (157–159). The incidence is higher in older patients and in those who have prolonged periods of CPB. The relationships between procedure type, blood pressure and/or temperature during bypass, number of microemboli, and neurobehavioral outcome are unclear (160). Avoidance of prolonged hypotension during CPB, minimizing manipulation of the atherosclerotic ascending aorta, and avoiding perioperative hyperthermia are recommended (161). Elimination of the use of CPB ("off-pump" surgery) may be associated with a reduction in the incidence of cognitive decline (162).

When postoperative neurobehavioral dysfunction is identified, the treatment is supportive. The patient should be closely observed to prevent self-injury, and the patient's family should be cautiously reassured that the cognitive defect improves with time in most patients. The late outcome of cognitive decline in coronary bypass patients is, however, variable, and persistent changes in certain testing domains may occur (163).

PERIPHERAL NERVE INJURY

Peripheral nerve injuries may occur during open-heart surgery. The most common injuries are to the upper extremity nerve supply, particularly the brachial plexus, although the risk of prolonged symptoms from this complication is well less than 1%. The mechanism of injury to the brachial plexus is not certain but is probably due to traction on the sternal halves, with stretching of the lower nerve roots (C8-T1) (164). The most common form of brachial plexopathy is that of ulnar neuropathy, and this occurs more often in older patients, men, and diabetic individuals (165).

Efforts to prevent these injuries have included opening the sternum only as wide as necessary, positioning the retractor low in the split sternum, use of the hands-up position, and maintenance of neutral head position, although consistent relationships between positioning and the development of brachial plexus injury have not been demonstrated. The usual presentation of this complication is numbness, sometimes with tingling, of the fifth finger and the medial portion of the fourth finger of the involved hand. Nerve conduction studies and electromyelography may be performed, although there is no specific treatment available. Reassurance of the patient is indicated, and for some patients, this is reinforced when it is heard also from a consulting neurologist. The overall prognosis is very good, with resolution of the symptoms in most patients. More than 75% of affected patients become asymptomatic within 4 months.

Saphenous neuropathy is the result of injury to the saphenous nerve, usually in the distal leg, which occurs in association with harvesting of the saphenous vein. It is characterized by anesthesia, hyperesthesia, and pain along the medial side of the calf and foot. Common early after surgery, the symptoms may persist for >18 months in a small proportion of affected patients. Most often, the problem is not serious, resolves without specific treatment, and requires only reassurance of the patient.

Patients who undergo radial artery harvesting for coronary bypass surgery may experience postoperative neurologic deficits involving the hand. In one study, 5% of patients reported decreased thumb strength and 18% described sensation abnormalities (166). In our experience, the incidence is considerably lower. The most common complaint is skin numbness at the base of the thumb. Significant associations between the self-reported neurologic complications and diabetes, peripheral vascular disease, elevated creatinine levels, and smoking were demonstrated. The majority of patients with hand neurologic abnormalities following radial artery removal recover within months after the operation.

Another interesting, but rare, peripheral nerve complication may occur in patients who undergo cardiac surgery. Known to occur following both coronary bypass and valve procedures, *meralgia paresthetica* is characterized by a focal region of numbness and paresthesia on the anterolateral aspect of the thigh. The syndrome results from an injury to the lateral femoral cutaneous nerve, likely secondary to positioning of the legs during the operation. The symptoms usually resolve over time, although in rare patients, surgical division of the nerve may be required (167).

COMPLICATIONS OF SAPHENOUS VEIN HARVESTING

Although the use of one or both internal mammary arteries as conduit for myocardial revascularization provides superior long-term results, it is still often necessary to use segments of the greater saphenous vein for additional conduits in patients who undergo multivessel CABG procedures. Leg wound complications, predominantly minor, occur in nearly one-fourth of patients in whom the saphenous vein is harvested. Serious complications, requiring major surgical procedures, occur in <1%. Meticulous surgical technique and a good understanding of the anatomy of the leg's venous drainage are important ways for the surgeon to avoid such problems. Risk factors associated with an increased incidence of leg wound problems include female gender, peripheral vascular disease, diabetes, and postoperative intraaortic balloon pump use (107). Careful preoperative evaluation of the leg to denote the presence of arterial insufficiency, use of small noncontiguous incisions (with or without the aid of a lighted endoscope), avoidance of hematomas, and careful attention to proper incision closure technique are important factors in reducing the incidence of vein harvest site problems. For difficult patients (such as those with previous vein stripping, thrombophlebitis, or obesity), preoperative duplex ultrasound scanning with marking of the skin overlying the identified vein can provide a "map" to guide the surgeon in the operating room (168). Endoscopic vein-harvesting techniques may be associated with reduced complication rates (169,170).

The most common complications of saphenous vein removal are infection, separation of the wound, cellulitis, lymphangitis, lymphocele or lymph drainage from the wound, and abscess formation. Postoperatively, some degree of distal leg edema is common; this usually resolves over a few weeks. Thus, patients are advised to keep the donor leg elevated when not ambulating. If the wound becomes infected, antibiotics are administered, and open packing of the wound is performed as necessary. Although problems with the leg wound may seem trivial compared with the surgery performed directly on the heart, serious leg wound complications can lead to significant morbidity, patient discomfort, and prolonged hospitalization. Rarely, major surgical reconstruction or even amputation may be required.

COMPLICATIONS RELATED TO USE OF THE RADIAL ARTERY

Use of the radial artery as bypass graft conduit is increasing due to apparent improved midterm patency results that are comparable with those of other arterial grafts (171). Preoperative evaluation generally involves the use of the Allen test or various modifications to ensure adequate collateral perfusion of the hand via the ulnar artery. With proper selection, ischemic complications are very rare. In one large series of >6,600 patients with radial artery grafts, only two patients experienced fingertip ischemia (172). As discussed previously, however, neurologic complaints (usually numbness at the base of the thumb) are not rare, but these usually resolve with time. Other potential complications include forearm hematoma, compartment syndrome, stitch abscesses, skin dehiscence, and infection. Overall, the incidence of nonneurologic complications, mostly minor, is <5% (173).

COMPLICATIONS RELATED TO INTERNAL MAMMARY ARTERY MOBILIZATION

One or both of the internal mammary (thoracic) arteries are utilized in >90% of the coronary revascularization procedures performed at our institutions because of the proven long-term benefits of this conduit as compared with saphenous vein aortocoronary bypass grafts. It is remarkable that only rarely do the mobilization and distal division of this artery (which is the major blood supply to the sternum) contribute to wound or other postoperative complications.

In some, but not all, reports, the use of bilateral internal mammary arteries in diabetic patients has been associated with an increased risk of sternal wound infections (87,174,175). Thus, the decision to use both mammary arteries in the diabetic patient must be made with consideration of the associated risks and benefits.

Postoperative respiratory insufficiency may be worsened by the effects of mammary artery mobilization, likely as the result of injury to the phrenic nerve. Careful dissection and avoidance of thermal injury to the nerve during mobilization of the artery are important.

DEEP VENOUS THROMBOSIS AND PULMONARY EMBOLISM

The incidences of deep venous thrombosis and pulmonary embolism following cardiac surgery are lower than those for other major surgical procedures. It is recognized, however, that the majority of episodes of deep venous thrombosis are silent, with clinically apparent deep venous thrombosis occurring in <2% of patients. The incidence of fatal pulmonary embolism following cardiac surgery has been reported to be as high as 0.5% (176).

Postoperative pulmonary emboli are more common in patients with postoperative atrial fibrillation or perioperative myocardial infarction. Delayed recovery and prolonged immobility are likely contributors in many affected patients. The most common presentation is catastrophic hemodynamic collapse due to a large embolus. Smaller emboli result in respiratory insufficiency with unexplained hypoxemia. For hypoxic patients in whom a pulmonary embolism is suspected, a ventilation–perfusion lung scan should be performed, although the accuracy of this test is diminished in the postoperative patient who commonly has atelectasis. If normal, then pulmonary embolism is highly unlikely. Patients with a "high probability" scan very likely have a pulmonary embolism, and if the clinical probability appears high, treatment should be initiated. If the ventilation–perfusion scan is high probability but the clinical probability is intermediate or low, spiral CT or pulmonary angiography should be performed for confirmation. Those with "low" or "intermediate" probability scans and positive venous (duplex) ultrasound examinations have a significant chance of pulmonary embolism. If the ventilation–perfusion scan is low or intermediate probability and the venous duplex scan is positive, treatment should be begun. If the venous duplex scan is negative, spiral CT scanning or pulmonary angiography is in order (177).

Treatment of pulmonary embolism is initiated by systemic heparinization for 5 to 10 days with overlapping warfarin anticoagulation for 4 to 5 days (178). The warfarin is then continued for at least 6 months. LMWH may be used instead of unfractionated heparin. For very desperately ill patients, an emergency embolectomy may be lifesaving (179). There is no role for systemic thrombolytic therapy for deep venous thrombosis or pulmonary embolism in patients who have recently undergone cardiac surgery due to the high risk of serious bleeding problems. Patients with contraindications to anticoagulation or patients who experience recurrence of pulmonary emboli despite anticoagulation are candidates for placement of an inferior vena caval filter.

Generally, patients undergoing coronary bypass surgery without the use of CPB ("off pump") receive less anticoagulation than patients who undergo surgery using the heart–lung machine. The incidence of postoperative thrombotic complications in off-pump coronary artery operations is low, although some surgeons have recommended prophylactic administration of subcutaneous heparin (5,000 U) beginning 1 to 2 hours before surgery and then three times per day until the patient's discharge from the hospital (180).

REFERENCES

1. Munoz JJ, Birkmeyer, Dacey LJ, et al. Trends in rates of reexploration for hemorrhage after coronary artery bypass surgery. *Ann Thorac Surg* 1999;68:1321–1325.
2. Moulton MJ, Creswell LL, Mackey ME, et al. Reexploration for bleeding is a risk factor to adverse outcomes after cardiac operations. *J Thorac Cardiovasc Surg* 1996;111:1037–1046.
3. Magovern JA, Sakert T, Benckart DH, et al. A model for predicting transfusion after coronary artery bypass grafting. *Ann Thorac Surg* 1996;61:27–32.
4. Despotis GJ, Filos KS, Zoys TN, et al. Factors associated with excessive postoperative blood loss and hemostatic transfusion requirements: a multivariate analysis in cardiac surgical patients. *Anesth Analg* 1996;82:13–21.
5. Dietrich W, Dilthey G, Spannagl M, et al. Warfarin pretreatment does not lead to increased bleeding tendency during cardiac surgery. *J Cardiothorac Vasc Anesth* 1995;9:250–254.
6. Morris CD, Vega JD, Levy JH, et al. Warfarin therapy does not increase bleeding in patients undergoing heart transplantation. *Ann Thorac Surg* 2001;72:714–718.
7. Davies LK. Cardiopulmonary bypass in infants and children: how is it different? *J Cardiovasc Vasc Anesth* 1999;13:330–345.
8. Wilkes MM, Navickis RJ, Sibbald WJ. Albumin versus hydroxyethyl starch in cardiopulmonary bypass surgery: a meta-analysis of postoperative bleeding. *Ann Thorac Surg* 2001;72:527–534.
9. Mojcik CF, Levy JH. Aprotinin and the systemic inflammatory response after cardiopulmonary bypass. *Ann Thorac Surg* 2001; 71:745–754.
10. Asimakoloulos G, Taylor KM. Effects of cardiopulmonary bypass on leukocyte and endothelial adhesion molecules. *Ann Thorac Surg* 1998;66:2135–2144.
11. Ascione R, Williams S, Lloyd CT, et al. Reduced postoperative blood loss and transfusion requirement after beating-heart coronary operations: a prospective randomized trial. *J Thorac Cardiovasc Surg* 2001;121:689–696.
12. Puskas JD, Thourani VH, Marshal JJ, et al. Clinical outcomes, angiographic patency, and resource utilization in 200 consecutive off-pump coronary bypass patients. *Ann Thorac Surg* 2001; 71:1477–1484.
13. Despotis GJ, Hogue CW. Pathophysiology, prevention, and treatment of bleeding after cardiac surgery: a primer for cardiologists and an update for the cardiothoracic team. *Am J Cardiol* 1999;83:15B–30B.
14. Brieger DB, Mak K-H, Kottke-Marchant KL, et al. Heparin-induced thrombocytopenia. *J Am Coll Cardiol* 1998;31:1449–1459.

15. Francis JL, Palmer GJ, Moroose R, et al. Comparison of bovine and porcine heparin in heparin antibody formation after cardiac surgery. *Ann Thorac Surg* 2003;75:17–22.
16. Lewis BE, Wallis DE, Berkowitz SD, et al. Agatroban anticoagulant therapy in patients with heparin-induced thrombocytopenia. *Circulation* 2001;103:1838–1843.
17. Greinacher A, Lubenow N, Recombinant hirudin in clinical practice. *Circulation* 2001;103:1479–1487.
18. Follis F, Schmidt CA. Cardiopulmonary bypass in patients with heparin-induced thrombocytopenia and thrombosis. *Ann Thorac Surg* 2000;70:2173–2181.
19. King SB. Optimizing antiplatelet therapy in coronary intervention. *Clin Cardiol* 2000;23(suppl VI):VI8–VI13.
20. Fry JA, Grines CL. Optimization of platelet therapy. *Semin Intervent Cardiol* 2000;5:117–128.
21. Patrono C, Coller B, Dalen JE, et al. Platelet-active drugs: the relationships among dose, effectiveness, and side effects. *Chest* 2001;119:39S–63S.
22. Sethis GK, Copeland JG, Goldman S, et al. Implications of preoperative administration of aspirin in patients undergoing coronary artery bypass grafting. *J Am Coll Cardiol* 1990;15:15–20.
23. Bashein G, Nessly ML, Rice AL, et al. Preoperative aspirin therapy and reoperation for bleeding after coronary artery bypass surgery. *Arch Intern Med* 1991;151:89–93.
24. Reich DL, Patel GC, Vela-Cantos F, et al. Aspirin does not increase homologous blood requirements in elective coronary bypass surgery. *Anesth Analg* 1994;79:4–8.
25. Ferraris VA, Ferraris SP, Oji J, et al. Aspirin and postoperative bleeding after coronary artery bypass grafting. *Ann Surg* 2002; 235:820–827.
26. Dacey LJ, Munoz JJ, Johnson ER, et al. Effect of preoperative aspirin use on mortality in coronary artery bypass grafting patients. *Ann Thorac Surg* 2000;70:1986–1990.
27. Mangano DT. Multicenter Study of Perioperative Ischemia Research Group. Aspirin and mortality from coronary bypass surgery. *N Engl J Med* 2002;347:1309–1317.
28. Murkin JM, Lux J, Shannon NA, et al. Aprotinin significantly decreases bleeding and transfusion requirements in patients receiving aspirin and undergoing cardiac operations. *J Thorac Cardiovasc Surg* 1994;107:554–561.
29. Bidstrup BP, Hunt BJ, Sheikh S, et al. Amelioration of the bleeding tendency of preoperative aspirin after coronary bypass grafting. *Ann Thorac Surg* 2000;69:541–547.
30. Goldman S, Copeland J, Moritz T, et al. Starting aspirin therapy after operation: effects on early graft patency. *Circulation* 1991; 84:520–526.
31. Quinn MJ, Fitzgerald DJ. Ticlopidine and clopidogrel. *Circulation* 1999;100:1667–1672.
32. Thebault JJ, Kieffer G, Cariou R. Single-dose pharmacodynamics of clopidogrel. *Semin Thromb Hemost* 1999;25(suppl 2):3–8.
33. Hongo RH, Ley J, Dick Se, et al. The effect of clopidogrel in combination with aspirin when given before coronary artery bypass grafting. *J Am Coll Cardiol* 2002;40:231–237.
34. Lemmer JH Jr, Metzdorff MT, Krause AH Jr, et al. Emergency coronary artery bypass graft surgery in abciximab-treated patients. *Ann Thorac Surg* 2000;69:90–95.

35. Singh M, Nuttall GA, Ballman KV, et al. Effect of abciximab on the outcome of emergency coronary artery bypass grafting after failed percutaneous coronary intervention. *Mayo Clin Proc* 2001; 76:784–788.
36. Lincoff AM, LeNarz LA, Despotis GJ, et al. Abciximab and bleeding during coronary surgery: results from the EPILOG and EPISTENT trials. *Ann Thorac Surg* 2000;70:516–526.
37. Lemmer JH Jr. Clinical experience in coronary bypass surgery for abciximab-treated patients. *Ann Thorac Surg* 2000;70:S33–S37.
38. Dyke CM, Bhatia D, Lorenz TJ, et al. Immediate coronary artery bypass surgery after platelet inhibition with eptifibatide: results from PURSUIT. *Ann Thorac Surg* 2000;70:866–872.
39. Genoni M, Zeller D, Bertel O, et al. Tirofiban therapy does not increase the risk of hemorrhage after emergency coronary surgery. *J Thorac Cardiovasc Surg* 2001;122:630–632.
40. Bizzarri F, Scolletta S, Tucci E, et al. Perioperative use of tirofiban hydrochloride (Aggrastat) does not increase surgical bleeding after emergency or urgent coronary artery bypass grafting. *J Thorac Cardiovasc Surg* 2001;122:1181–1185.
41. Despotis GJ, Skubas NJ, Goodnough LT. Optimal management of bleeding and transfusion in patients undergoing cardiac surgery. *Semin Thorac Cardiovasc Surg* 1999;11:84–104.
42. Hirsh J, Warkentin TE, Shaughnessy SG, et al. Heparin and low-molecular-weight heparin: mechanisms of action, pharmacokinetics, dosing, monitoring, efficacy, and safety. *Chest* 2001; 119:64S–94S.
43. Lemmer JH Jr, Despotis GJ. Antithrombin III concentrate to treat heparin resistance in patients undergoing cardiac surgery. *J Thorac Cardiovasc Surg* 2002;123:213–217.
44. Depotis GJ, Gravlee, Filos K, et al. Anticoagulation monitoring during cardiac surgery. *Anesthesiology* 1999;91:1122–1151.
45. Clark SC, Vitale N, Zacharias J, et al. Effect of low molecular weight heparin (Fragmin) on bleeding after cardiac surgery. *Ann Thorac Surg* 2000;69:762–765.
46. Jones HU, Muhlestein JB, Jones KW, et al. Preoperative use of enoxaparin compared with unfractionated heparin increases the incidence of re-exploration for postoperative bleeding after open-heart surgery in patients who present with an acute coronary syndrome: clinical investigation and reports. *Circulation* 2002; 106(suppl I):I19–I22.
47. Henry TD, Satran D, Knox LL, et al. Are activated clotting times helpful in the management of anticoagulation with subcutaneous low-molecular-eight heparin? *Am Heart J* 2001;142:590–593.
48. Mannucci PM. Hemostatic drugs. *N Engl J Med* 1998;339: 245–253.
49. Peters DC, Noble S. Aprotinin: an update of its pharmacology and therapeutic use in open heart surgery and coronary bypass surgery. *Drugs* 1999;57:233–260.
50. Hardy J-F. Pharmacological strategies for blood conservation in cardiac surgery: erythropoietin and antifibrinolytics. *Can J Anaesth* 2001;48:S24–S31.
51. Fiser SM, Tribble CG, Kern JA, et al. Cardiac reoperation in the intensive care unit. *Ann Thorac Surg* 2001;71:1888–1893.
52. Russo AM, O'Connor WH, Waxman HL. Atypical presentations and echocardiographic findings in patients with cardiac tampon-

ade occurring early and late after cardiac surgery. *Chest* 1993; 104:71–78.

53. Cheitlin MD, Alpert JS, Armstrong WF, et al. ACC/AHA Guidelines for the Clinical Application of Echocardiography: a report of the American College of Cardiology/American Heart Association Task Force on Practice Guidelines. *Circulation* 1997; 95:1686–1744.
54. Kuvin JT, Harati NA, Pandian NG, et al. Postoperative tamponade in the modern surgical era. *Ann Thorac Surg* 2002;74: 1148–1153.
55. Mangi AA, Palacios IF, Torchiana DF. Catheter pericardiocentesis for delayed tamponade after cardiac valve operation. *Ann Thorac Surg* 2002;73:1479–1483.
56. Tsang TSM, Barnes ME, Hayes SN, et al. Clinical and echocardiographic characteristics of significant pericardial effusions following cardiothoracic surgery and outcomes of echo-guided pericardiocentesis for management: Mayo Clinic experience 1979–1988. *Chest* 199;116:322–331.
57. Chertow GM, Lazarus JM, Christiansen, et al. Preoperative renal risk stratification. *Circulation* 1997;95:878–884.
58. Conlon PJ, Stafford-Smith M, White WD, et al. Acute renal failure following cardiac surgery. *Nephrol Dialysis Transplant* 1999; 14:1158–1162.
59. Mangano CM, Diamondstone LS, Ramsay JG, et al. Renal dysfunction after myocardial revascularization: risk factors, adverse outcomes, and hospital resource utilization. *Ann Intern Med* 1998;128:194–203.
60. Schweizer A, Hohn L, Morel DR, et al. Aprotinin does not impair renal haemodynamics and function after cardiac surgery. *Br J Anaesth* 2000;84:16–22.
61. Lemmer JH, Stanford W, Bonney SL, et al. Aprotinin for coronary artery bypass grafting: effect on postoperative renal function. *Ann Thorac Surg* 1995;59:132–136.
62. Ascione R, Lloyd CT, Underwood MJ, et al. On-pump versus off-pump coronary revascularization: evaluation of renal function. *Ann Thorac Surg* 1999;68:493–498.
63. Luciani GB, Nichani S, Chang AC, et al. Continuous versus intermittent furosemide infusion in critically ill infants after open heart operations. *Ann Thorac Surg* 1997;64:1133–1139.
64. Copeland JG, Campbell DW, Plachetka JR, et al. Diuresis with continuous infusion of furosemide after cardiac surgery. *Am J Surg* 1983;146:796–799.
65. Thadhani R, Pascual M, Bonventre JV. Acute renal failure. *N Engl J Med* 1996;334:1448–1460.
66. Aronson S, Blumenthal R. Perioperative renal dysfunction and cardiovascular anesthesia: concerns and controversies. *J Cardiothorac Vasc Anesth* 1998;12:567–586.
67. Australian and New Zealand Intensive Care Society Clinical Trials Group. Low-dose dopamine in patients with early renal dysfunction: a placebo-controlled randomized trial. *Lancet* 2000;356: 2139–2143.
68. Woo EBC, Tang ATM, Gamel AE, et al. Dopamine therapy for patients at risk of renal dysfunction following cardiac surgery: science or fiction? *Eur J Cardiothorac Surg* 2002;22:106–111.

69. Marik PE. Low-dose dopamine: a systematic review. *Intensive Care Med* 2002;28:877–893.
70. Dittrich S, Dahnert I, Vogel M, et al. Peritoneal dialysis after infant open heart surgery; observations in 27 patients. *Ann Thorac Surg* 1999;68:160–163.
71. Forni LG, Hilton PJ. Continuous hemofiltration in the treatment of acute renal failure. *N Engl J Med* 1997;336:1303–1309.
72. Ostermann ME, Taube D, Morgan CJ, et al. Acute renal failure following cardiopulmonary bypass: a changing picture. *Intensive Care Med* 2000;26:565–571.
73. Bent P, Tan HK, Bellomo R, et al. Early and intensive continuous hemofiltration for severe renal failure after cardiac surgery. *Ann Thorac Surg* 2001;71:832–837.
74. Rebollo MH, Bernal JM, Llorca J, et al. Nosocomial infections in patients having cardiovascular operations: a multivariate analysis of risk factors. *J Thorac Cardiovasc Surg* 1996;112:908–913.
75. Francel TJ, Kouchoukos NT. A rational approach to wound difficulties after sternotomy: the problem. *Ann Thorac Surg* 2001;72:1411–1418.
76. Carrel TP, Aisinger E, Vogt M, et al. Pneumonia after cardiac surgery is predictable by tracheal aspirates but cannot be prevented by prolonged antibiotic prophylaxis. *Ann Thorac Surg* 2001;72:143–148.
77. Lynch JP. Hospital-acquired pneumonia. *Chest* 2001;119: 373S–384S.
78. Leal-Noval SR, Marquez-Vacaro JA, Garcia-Curiel A, et al. Nosocomial pneumonia in patients undergoing heart surgery. *Crit Care Med* 2000;28:935–940.
79. Abramowicz M, ed. The choice of antibacterial drugs. *Med Lett* 2001;69–78.
80. Losanoff JE, Richman BW, Jones JW. Disruption and infection of median sternotomy: a comprehensive review. *Eur J Cardiothorac Surg* 2002;21:831–839.
81. Braxton JH, Marrin CAS, McGrath PD, et al. Mediastinitis and long-term survival after coronary artery bypass graft surgery. *Ann Thorac Surg* 2000;70:2004–2007.
82. Milano CA, Kesler K, Archibald N, et al. Mediastinitis after coronary artery bypass graft surgery. *Circulation* 1995;92:2245–2251.
83. Carrier M, Perrault LP, Pellerin M, et al. Sternal wound infection after heart transplantation: incidence and results with aggressive surgical treatment. *Ann Thorac Surg* 2001;72:719–724.
84. Loop FD, Lytle BW, Cosgrove DM, et al. Sternal complications after isolated coronary artery bypass grafting: early and late mortality, morbidity, and cost of care. *Ann Thorac Surg* 1990;49: 179–187.
85. Borger MA, Rao V, Weisel RD, et al. Deep sternal wound infection: risk factors and outcomes. *Ann Thorac Surg* 1998;65: 1050–1056.
86. Parisian Mediastinitis Study Group. Risk factors for deep sternal wound infection after sternotomy: a prospective, multicenter study. *J Thorac Cardiovasc Surg* 1996;111:1200–1207.
87. Lytle BW, Blackstone EH, Loop FD, et al. Two internal thoracic artery grafts are better than one. *J Thorac Cardiovasc Surg* 1999;117:855–872.

88. Curtis JJ, Clark NC, McKenney CA, et al. Tracheostomy: a risk factor for mediastinitis after cardiac operation. *Ann Thorac Surg* 2001;72:731–734.
89. Ko W, Lazenby D, Zelano JA, et al. Effects for shaving methods and intraoperative irrigation on suppurative mediastinitis after bypass operations. *Ann Thorac Surg* 1992;53:301–305.
90. Hall JC, Christiansen K, Carter MJ, et al. Antibiotic prophylaxis in cardiac operations. *Ann Thorac Surg* 1993;56:916–922.
91. Nooyen SMH, Overbeek BP, de la Riviere AB, et al. Prospective randomized comparison of single-dose versus multiple-dose cefuroxime for prophylaxis in coronary artery bypass grafting. *Eur J Clin Microbiol Infect Dis* 1994;13:1033–1037.
92. Mossad SB, Serkey JM, Longworth DL, et al. Coagulase-negative staphylococcal sternal wound infections after open heart operations. *Ann Thorac Surg* 1997;63:395–401.
93. Finkelstein R, Rabino G, Mashiah T, et al. Vancomycin versus cefazolin prophylaxis for cardiac surgery in the setting of a high prevalence of methicillin-resistant staphylococcal infections. *J Thorac Cardiovasc Surg* 2002;123:326–332.
94. Abramowicz M, ed. Antimicrobial prophylaxis in surgery. *Med Lett* 1999;41:75–80.
95. Olsen MA, Lock-Buckley P, Hopkins D, et al. The risk factors for deep and superficial chest surgical-site infections after coronary artery bypass graft surgery are different. *J Thorac Cardiovasc Surg* 2002;124:136–145.
96. Furnary AP, Zerr KJ, Grunkemeier GL, et al. Continuous intravenous insulin infusion reduces the incidence of deep sternal wound infection in diabetic patients after cardiac surgical procedures. *Ann Thorac Surg* 1999;67:352–362.
97. Tegnell A, Aren C, Ohman L. Coagulase-negative staphylococci and sternal infections after cardiac operation. *Ann Thorac Surg* 2000;69:1104–1109.
98. Misawa Y, Fuse K, Hasegawa T. Infectious mediastinitis after cardiac operations: computed tomographic findings. *Ann Thorac Surg* 1998;65:622–624.
99. El Oakley RM, Wright JE. Postoperative mediastinitis: classification and management. *Ann Thorac Surg* 1996;61:1030–1036.
100. Rand Cochran RP, Aziz S, Hofer BO, et al. Prospective trial of catheter irrigation and muscle flaps for sternal wound infection. *Ann Thorac Surg* 1998;65:1046–1049.
101. Gamel AE, Yonan NA, Hassan R, et al. Treatment of mediastinitis: early modified Robicsek closure and pectoralis major advancement flaps. *Ann Thorac Surg* 1998;65:41–44.
102. Jones G, Jurkiewicz MJ, Bostwick J, et al. Management of the infected median sternotomy wound with muscle flaps. The Emory 20-year experience. *Ann Surg* 1997;225:766–776.
103. Hugo NE, Asçherman JA, Patsis MC, et al. Single-stage management of 74 consecutive sternal wound complications with pectoralis major myocutaneous advancement flaps. *Plast Reconstr Surg* 1994;93:1433–1441.
104. Erez E, Katz M, Sharoni E, et al. Pectoralis major muscle flap for deep sternal wound infection in neonates. *Ann Thorac Surg* 2000;69:572–577.
105. Francel TJ, Kouchoukos NT. A rational approach to wound difficulties after sternotomy: reconstruction and long-term results. *Ann Thorac Surg* 2001;72:1419–1429.

106. Suen HC, Barner HB. Repair of right ventricular rupture complicating mediastinitis. *Ann Thorac Surg* 1998;66:2115–2116.
107. Paletta CE, Huang DB, Fiore AC, et al. Major leg wound complications after saphenous vein harvest for coronary revascularization. *Ann Thorac Surg* 2000;70:492–497.
108. Kac G, Durain E, Amrein C, et al. Colonization and infection of pulmonary artery catheter in cardiac surgery patients: epidemiology and multivariate analysis of risk factors. *Crit Care Med* 2001;29:971–975.
109. Merrer J, De Jonghe B, Golliot F, et al. Complications of femoral and subclavian venous catheterization in critically ill patients. *JAMA* 2001;286:700–707.
110. Christenson JT, Schmuziger M, Maurice J, et al. Gastrointestinal complications after coronary artery bypass grafting. *J Thorac Cardiovasc Surg* 1994;108:899–906.
111. Zacharias A, Schwann TA, Parenteau GL, et al. Predictors of gastrointestinal complications in cardiac surgery. *Tex Heart Inst J* 2000;27:93–99.
112. Simic O, Strathausen S, Hess W, et al. Incidence and prognosis of abdominal complications after cardiopulmonary bypass. *Cardiovasc Surg* 1999;7:419–424.
113. Aouifi A, Piriou V, Bastien O, et al. Severe digestive complications after heart surgery using extracorporeal circulation. *Can J Anaesth* 1999;46:114–121.
114. Lam NP, Le P-D T, Crawford SY, et al. National survey of stress ulcer prophylaxis. *Crit Care Med* 1999;27:98–103.
115. van der Voort PHJ, Zandstra DF. Pathogenesis, risk factors, and incidence of upper gastrointestinal bleeding after cardiac surgery: is specific prophylaxis in routine bypass procedures needed? *J Cardiothorac Vasc Anesth* 2000;14:293–299.
116. Tryba M, Cook D. Current guidelines on stress ulcer prophylaxis. *Drugs* 1997;54:581–596.
117. Rosen HR, Vlahakes GJ, Rattner DW. Fulminant peptic ulcer disease in cardiac surgical patients: pathogenesis, prevention, and management. *Crit Care Med* 1992;20:354–359.
118. Rady MY, Kodavatiganti R, Ryan T. Perioperative predictors of acute cholecystitis after cardiovascular surgery. *Chest* 1998;114:76–84.
119. Rattner DW, Gu ZY, Vlahakes GJ, et al. Hyperamylasemia after cardiac surgery. Incidence, significance, and management. *Ann Surg* 1989;209:279–283.
120. Gan TJ. Postoperative nausea and vomiting—can it be eliminated? *JAMA* 2002;1233–1236.
121. Ferraris VA, Ferraris SP, Moritz DM, et al. Oropharyngeal dysphagia after cardiac operations. *Ann Thorac Surg* 2001;71:1792–1796.
122. Gundry SR, Borkon AM, McIntosh CL, et al. Candida esophagitis following cardiac operation and short-term antibiotic prophylaxis. *J Thorac Cardiovasc Surg* 1980;80:661–668.
123. Thompson DF, Landry JP. Drug-induced hiccups. *Ann Pharmacother* 1997;31:367–369.
124. Friedman NL. Hiccups: a treatment review. *Pharmacotherapy* 1996;16:986–995.
125. Roach GW, Kanchuger M, Mangano CM, et al. Adverse cerebral outcomes after coronary bypass surgery. *N Engl J Med* 1996;335:1857–1863.

126. Puskas JD, Winston D, Wright CE, et al. Stroke after coronary artery operation: incidence, correlates, outcome, and cost. *Ann Thorac Surg* 2000;69:1053.
127. Taggart DP, Westaby S. Neurological and cognitive disorders after coronary artery bypass grafting. *Curr Opin Cardiol* 2001; 16:217–276.
128. Mickleborough LL, Walker PM, Takagi Y, et al. Risk factors for stroke in patients undergoing coronary artery bypass grafting. *J Thorac Cardiovasc Surg* 1996;112:1250–1259.
129. McKhann GM, Goldsborough MA, Borowicz LM, et al. Predictors of stroke risk in coronary artery bypass patients. *Ann Thorac Surg* 1997;63:516–521.
130. Almassi GH, Sommer T, Moritz TE, et al. Stroke in cardiac surgical patients: determinants and outcome. *Ann Thorac Surg* 1999;68:391–398.
131. John R, Choudhri AF, Weinberg AD, et al. Multicenter review of preoperative risk factors for stroke after coronary artery bypass grafting. *Ann Thorac Surg* 2000;69:30–36.
132. Liddicoat JR, Redmond JM, Vassileva CM, et al. Hypothermic circulatory arrest in octogenarians: risk of stroke and mortality. *Ann Thorac Surg* 2000;69:1048–1052.
133. Diegeler A, Hirsch R, Schneider F, et al. Neuromonitoring and neurocognitive outcome in off-pump versus conventional coronary bypass operation. *Ann Thorac Surg* 2000;69:1162–1166.
134. Yokoyama T, Baumgartner FJ, Gheissari A, et al. Off-pump versus on-pump coronary bypass in high-risk subgroups. *Ann Thorac Surg* 2000;70:1546–1550.
135. Iglesia I, Murkin JM. Beating heart surgery or conventional CABG: are neurologic outcomes different? *Semin Thorac Cardiovasc Surg* 2001;13:158–169.
136. Van Dijk D, Jansen EWL, Hijman R, et al. Cognitive outcome after off-pump and on-pump coronary artery bypass surgery: a randomized trial. *JAMA* 2002;287:1405–1412.
137. Smith PK, Muhlbaier LH. Aprotinin: safe and effective only with the full-dose regimen. *Ann Thorac Surg* 1996;62:1575–1577.
138. Grigore Am, Grocott HP, Mathew JP, et al. The rewarming rate and increased peak temperature alter neurocognitive outcome after cardiac surgery. *Anesth Analg* 2002;94:4–10.
139. Cook DJ. Cerebral hyperthermia and cardiac surgery: consequences and prevention. *Semin Thorac Cardiovasc Surg* 2001; 13:176–183.
140. Furster V, Ryden LE, Asinger RW, et al. ACC/AHA/ESC Guidelines for the Management of Patients with Atrial Fibrillation. *J Am Coll Cardiol* 2001;38:1231–1265.
141. Barbut D, Lo Y-W, Gold JP, et al. Impact of embolization during coronary artery bypass grafting on outcome and length of stay. *Ann Thorac Surg* 1997;63:998–1002.
142. Salazar JD, Wityk RJ, Grega MA, et al. Stroke after cardiac surgery: short- and long-term outcomes. *Ann Thorac Surg* 2001; 72:1195–1202.
143. Wareing TH, Davila-Roman VG, Daily BB, et al. Strategy for the reduction of stroke incidence in cardiac surgical patients. *Ann Thorac Surg* 1993;55:1400–1408.
144. Fukuda I, Gomi S, Watanabe K, et al. Carotid and aortic screening for coronary artery bypass grafting. *Ann Thorac Surg* 2000; 70:2034–2039.

145. Borger MA, Fremes SE. Management of patients with concomitant coronary and carotid vascular disease. *Semin Thorac Cardiovasc Surg* 2001;13:192–198.
146. Zacharias A, Schwann TA, Riordan CJ, et al. Operative and 5-year outcomes of combined carotid and coronary revascularization: review of a large contemporary experience. *Ann Thorac Surg* 2002;73:491–498.
147. Trehan N, Mishra M, Kasliwal RR, et al. Surgical strategies in patients at high risk of stroke undergoing coronary artery bypass grafting. *Ann Thorac Surg* 2000;70:1037–1045.
148. Beique FA, Joffe D, Tousignant G, et al. Echocardiographic-based assessment and management of atherosclerotic disease of the thoracic aorta. *J Cardiovasc Vasc Anesth* 1998;12:206–220.
149. Cleveland JC, Shroyer ALW, Chen AY, et al. Off-pump coronary artery bypass grafting decreases risk-adjusted mortality and morbidity. *Ann Thorac Surg* 2001;72:1282–1289.
150. Kincaid EH, Jones TJ, Stump DA, et al. Processing scavenged blood with a cell saver reduces cerebral lipid microembolization. *Ann Thorac Surg* 2000;1296–1300.
151. Mills NL, Ochsner. Massive air embolism during cardiopulmonary bypass. *J Thorac Cardiovasc Surg* 1980;80:708–717.
152. Ziser A, Adir Y, Lavon H, et al. Hyperbaric oxygen therapy for massive arterial air embolism during cardiac operations. *J Thorac Cardiovasc Surg* 1999;117:818–821.
153. Shahian DM, Speert PK. Symptomatic visual deficits after open heart operations. *Ann Thorac Surg* 1989;48:275–279.
154. Shapira OM, Kimmel WA, Lindsey PS, et al. Anterior ischemic optic neuropathy after open heart operations. *Ann Thorac Surg* 1996;61:660–666.
155. Floyd TF, Cheung AT, Stecker MM. Postoperative neurologic assessment and management of the cardiac surgical patient. *Semin Thorac Cardiovasc Surg* 2000;12:337–348.
156. McKhann GM, Grega MA, Borowicz LM, et al. Encephalopathy and stroke after coronary artery bypass grafting. *Arch Neurol* 2002;59:1422–1428.
157. Newman MF, Kirchner JL, Phillips-Bute B, et al. Longitudinal assessment of neurocognitive function after coronary artery bypass surgery. *N Engl J Med* 2001;344:395–402.
158. Mahanna EP, Blumenthal JA, White WD, et al. Defining neuropsychological dysfunction after coronary artery bypass grafting. *Ann Thorac Surg* 1996;61:1342–1347.
159. Hammon JW, Stump DA, Butterworth JB, et al. Approaches to reduce neurologic complications during cardiac surgery. *Semin Thorac Cardiovasc Surg* 2001;13:184–191.
160. Hammon JW, Stump DA, Kon ND, et al. Risk factors and solutions for the development of neurobehavioral changes after coronary artery bypass grafting. *Ann Thorac Surg* 1997;63:1613–1618.
161. Nathan HJ, Wells GA, Munson JL, et al. Neuroprotective effect of mild hypothermia in patients undergoing coronary artery surgery with cardiopulmonary bypass. *Circulation* 2001;104 (suppl I):I85–I91.
162. Taggart DP, Browne SM, Halligan, et al. Is cardiopulmonary bypass still the cause of cognitive dysfunction after cardiac operations? *J Thorac Cardiovasc Surg* 1999;118:414–420.

163. McKhann GM, Goldsborough MA, Borowicz LM, et al. Cognitive outcome after coronary artery bypass; a one-year prospective study. *Ann Thorac Surg* 1997;63:510–515.
164. Sharma AD, Parnley CL, Seeram G, et al. Peripheral nerve injuries during cardiac surgery: risk factors, diagnosis, prognosis, and prevention. *Anesth Analg* 2000;91:1358–1369.
165. Warner MA, Warner ME, Martin JT. Ulnar neuropathy: incidence, outcome, and risk factors in sedated or anesthetized patients. *Anesthesiology* 1994;81:1332–1340.
166. Denton TA, Trento L, Cohen M, et al. Radial artery harvesting for coronary bypass operations: neurologic complications and their potential mechanisms. *J Thorac Cardiovasc Surg* 2001; 121:951–956.
167. Ivins GK. Meralgia paresthetica, the elusive diagnosis: clinical experience in 14 adult patients. *Ann Surg* 2000;232:281–286.
168. Lemmer JH Jr, Meng RL, Corson JD, et al. Preoperative saphenous vein mapping for coronary artery bypass. *J Cardiac Surg* 1988;3:237–240.
169. Carpino PA, Khabbaz KP, Bojar RM, et al. Clinical benefits of endoscopic vein harvesting in patients with risk factors for saphenectomy wound infections undergoing coronary artery bypass grafting. *J Thorac Cardiovasc Surg* 2000;119:69–76.
170. Hayward TZ, Hey LA, Newman LL, et al. Endoscopic versus open saphenous vein harvest: the effect on postoperative outcomes. *Ann Thorac Surg* 1999;68:2107–2111.
171. Amano QA, Hirose H, Takahashi A, et al. Coronary artery bypass grafting using the radial artery: midterm results in a Japanese institute. *Ann Thorac Surg* 2001;72:120–125.
172. Tatoulis J, Royse AG, Buxton BF, et al. The radial artery in coronary surgery: a 5-year experience-clinical and angiographic results. *Ann Thorac Surg* 2002;73:143–148.
173. Greene MA, Malias MA. Arm complications after radial artery procurement for coronary bypass operation. *Ann Thorac Surg* 2001;72:126–128.
174. Kouchoukos NT, Wareing TH, Murphy SF, et al. Risks of bilateral internal mammary artery bypass grafting. *Ann Thorac Surg* 1990;49:210–219.
175. Gurevitdch J, Paz Y, Shapira I, et al. Routine use of bilateral skeletonized internal mammary arteries for myocardial revascularization. *Ann Thorac Surg* 1999;68:406–412.
176. Shammas NW. Pulmonary embolus after coronary artery bypass surgery: a review of the literature. *Clin Cardiol* 2000;23:637–644.
177. Ehsan M, Prow HW, Clagett GP. Diagnosing acute pulmonary embolism in surgical patients. *Surg Rounds* 2001:67–78.
178. Hyers TM, Agnelli G, Hull RD, et al. Antithrombotic therapy for venous thromboembolic disease. *Chest* 2001;119:176S–193S.
179. Putnam JB, Lemmer JH, Rocchini PA, et al. Embolectomy for acute pulmonary artery occlusion following Fontan procedure. *Ann Thorac Surg* 1988;45:335–336.
180. Cartier R, Robitaille D. Thrombotic complications in beating heart operations. *J Thorac Cardiovasc Surg* 2001;121:920–922.

Late Postoperative Management

CARDIAC REHABILITATION

For most patients, the goal of undergoing cardiac surgery is to permit their return to as normal a lifestyle as possible, including employment when appropriate. Cardiac rehabilitation has assumed greater importance in the modern era, where patients with more advanced disease are undergoing heart surgery and where the disability that must be overcome after some operations (e.g., cardiac transplantation for severe heart failure) is considerable. Advanced patient age, concomitant diseases, and reduced transfusions with the resultant postoperative anemia are factors that further complicate the rehabilitative process. Cardiac rehabilitation should be offered to all eligible patients (1).

A well-organized program for cardiac rehabilitation addresses both the physical and the emotional needs of the postoperative patient and begins with instruction in the preoperative period (2). An important element in cardiac rehabilitation is developing a positive patient attitude, starting with the assumption that rehabilitation to an active lifestyle is the norm. The basic principle of cardiac rehabilitation is to offer the patients graded exercise in a supervised environment up to the limit of their cardiac function. With continued conditioning, many of these patients, particularly those with heart failure that has been improved or corrected, should experience considerable improvement in exercise capacity over their preoperative status. This may, however, require a considerable effort over a period of time; a well-organized cardiac rehabilitation program should recognize and develop that goal. For most patients, postoperative cardiac rehabilitation begins, in the hospital, a process that will continue when they are at home. Most initial rehabilitation programs for postoperative patients achieve only low-level exercise and low-level caloric expenditure during the inpatient portion of the program (3).

Ambulation is initiated as early as possible in the hospital after surgery. This is to decrease the amount of "deconditioning" and lack of mobility that occur with bedrest, to optimize pulmonary toilet and minimize atelectasis, and to decrease venous stasis in the lower extremities, consequently lowering the risk of phlebitis. In addition, it has been demonstrated that patients achieve a better quality of life by 3 months following surgery if ambulation and rehabilitation are started early after surgery during the acute hospitalization (4). The program of ambulation varies from hospital to hospital, but, in general, it should progress to supervised stair climbing or exercise on a stationary bicycle before discharge. From both physical and emotional perspectives, the inpatient ambulation and rehabilitation program should introduce and prepare the patient for the outpatient program. As there is an emphasis on shortening the length of the hospital stay, generating a positive attitude toward rehabilitation and de-emphasizing cardiac illness may be important factors in reducing the number of postoperative in-hospital days. Similarly, this approach should help increase the likelihood that previously employed patients will return to their jobs (5).

For patients who have undergone coronary artery bypass graft (CABG) procedures, a postoperative exercise stress test is sometimes used to provide objective evidence that ischemia has been relieved, so that patients may pursue a more aggressive outpatient rehabilitative process with greater confidence. In patients with relatively straightforward anatomic considerations and an average level of activity, rehabilitation can be undertaken safely without a stress test (6). However, an electrocardiographic (ECG) exercise stress test may be useful for those patients who, after initial rehabilitation, will begin heavier forms of exercise such as jogging; for those patients who had silent ischemia before surgery; and for those patients with particularly severe distal coronary arterial disease. In some series, positive postoperative studies were noted in up to 10% of patients and can influence the decision to restart anti-ischemic medications, to recatheterize, or to limit exercise. The stress test is performed approximately 2 or 3 months after surgery when patients are freely ambulatory and can perform the test to their comfortable limit of fatigue. This time interval permits resolution of postoperative anemia and return of normal chest wall mechanics to allow optimal exercise performance during the test. ECG stress testing is about 70% sensitive and 80% specific for the recognition of exercise-induced myocardial ischemia.

GRAFT PATENCY AFTER CORONARY ARTERY BYPASS GRAFTING

It is recognized that CABG is palliative and that atherosclerosis in the native coronary arteries often progresses. Approximately 10% of saphenous vein bypass grafts will be occluded at the end of the first postoperative year; hence, for patients who have received more than one saphenous vein graft, the likelihood of having at least one occluded graft increases. Graft occlusion is a complex subject, but factors that influence short-term graft patency include the technical quality of proximal and distal anastomoses, the size and quality of the coronary artery, injury to the conduit before implantation, and low-flow rates at the time of surgery (<40 mL per minute). Vein graft intimal hyperplasia and recurrent atherosclerosis influence long-term patency. By 5 years after coronary bypass grafting, approximately 20% of saphenous vein grafts are occluded, and by 10 years, 40% are occluded (7–9).

It is now standard practice to employ measures to enhance graft patency. From the surgical standpoint, this has included maximal use of arterial conduits because of their superior long-term patency rate as compared with vein grafts. Postoperative efforts have concentrated in two areas: platelet inhibitor drug treatment and atherosclerosis risk factor modification. Antiplatelet drugs can enhance graft patency; in particular, aspirin has been demonstrated to improve graft patency rates (10,11). For this purpose, aspirin should be given within 6 hours of surgery (by rectal suppository) as long as the patient is not bleeding (12). When the patient is taking oral medications, enteric-coated aspirin is instituted. Although no data are available documenting aspirin's beneficial effects on graft patency beyond 1 year, it is our practice to continue aspirin therapy indefinitely in part because of its effectiveness in decreasing the rate of future myocardial infarction (13).

With the recognition that recurrent atherosclerosis can occur both in the native circulation as well as in bypass grafts, there is now an increasing emphasis on postoperative atherosclerosis risk factor modification. The risk factors known to accelerate atherosclerosis that can be controlled or modified include smoking, obesity, hyperlipidemia, hypertension, and diabetes. Younger patients with accelerated atherosclerosis and no other significant common risk factors should be screened either before or 2 to 3 months after surgery for uncommon causes of premature atherosclerosis, such as coagulation system disorders or elevated homocysteine level. Emphasizing the importance of eliminating controllable risk factors (such as smoking and atherogenic diet) and treating treatable risk factors (such as hypertension and diabetes) are prominent parts of the cardiac rehabilitation process. The initial treatment of all hyperlipidemias includes weight loss, dietary modification with respect to fat intake, and aerobic exercise. In general, patients with an abnormal lipid profile on further postoperative follow-up despite these measures should have further treatment. Patients with diabetes mellitus and coronary artery disease have an impaired long-term prognosis, and optimization of their risk factors and pharmacologic treatment regimen is important (14).

With the availability of effective lipid-lowering medications such as the *statins* (hydroxymethylglutaryl–coenzyme A reductase inhibitors) and the *fibrates,* a greater degree of control over lipid metabolism is now possible (15–17). In particular, low-density lipoprotein–cholesterol should be kept below 100 mg/dL, with some advocating that it should be <80 mg/dL, particularly in younger patients. When possible, CABG patients undergo lipid profile [total cholesterol, triglycerides, high-density lipoprotein (HDL)–cholesterol, low-density lipoprotein–cholesterol] evaluation prior to surgery, and if results are abnormal, diet and/or drug therapy is instituted at the time of discharge. If the patient was already taking medication for hyperlipidemia preoperatively, the drug regimen is restarted at the time of discharge. Although relatively safe, long-term treatment with lipid-lowering drugs does require careful follow-up. The most serious common side effect of statin therapy is an increase in hepatic serum aminotransferase (i.e., AST and ALT) enzyme levels; this may occur in up to 3% of treated patients. Thus, liver function testing is required at 6 to 12 weeks after initiation of statin therapy (or increase in dosage) and then repeated every 3 to 6 months for at least the first year of therapy (18). Statins may potentiate the effect of warfarin and should be used with care in patients with known liver disease. Another statin side effect is uncomplicated myalgia; much more rare is severe rhabdomyolysis with renal failure. Other medications to treat dyslipidemias include the *fibrates* (often used for hypertriglyceridemia) and *niacin.* Attention has also focused on the role of HDL–cholesterol as an important predictor of survival following coronary revascularization, with low-HDL–cholesterol (<35 mg/dL) a predictor of decreased survival. Weight loss, aerobic exercise, and medications such as niacin and gemfibrazole may be of value in this setting (19,20).

COMPLICATIONS OF PROSTHETIC VALVES

Infection

Bacterial endocarditis is a potential risk in any patient who has undergone cardiac surgery, even after isolated mitral valve repair (21–24). Dental procedures, particularly those involving the gums (including professional cleaning), and certain surgical and endoscopic procedures carry the highest incidence of associated bacteremia. Accordingly, patients undergoing these and related procedures should be considered for effective antibiotic prophylaxis (25–28). Because the risk of endocarditis for patients who have undergone prior cardiac procedures varies based on the nature of the procedure, guidelines regarding antibiotic prophylaxis have been developed. For example, patients who underwent prior CABG or uncomplicated atrial septal defect repair >6 months previously are at very low risk of subsequent endocarditis, and accordingly, prophylaxis is not indicated. In contrast, those with previously placed prosthetic valves do require prophylactic antibiotic treatment whenever undergoing procedures that may cause bacteremia. Appendix 2 shows the American Heart Association recommendations for the prevention of bacterial endocarditis (25). Patients who are at risk and who sustain open injuries must have meticulous wound care and be monitored carefully for potential wound infections; the threshold to treat suspected early cellulitis should be lower than that for patients who are not at risk for endocarditis.

Historically, *prosthetic valve endocarditis* (PVE) has been a highly lethal disease. However, with contemporary antibiotics and an aggressive surgical approach to patients with antibiotic-resistant endocarditis, the current potential for cure has become greater (28,29). Any patient with a prosthetic valve who is febrile without an easily identifiable source must be considered as possibly having PVE (27,30). These patients should undergo multiple blood cultures, ideally during the onset of a fever spike. The physical examination may reveal evidence of heart failure, new paravalvular leaks (regurgitant murmur), and/or evidence of metastatic infection. Echocardiography, most often transesophageal, is an important feature of making the diagnosis as this can demonstrate leakage around the valve and the presence of vegetations.

The treatment plan for PVE depends on the features of the presentation. Patients with fever and positive blood cultures but no hemodynamic deterioration are initially treated with high-dose antibiotic therapy. The drug is selected on the basis of culture data and optimized according to blood levels and quantitative bactericidal studies. If treatment results in fever resolution and if there is no evidence of prosthetic valve dysfunction, metastatic infection, or emboli, the antibiotics are continued for 6 weeks. Following this, the antibiotics are discontinued, and patients are observed and recultured if recurrent fever occurs.

Due to the presence of foreign material (the sewing ring of the prosthesis), PVE is less likely to be cured by antibiotics alone than is native valve endocarditis, particularly in cases that involve virulent organisms such as *Staphylococcus* sp. or fungi (31). Whereas the antibiotic cure rate for PVE caused by *Streptococcus viridans* may be as high as 80%, PVE due to *Staphylococcus* is cured by antimicrobial treatment alone in <25% of patients (32).

Antimicrobial treatment of fungal endocarditis fails in 99% of PVE cases. In PVE due to the more virulent organisms, erosion of the cardiac tissues is more common, resulting in paravalvular leaks, abscess formation, and detachment of the valve or a recently placed intracardiac patch. Conduction system abnormalities (e.g., heart block) or a fistula from the aorta to the right atrium may develop in patients with aortic valve PVE, especially if caused by *Staphylococcus*. Thus, early operation is usually indicated for the patients with PVE caused by organisms that are unlikely to be successfully treated with antimicrobial drugs. The occurrence of emboli despite antibiotic therapy is another indication for surgery. In virtually all instances of fungal endocarditis, early reoperation is required.

In patients with PVE receiving warfarin anticoagulation, we generally convert to heparin anticoagulation while the patient is hospitalized in case urgent operation is needed. Stroke is a significant risk in patients with PVE, and it is not always prevented by anticoagulation (33).

Echocardiography, in particular transesophageal echocardiography, can delineate the anatomy and provide the detail needed for surgery (34). If the PVE patient is being considered for surgery and possibly has coronary artery disease, coronary angiography may be needed. If, however, aortic valve vegetations are present, there is a risk of creating emboli; therefore, care must be taken in engaging the coronary ostia. In general, when surgery is needed for PVE, the infection often extends beyond the prosthesis, and surgery must be aggressive to extirpate all infected tissue. The infected valve may be successfully replaced with a mechanical valve or a tissue valve, depending on the patient's age and other factors affecting life expectancy (such as coronary artery disease, ventricular function, renal failure) (35). There has been considerable success using cryopreserved allografts for the treatment of PVE, even under emergency conditions, particularly in patients in whom considerable tissue destruction has occurred (36–38).

Deterioration of Tissue Prosthetic Valves

Glutaraldehyde-fixed xenograft (porcine) bioprosthetic valves offer patients the advantage of a low thromboembolic rate without the need for systemic anticoagulation (39). Although primary failure of tissue valves can occur early, the rate of failure generally begins to increase about 5 years after implantation. Younger patients, particularly those under 40 years old, suffer deterioration of bioprosthetic valves more rapidly, and in children, valve survival can be quite short (2 to 3 years) (40,41). Bovine pericardial bioprostheses appear to have greater durability than porcine aortic bioprostheses, with freedom from structural valve deterioration at 94% 10 years after implantation and at 77% 15 years after implantation (42). These findings suggest that this type of aortic prosthesis is appropriate for adults older than 65 years, with some surgeons implanting this prosthesis in patients in their early 60s (43). In the mitral position, porcine bioprosthetic valves may deteriorate prematurely in patients over a wide range of ages, including in the elderly (44). Thus, we usually use mechanical valves in the mitral position even in older patients unless the patient has a predictably limited expected lifespan. If there is a contraindication to long-term warfarin anticoagulation, it is necessary to use bioprosthetic aortic and mitral prostheses. The longevity of patients who have both valvular and coronary artery disease is usually determined by the natural history of the coronary atherosclerosis. Thus, in patients undergoing combined valve replacement and CABG, bioprosthetic valves are often used. This is because their long-term survival is more likely limited by the coronary artery disease (especially when extensive) than by future valve deterioration.

Tissue prostheses are subject to leaflet calcification or fracture, resulting in valve regurgitation or, less commonly, stenosis. Valve failure may occur as a gradual process over a few years, and in these patients, symptoms develop slowly. Or it may occur in a more acute fashion with the rather sudden onset of symptoms. Most commonly, the presentation is that of congestive heart failure.

Malfunction of Mechanical Valves

Low-profile mechanical valves incorporating pyrolytic carbon components are the most commonly used mechanical valve prostheses in the United States. The present generation of valves offers patients relatively low thromboembolic rates—less than those observed in prior decades with earlier mechanical prostheses (45); contemporary valves also have excellent flow characteristics, even in smaller sizes. In contrast to the experience with caged ball and tilting disk valves implanted in the 1960s and 1970s, contemporary mechanical valves are not subject to problems related to pannus ingrowth.

If inadequate anticoagulation is allowed to persist, contemporary mechanical prostheses are prone to thrombosis. This may present as either stroke or peripheral emboli or with prosthetic valve dysfunction. Bileaflet carbon prostheses can thrombose, especially in the mitral position. Because closing forces are greater than opening forces in the mitral position, if bileaflet valve thrombosis occurs, it often presents as one of the two leaflets failing to open, producing prosthetic stenosis. Thrombolytic therapy can be used to treat prosthetic valve thrombosis, especially in very ill patients who are at high risk for surgery. There is, however a significant risk of clot embolization (about 20%) and rethrombosis (46,47). Hence, unless there is a significant contraindication to surgery, reoperation is most often indicated. This topic is also discussed in Chapter 1.

Paravalvular Leaks

In the early decades of cardiac surgery, paravalvular leaks were recognized with some frequency, estimated at 14% for valves placed in the aortic position and at 9% for valves placed in the mitral position (48). However, with improved surgical techniques (including the use of pledget-reinforced sutures) and with the decreasing frequency of patients undergoing valve surgery for advanced rheumatic heart disease (with associated annular calcification), the incidence of significant paravalvular leaks has been reduced to <1%. The use of intraoperative transesophageal echocardiography (after weaning the patient from bypass but before closing the chest) provides for detection of paravalvular leaks in the operating room that may be a result of technical factors, which can be corrected at the time of primary implantation.

Occasionally, paravalvular leaks, particularly around mitral prostheses, may be silent. Trauma to the red blood cells can result in hemolytic anemia; this may be the only clue that a paravalvular leak is present. Patients with persistent anemia after valve replacement should be evaluated by echocardiography for paravalvular leaks. Laboratory evaluation will often demonstrate fragmented erythrocytes and elevated lactate dehydrogenase level. Significant anemia, particularly if there is a transfusion requirement or hemodynamic compromise, mandates reoperation. Although it is tempting to close paravalvular leaks by primary suture, their boundaries are often rigid, consisting of the prosthetic sewing ring and a fibrotic or calcified annulus. Unless primary suture closes the defect with little tension, consideration must be given to closing a paravalvular leak with a patch or by rereplacement, often increasing the size of the prosthesis.

Subclinical hemolysis may also occur due to a prosthetic valve, even in the absence of a paravalvular leak. This is most common with the mechanical prostheses with a low incidence in stented tissue valves. The presence of subclinical hemolysis is evidenced by elevated lactic dehydrogenase levels, although in the absence of a paravalvular leak, anemia does not usually occur (49).

Thromboembolism

Patients with prosthetic valves are at risk for thrombotic complications, and the risk is greater for valves in the mitral position than the aortic. Whereas the risk is <1% per year for patients with biological (tissue) valves, mechanical valves are at higher risk and, thus, require lifelong warfarin anticoagulation. For patients with mechanical valves, good long-term anticoagulation control (minimizing variability in the degree of anticoagulation) is associated with improved long-term survival (50). Even with "adequate" warfarin treatment, the incidence of thromboemboli in patients with mechanical valves is 1% to 2% per year (51). Previously, the prothrombin time was used to express the degree of anticoagulation. However, this laboratory test uses thromboplastin, and variability in thromboplastin responsiveness to warfarin-induced reductions in vitamin K-dependent clotting factors causes variability in prothrombin time determinations. To compensate for this variability in thromboplastin activity, the international normalized ratio (INR) was developed (52). The optimum INR range for prosthetic valves has been the subject of numerous studies, reviews, and consensus committees (53–55). Currently recommended guidelines are shown in Table 6-1. These recommendations take into account the type of valve (mechanical versus tissue) and the presence or absence of additional risk factors such as prior thromboembolism and atrial fibrillation. Patients with prosthetic heart valves receiving warfarin may also be treated with aspirin. This combined therapy reduces the rate of thromboembolism and total mortality but increases the rate of bleeding complications somewhat (56). Low-dose aspirin (80 to 100 mg daily) may have a lower bleeding rate than conventional dose. Aspirin therapy, in addition to warfarin, should be considered for all patients with mechanical prostheses who have additional risk

Table 6-1. Antithrombotic therapy[a]—prostheticheart valves

	Mechanical Prosthetic Valves			Biological Prosthetic Valves		
	Warfarin, INR 2–3	Warfarin, INR 2.5–3.5	Aspirin, 50–100 mg	Warfarin, INR 2–3	Warfarin, INR 2.5–3.5	Aspirin, 50–100 mg
First 3 mo after valve replacement		+	+		+	+
After first 3 mo						
Aortic valve	+		+			+
Aortic valve + risk factor[b]		+	+	+		
Mitral valve		+	+			+
Mitral valve + risk factor		+	+		+	+

INR, international normalized ratio.
[a]Depending on the clinical status of patient, antithrombotic therapy must be individualized.
[b]Risk factors: atrial fibrillation, previous thromboembolus, left ventricular dysfunction, hypercoagulable state.
From O'Rourke RA, Fuster V, Alexander RW, et al., eds. *Hurst's the heart manual of cardiology,* 10th ed. New York: McGraw Hill, 2001: 491, with permission.

factors such as a prosthesis in the mitral position, thromboembolism on warfarin alone, atrial fibrillation, coronary artery disease, large left atrium, documented left atrial thrombus, or more than one prosthetic valve. Generally, patients with previously implanted ball-in-cage mechanical prostheses are maintained with an INR of at least 3.0 in addition to daily aspirin.

Patients who receive tissue prosthetic valves and who are in sinus rhythm do not require lifelong warfarin treatment. They are, however, at increased risk for thrombus formation during the first 3 months following valve implantation, especially for mitral prostheses. Thus, unless contraindications exist, anticoagulation for 3 months is generally recommended, although this opinion is not universal (55,57,58). Long-term (after the initial 3 months has passed) aspirin therapy is recommended. If the patient with a bioprosthetic valve does have atrial fibrillation, continued warfarin therapy is usually indicated on that basis (59).

Anticoagulation treatment for patients with prosthetic valves begins when the patients are able to take medications orally. We do not use a loading dose of warfarin as it is undesirable for postoperative patients to exceed their INR goal and there is the potential for causing a temporary prothrombotic state (60). If the patient's maintenance dose is known from prior warfarin therapy, this is initiated postoperatively. For patients who are receiving warfarin for the first time, we generally start with a dose of 2.5 to 5.0 mg per day and follow the INR daily during the early postoperative period (61). The lower initial dose is used in patients who have had elevated right-sided filling pressures, any evidence of hepatic dysfunction, or long-standing cardiac cachexia. The dose is then increased by 1.0 to 2.5 mg every day or every other day until the INR begins to rise. After discharge, the INR is checked regularly (initially two to three times per week, then weekly) until a stable level is demonstrated, at which time the interval between determinations may be lengthened. With continued patient recovery and, in particular, improvement in postoperative nutrition, the dose may need to be increased gradually above the amount needed during the early postoperative period.

The response of patients to warfarin is quite variable, and patients with hereditary resistance have been described (62). Generally, the onset of action is not until at least 24 hours after the first dose, and the full effect is not reached for 72 to 96 hours. Many drugs may interfere with warfarin anticoagulation (and alter the INR) either by depressing or accelerating hepatic metabolism or by enhancing or interfering with warfarin–protein binding; patients must be aware of these (Table 6-2). Patients should also be aware that dietary intake of vitamin K may affect the INR; they should be urged to be relatively consistent in their dietary habits. Foods containing relatively large amounts of vitamin K include broccoli, cabbage, collard greens, mustard greens, peas, spinach, and pickles (63).

LONG-TERM ISSUES IN PATIENTS RECEIVING WARFARIN

Patients taking warfarin are at risk for hemorrhage, either related to excessive anticoagulation or secondary to other medical conditions. Management of the excessively prolonged INR anti-

Table 6-2. Drug interactions with warfarin

Drug	Effect on Anticoagulation
Acetaminophen	Increase
Allopurinol	Increase
Amiodarone	Increase
Barbiturate	Decrease
Carbamazepine	Decrease
Cholestyramine	Decrease
Cimetidine	Increase
Ciprofloxacin	Increase
Clofibrate	Increase
Dicloxacillin	Decrease
Gemfibrozil	Increase
Griseofulvin	Decrease
Lovastatin	Increase
Metronidazole	Increase
Nafcillin	Decrease
Neomycin	Increase
Omeprazole	Increase
Phenytoin	Decrease
Propafenone	Increase
Propoxyphene	Increase
Quinidine	Increase
Sucralfate	Decrease
Vitamin E	Increase
Vitamin K	Decrease
Zafirlukast	Increase

Note: This list includes many of the drugs that might be administered to heart surgery patients, but does not include all drugs that are known to affect warfarin's action.

coagulation takes into account magnitude of the INR and whether or not there is bleeding present (64). If the INR is above therapeutic but below 5.0, a dose or two of warfarin is omitted, and the INR is rechecked; dosage adjustment is probably in order. If the INR exceeds 5.0 without bleeding but the patient is at risk for bleeding or if urgent surgery is required, a small oral dose of vitamin K (1 to 2.5 mg) may be given. It will take about 24 hours for the INR to be reduced. If the INR exceeds 9.0 without bleeding, warfarin should be held, a larger dose of oral vitamin K (3 to 5 mg) may be given, and when the INR is within therapeutic range, warfarin may be restarted at a lower dose with more frequent INR monitoring. In general, if serious bleeding is not present, oral vitamin K is preferred to the intravenous route (64). If the INR is very elevated and serious bleeding is present, intravenous vitamin K, 10 mg, is given by slow infusion and is supplemented with fresh frozen plasma or prothrombin complex concentrate, as dictated by the clinical circumstance. Vitamin K is avoided, if at all possible, in patients who have mechanical prosthetic valves in place as rapid normalization of the INR may precipitate valve thrombosis. Following correction of the INR (and management of bleeding), reinstitution of anticoagulation may be begun with heparin infusion; this may require additional time to overcome resistance to warfarin caused by the previously administered vitamin K.

Pregnancy presents a special problem in patients who require warfarin anticoagulation for prosthetic heart valves. Warfarin is teratogenic in a dose-dependent manner (65). The teratogenic effect can be prevented if warfarin is omitted during the first 12 weeks of gestation (to avoid embryopathy) and near term (to avoid delivery of an anticoagulated baby) (66,67). During these times, anticoagulation can be achieved using an aggressive adjusted-dose unfractionated subcutaneous heparin protocol (monitoring the activated prothrombin time or the anti-Xa heparin level) or by using a weight-adjusted subcutaneous low molecular weight heparin protocol (monitoring anti-Xa levels to adjust the dose). Neither form of heparin appears to cross the placenta. With use of this regimen, warfarin treatment is used beginning week 13 and up to the middle of the last trimester. Alternative regimens include the use of subcutaneous unfractionated heparin or low molecular weight heparin throughout the entire pregnancy. Of note, low-dose aspirin appears to be safe during the second and third trimesters of pregnancy.

PERICARDITIS AND DELAYED PERICARDIAL TAMPONADE

Delayed postoperative pericardial effusions can occur in any patient who has undergone cardiac surgery (68,69), whether the pericardium was left open or closed and even if the pleural spaces were entered during sternotomy. The boundaries of the pericardial space will seal in the first 1 to 2 weeks after surgery; thus, despite what appears to be adequate drainage at the time of operation, the pericardial space can once again become "closed." Serous or serosanguinous effusions can occur from pericarditis. Sometimes, the presence of evolving pericarditis may be suggested while patients are in the hospital by the presence of pain, a pericardial rub, and/or fever after surgery. Such patients are treated with a nonsteroidal antiinflammatory agent such as indomethacin. Indomethacin does have the potential for renal toxicity, and therefore, the patient's creatinine level should be checked, especially if heart failure is present. Pericarditis and pericardial effusions may also develop in the weeks after surgery. When seeing the patient postoperatively, the surgeon must be alert to nonspecific complaints such as malaise, slow progress, lack of energy, or sometimes nausea and anorexia. Heart sounds may be muffled on examination. The neck veins may be distended, and paradox may be present when the blood pressure is determined. The QRS voltage of the ECG may be diminished. Fluid retention and weight gain may occur despite use of diuretics, and blood urea nitrogen level may be elevated out of proportion to the creatinine level and the fluid status. If pericarditis is suspected, an echocardiogram is in order.

In some patients, particularly those taking warfarin, bleeding into the pericardial space can occur (70). In such instances, the pericardial effusion can progress rapidly to subacute tamponade, necessitating urgent hospitalization. In addition, pericardial effusions can increase venous pressure, resulting in hepatic congestion, increased sensitivity to warfarin, and, consequently, out-of-range anticoagulation. Most pericardial effusions and delayed tamponade may be managed by percutaneous drainage with pericardial catheters, antiinflammatory treatment as indicated, and adjustment of the INR if excessively prolonged (71). In the case of recurrent effusions refractory to medical therapy and repeated percutaneous drainage, creation of a pericardial "window" may be indicated. This surgically created pericardial defect allows for drainage of the pericardial fluid into the pleural space where there are more room and surface area for absorption. In very unusual cases, delayed pericardial tamponade may be the result of chylous effusions (72). These are managed by prolonged drainage, institution of a low-fat or no-fat diet, or, if needed, intravenous hyperalimentation. Once discharged from the hospital after treatment of delayed pericardial effusions, the patient undergoes follow-up echocardiograms to ensure that the effusions have not recurred.

A late complication of postoperative pericarditis is pericardial constriction (73). In this condition, the heart becomes encased by the thickened, noncompliant pericardium with resultant impaired diastolic filling of the ventricles and venous congestion. The patient presents with fatigue, dyspnea, weight gain, ascites, liver enlargement, and edema. Echocardiography (to demonstrate abnormal ventricular filling), computed tomography (to evaluate pericardial thickness), and cardiac catheterization are used to make the diagnosis (74). Treatment of constrictive pericarditis usually involves pericardiectomy, a procedure of significant morbidity and mortality, but long-term relief of symptoms is achieved in most patients (75).

REFERENCES

1. Eagle KA, Guyton RA, Davidoff R, et al. ACC/AHA Guidelines for Coronary Artery Bypass Graft Surgery: a report of the American Heart Association/American College of Cardiology Task Force on Practice Guidelines (Committee to Revise the 1991 Guidelines for Coronary Artery Bypass Surgery). *J Am Coll Cardiol* 1999;34: 1262–1346.
2. Cupples SA. Effects of timing and reinforcement of preoperative education on knowledge and recovery of patients having coronary bypass graft surgery. *Heart Lung* 1991;20:654–660.
3. Savage PD, Brochu M, Scott P, et al. Low caloric expenditure in cardiac rehabilitation. *Am Heart J* 2000;140:527–533.
4. Myles PS, Hunt JO, Fletcher H, et al. Relation between quality of recovery in hospital and quality of life at 3 months after cardiac surgery. *Anesthesiology* 2001;95:862–867.
5. Liddle HV, Jensen R, Clayton PD. The rehabilitation of coronary surgical patients. *Ann Thorac Surg* 1981;34:374.
6. McConnell TR, Klinger TA, Gardner JK, et al. Cardiac rehabilitation without exercise tests for post-myocardial infarction and post-bypass surgery patients. *J Cardiopulm Rehabil* 1998;18:458–463.
7. Lawrie GM, Morris GC Jr, Earle N. Long-term results of coronary bypass surgery. Analysis of 1698 patients followed 15 to 20 years. *Ann Surg* 1991;213:377–385.
8. FitzGibbon GM, Leach A, Keon WJ, et al. Coronary bypass graft patency. Angiographic study of 1179 vein grafts early, one year,

and five years after operation. *J Thorac Cardiovasc Surg* 1986;91: 773–778.
9. FitzGibbon GM, Leach AJ, Kafka HP, et al. Coronary bypass graft fate: long-term angiographic study. *J Am Coll Cardiol* 1991;17: 1075–1080.
10. Fuster V, Chesbro JH. Role of platelets and platelet inhibition in aortocoronary artery vein graft disease. *Circulation* 1986;73: 227–232.
11. Goldman S, Copeland J, Moritz T, et al. Saphenous vein graft patency 1 year after coronary bypass surgery and effects of antiplatelet therapy. Results of a Veterans Administration Cooperative Study. *Circulation* 1989;80:1190–1197.
12. Goldman S, Copeland J, Moritz, et al. Starting aspirin therapy after operation: effects on early graft patency. *Circulation* 1991;84: 520–526.
13. Final report on the aspirin component of the ongoing Physicians' Health Study. Steering Committee of the Physicians' Health Study Research Group. *N Engl J Med* 1989;321:129–135.
14. Marso SP. Optimizing the diabetic formulary: beyond aspirin and insulin. *J Am Coll Cardiol* 2002;40:652–661.
15. Bates ER. Raising high-density lipoprotein cholesterol and lowering low-density lipoprotein cholesterol as adjunctive therapy to coronary artery revascularization (Review). *Am J Cardiol* 2000;86: 28L–34L.
16. Foody JM, Ferdinand FD, Pearce GL, et al. HDL cholesterol level predicts survival in men after coronary artery bypass graft surgery: 20-year experience from The Cleveland Clinic. *Circulation* 2000; 102(suppl III):III90–III94.
17. White CW, Gobel FL, Campeau L, et al. Effect of an aggressive lipid-lowering strategy on progression of atherosclerosis in the left main coronary artery form patients in the post coronary bypass graft trial. *Circulation* 2001;104:2660–2665.
18. McEvoy GK, ed. *Antilipemic agents. American Hospital Formulary Services drug information 2002.* Bethesda: American Society of Health-System Pharmacists, 2002:1755–1769.
19. Frick MH, Syvanne M, Nieminen MS, et al. Prevention of the angiographic progression of coronary and vein-graft atherosclerosis by gemfibrazole after coronary bypass surgery in men with low levels of HDL cholesterol. Lopid Coronary Angiography Trial (LOCAT) Study Group. *Circulation* 1997;96:2137–2143.
20. Sprecher DL. Raising high-density lipoprotein cholesterol with niacin and fibrates: a comparative review (Review). *Am J Cardiol* 2000;86:46L–50L.
21. Kaplan EL, Rich H, Gersony W, et al. A collaborative study of infective endocarditis in the 1980s. Emphasis on infections in patients who have undergone cardiovascular surgery. *Circulation* 1979; 59:327.
22. Mylonakis E, Calderwood SB. Infective endocarditis in adults. *N Engl J Med* 2001;345:1318–1330.
23. Bayer AS, Bolger AF, Taubert KA, et al. Diagnosis and management of infective endocarditis and its complications. AHA scientific statement. *Circulation* 1998;98:2936–2948.
24. Gillinov MA, Faber NC, Sabik JF, et al. Endocarditis after mitral valve repair. *Ann Thorac Surg* 2002;73:1813–1816.

25. Dajani AS, Taubert KA, Wilson W, et al. Prevention of bacterial endocarditis: recommendations by the American Heart Association. AHA statement. *Circulation* 1997;96:358–366.
26. Imperiale TF, Horwitz RI. Does prophylaxis prevent postdental infective endocarditis? *Am J Med* 1990;88:131–136.
27. Heimberger TS, Duma RJ. Infection of prosthetic heart valves and cardiac pacemakers. *Infect Dis Clin North Am* 1989;3:221–245.
28. Karchmer AW. Prosthetic valve endocarditis: a continuing challenge for infection control. *J Hosp Infect* 1991;18(suppl A):355–366.
29. Gordon SM, Serkey JM, Longworth DL, et al. Early onset prosthetic valve endocarditis: the Cleveland Clinic experience 1992–1997. *Ann Thorac Surg* 2000;69:1388–1392.
30. Masur H, Johnson WD Jr. Prosthetic valve endocarditis. *J Thorac Cardiovasc Surg* 1980;80:31–37.
31. Tornos P, Sanz E, Permanyer-Miralda G, et al. Late prosthetic endocarditis. Immediate and long-term prognosis. *Chest* 1992; 101:37–41.
32. Naidu R, O'Rourke RA. Infective endocarditis. In: O'Rourke RA, Fuster V, Alexander RW, et al., eds. *Hurst's the heart manual of cardiology,* 10th ed. New York: McGraw-Hill, 2001:593–615.
33. Davenport J, Hart RG. Prosthetic valve endocarditis 1976–1987. Antibiotics, anticoagulation, and stroke. *Stroke* 1990;21:993–999.
34. Daniel WG, Mugge A, Martin RP, et al. Improvement in the diagnosis of abscesses associated with endocarditis by transesophageal echocardiography. *N Engl J Med* 1991;324:795–800.
35. Moon MR, Moller DC, Moore KA, et al. Treatment of endocarditis with valve replacement; the question of tissue versus mechanical prosthesis. *Ann Thorac Surg* 2001;71:1164–1171.
36. David TE. The surgical treatment of patients with prosthetic valve endocarditis (Review). *Semin Thorac Cardiovasc Surg* 1995;7: 47–53.
37. Lupinetti FM, Lemmer JH Jr. Emergency aortic valve replacement for endocarditis: comparison of allografts and prosthetic valves. *Am J Cardiol* 1991;68:637–641.
38. Sabik JF, Lytle BW, Blackstone EH, et al. Aortic root replacement with cryopreserved allograft for prosthetic valve endocarditis. *Ann Thorac Surg* 2002;74:650–659.
39. Burdon TA, Miller DC, Oyer PE, et al. Durability of porcine valves at fifteen years in a representative North American population. *J Thorac Cardiovasc Surg* 1992;103:231–251.
40. Dunn JM. Porcine valve durability in children. *Ann Thorac Surg* 1981;32:357.
41. Fiddler GI, Gerlis LM, Path FRC, et al. Calcification of glutaraldehyde-preserved porcine and bovine xenograft valves in young children. *Ann Thorac Surg* 1983;35:257.
42. Banbury MK, Cosgrove DM III, White JA, et al. Age and valve size effect on the long-term durability of the Carpentier–Edwards aortic pericardial bioprosthesis. *Ann Thorac Surg* 2001;72:753–757.
43. Hammermeister K, Sethi GK, Henderson WG, et al. Outcomes 15 years after valve replacement with a mechanical versus a bioprosthetic valve: final report of the Veterans Affairs Randomized Trial. *J Am Cardiol Coll* 2000;36:1152–1158.
44. Akins CW, Carroll DL, Buckley MJ, et al. Late results with Carpentier–Edwards porcine bioprosthesis. *Circulation* 1990; 82(suppl IV):IV65–IV74.

45. Antunes MJ. Clinical performance of St. Jude and Medtronic–Hall prostheses; a randomized comparative study. *Ann Thorac Surg* 1990;50:743–747.
46. Gupta D, Kothari SS, Bahl VK, et al. Thrombolytic therapy for prosthetic valve thrombosis: short- and long-term results. *Am Heart J* 2000;140:906–916.
47. Mantiega R, Carlos Souto C, Altes A, et al. Short-course thrombolysis as the first line of therapy for cardiac valve thrombosis. *J Thorac Cardiovasc Surg* 1998;115:780–784.
48. Kastor JA, Akbarian M, Buckley MJ, et al. Paravalvular leaks and hemolytic anemia following insertion of Starr–Edwards aortic and mitral valves. *J Thorac Cardiovasc Surg* 1968;56:279.
49. Mecozzi G, Milano AD, De Carlo M, et al. Intravascular hemolysis in patients with new-generation prosthetic heart valves: a prospective study. *J Thorac Cardiovasc Surg* 2002;123:550–556.
50. Butchart EG, Payne N, Li H-H, et al. Better anticoagulation control improves survival after valve replacement. *Ann Thorac Surg* 2002;123:715–723.
51. McAnulty JH, Rahimtoola SH. Antithrombotic therapy for valvular heart disease. In: O'Rourke RA, Fuster V, Alexander RW, et al., eds. *Hurst's the heart manual of cardiology*. New York: McGraw-Hill, 2001:483–492.
52. Hirsh J, Fuster V. Guide to anticoagulant therapy. Part 2. Oral anticoagulants. *Circulation* 1994;89:1469–1480.
53. Tiede DJ, Nishimura RA, Gastineau DA, et al. Modern management of prosthetic valve anticoagulation (Review). *Mayo Clin Proc* 1998;73:665–680.
54. Bonow RO, Carabello B, de Leon AC Jr, et al. ACC/AHA Guidelines for the Management of Patients with Valvular Heart Disease: executive summary. A report of the American College of Cardiology/American Heart Association Task Force on Practice Guidelines (Committee on Management of Patients with Valvular Heart Disease). *Circulation* 1998;98:1949–1984.
55. Stein PD, Alpert JS, Bussey HI, et al. Antithrombotic therapy in patients with mechanical and biological prosthetic heart valves. Sixth ACCP Consensus Conference on Antithrombotic Therapy. *Chest* 2001;119:220S–227S.
56. Massel D, Little SH. Risks and benefits of adding anti-platelet therapy to warfarin among patients with prosthetic heart valves: a meta-analysis. *J Am Coll Cardiol* 2001;37:569–578.
57. Heras M, Chesebro JH, Fuster V, et al. High risk of thromboemboli early after bioprosthetic cardiac valve replacement. *J Am Coll Cardiol* 1995;25:1111–1119.
58. Moinuddeen K, Quin J, Shaw R, et al. Anticoagulation is unnecessary after biological aortic valve replacement. *Circulation* 1998; 98(suppl):1195–1199.
59. Fuster V, Ryden LE, Asinger RW, et al. ACC/AHA/ESC Guidelines for the Management of Patients with Atrial Fibrillation: executive summary. *J Am Coll Cardiol* 2001;38:1231–1265.
60. Harrison L, Johnston M, Massicotte MP, et al. Comparison of 5-mg and 10-mg loading doses in initiation of warfarin therapy. *Ann Intern Med* 1997;126:133–136.
61. Ageno W, Turpie AG, Steidl L, et al. Comparison of a daily fixed 2.5-mg warfarin dose with a 5-mg, international normalized ratio adjusted, warfarin dose initially following heart valve replacement. *Am J Cardiol* 2001;88:40–44.

62. Hirsh J, Dalen JE, Anderson DR, et al. Oral anticoagulants: mechanism of action, clinical effectiveness, and optimal therapeutic range. Sixth ACCP Consensus Conference on Antithrombotic Therapy. *Chest* 2001;119:8S–21S.
63. Booth SL, Sadowski JA, Pennington JAT. Phylloquinone (vitamin K) content of food in the US Food and Drug Administrations Total Diet Study. *J Agric Food Chem* 1995;43:1574–1579.
64. Ansell J, Hirsh J, Dalen J, et al. Managing oral anticoagulant therapy. Sixth ACCP Consensus Conference on Antithrombotic Therapy. *Chest* 2001;119:22S–38S.
65. Vitale N, DeFeo M, DeSanto LS, et al. Dose-dependent fetal complications of warfarin in pregnant women with mechanical heart valves. *J Am Coll Cardiol* 1999;33:1637–1641.
66. Lee CN, Wu CC, Lin PY, et al. Pregnancy following cardiac prosthetic valve replacement. *Obstet Gynecol* 1994;83:353–356.
67. Ginsberg JS, Greer I, Hirsh J. Use of antithrombotic agents during pregnancy. Sixth ACCP Consensus Conference on Antithrombotic Therapy. *Chest* 2001;119:122S–131S.
68. Khan AH. The postcardiac injury syndrome. *Clin Cardiol* 1992; 15:67–72.
69. Ikaheimo MJ, Huikuri HV, Airaksinen KE, et al. Pericardial effusion after cardiac surgery: incidence, relation to the type of surgery, antithrombotic therapy, and early coronary bypass graft patency. *Am Heart J* 1988;116:97–102.
70. Ofori-Krakye SK, Tyberg TI, Geha AS, et al. Late cardiac tamponade after open heart surgery: incidence, role of anticoagulants in its pathogenesis and its relationship to postpericardiotomy syndrome. *Circulation* 1981;63:1323–1328.
71. Mangi AA, Palacios IF, Torchiana DF. Catheter pericardiocentesis for delayed tamponade after cardiac valve operation. *Ann Thorac Surg* 2002;73:1479–1483.
72. Thomas CS Jr, McGoon DC. Isolated massive chylopericardium following cardiopulmonary bypass. *J Thorac Cardiovasc Surg* 1971;61:945–948.
73. Killian DM, Furiasse JG, Scanlon PJ, et al. Constrictive pericarditis after cardiac surgery. *Am Heart J* 1989;118:563–568.
74. Myers RB, Spodick DH. Constrictive pericarditis: clinical and pathophysiologic characteristics. *Am Heart J* 1999;138:219–232.
75. Ling LH, Oh JK, Schaff HV, et al. Constrictive pericarditis in the modern era: evolving clinical spectrum and impact on outcome after pericardiectomy. *Circulation* 1999;100:1380–1386.

Management of Infants and Children

DIAGNOSTIC CONSIDERATIONS

A prompt and accurate anatomic diagnosis is essential for proper surgical management of the patient with congenital heart disease. Clinical presentation, physical examination, and even the chest x-ray film and electrocardiogram may be difficult to interpret or may only narrow minimally the diagnostic possibilities. For most patients, echocardiography can elucidate the anatomic basis for proper patient management.

Cardiac catheterization and angiocardiography were once the gold standard for congenital diagnosis. Whereas these techniques define anatomy angiographically, measure gradients, and quantify shunts, in some patients, such as very small infants, they may be technically more difficult, and certain risks are inevitable. Echocardiography, on the other hand, has none of the risks of cardiac catheterization. Although it may not define the anatomy of some malformations as well as catheterization, it is superior for others, and it permits frequent reassessments, including early intra- and postoperative evaluation, and for many lesions, high-quality echo eliminates the need for catheterization (1).

Brief Review of Common Lesions

Septal Defects

The most common congenital heart anomaly requiring operative correction is the ventricular septal defect (VSD). Preoperative evaluation is usually accomplished by echocardiography, which can assess the number and location of VSDs. VSDs in infants that have unrestricted blood flow through them produce systemic pulmonary hypertension and should be closed by 3 months of age to minimize the risk of postoperative pulmonary hypertension.

Most children and adults with atrial septal defects undergo operation based on echocardiography alone. Catheterization is sometimes considered if percutaneous closure is being considered, in which case defect sizing is performed with sizing balloons. In children with atrial or ventricular septal defects, the postoperative care is usually straightforward, although elevated pulmonary artery pressure may complicate the patient's course, particularly in those with VSDs that are closed beyond 3 or 4 months of age. In patients with unrestrictive VSDs who present late (older than 4 to 6 months), cardiac catheterization may be needed to assess the pulmonary circulation. Knowledge of whether the pulmonary vascular resistance falls in response to oxygen or vasodilators such as inhaled nitric oxide is helpful in planning the postoperative care.

Complete Atrioventricular Canal

Complete atrioventricular canal is accurately defined by echocardiography; this diagnostic modality gives critical information about atrioventricular valve anatomy and function. As in the case of VSDs, preoperative catheterization may be useful in evaluating the degree of the patient's pulmonary vascular resistance, particularly when repair is delayed beyond 4 or 5 months of age. The size of the two ventricles must be assessed to ascertain that they are "balanced" to permit repair with separate left and right ventricles. Postoperative care can be challenging if there is atrioventricular valve regurgitation or significant pulmonary hypertension in the postoperative period. These patients are especially prone to having spells of pulmonary vascular hypertensive crises postoperatively, and this must be planned for. This aspect of complete atrioventricular canal postoperative management is greatly aided by having a pulmonary artery catheter placed at the time of surgery, not only for the postoperative measurement of pulmonary artery pressure but also to permit blood sampling to measure pulmonary artery saturation and hence detect any residual shunts. Because atrioventricular valve function is sometimes an issue after correction, proper postoperative monitoring of atrial pressures is useful for assessing the mitral and tricuspid valves.

Tetralogy of Fallot

Tetralogy of Fallot sometimes requires cineangiography, particularly to define the anatomy of the pulmonary arteries and coronary arteries. Whereas much of this information can be ascertained by a high-quality echocardiogram, if there is any doubt as to whether or not an anomalous coronary artery crosses the right ventricular outflow tract or in cases of small pulmonary arteries, cineangiography may be needed. For the majority of patients with tetralogy of Fallot, primary complete repair is performed, unless there are very extenuating circumstances. In neonates with very small pulmonary arteries, occasionally a systemic-to-pulmonary shunt may be constructed to the central pulmonary arteries or right ventricular outflow tract reconstruction may be utilized, leaving the VSD open initially.

In the immediate postoperative period after complete repair, postoperative care requires particular attention to the function of the right ventricle, which usually has been incised to permit relief of outflow tract obstruction. Particularly when transannular outflow tract reconstruction has been performed, these patients sometimes experience low cardiac output early after surgery, during which they must be ventilated, carefully monitored, and supported with inotropic agents. In a prior era, some of these patients experienced severe low output after correction because of failure of the right ventricle. Particularly when corrections have been carried out early in the first few months of life, this potential problem may be managed by leaving open a patent foramen ovale. Thus, if right heart failure occurs after surgery, elevated right atrial pressure produces a right-to-left shunt at the atrial level. The result is some systemic desaturation with maintenance of good systemic ventricular output. As right ventricular function recovers during the first 3 to 5 days after surgery, this shunt diminishes with decreased right atrial pressure.

Postoperative management of tetralogy patients is facilitated by having a catheter introduced into the pulmonary artery across the right ventricular outflow tract. This permits blood sampling from the pulmonary artery to detect residual shunts and, at the time of line removal, permits the detection of any residual right ventricular outflow tract gradient. Obtaining this information in the postoperative period is useful during subsequent late follow-up.

Pulmonary Atresia with Ventricular Septal Defect

Pulmonary atresia with VSD may be considered a very severe form of tetralogy. Cardiac catheterization is useful in defining the ventricular anatomy and the size and location of the pulmonary arteries. When bronchial collaterals do not provide adequate pulmonary blood flow in the neonatal period, the patient is begun on prostaglandin E_1 (PGE_1) infusion to open the ductus arteriosus. Operation early in life consists of a shunt, with complete correction delayed until the child is much larger. In instances where a main pulmonary artery is present, initial palliation may also include a pulmonary valvotomy, an outflow tract patch, or a right ventricle-to-pulmonary artery conduit. Right ventricular outflow into the central pulmonary arteries can promote arterial growth. In these instances, postoperative care can be more complex because of the multiple sources of pulmonary blood flow.

Pulmonary Atresia with Intact Ventricular Septum

Pulmonary atresia with intact ventricular septum differs from pulmonary atresia with VSD in that the right ventricle is almost always very hypoplastic. PGE_1 again is useful in the newborn to stabilize the patient by increasing pulmonary blood flow. If the anatomy is suitable, valvotomy is performed both to improve pulmonary perfusion and, it is hoped, to stimulate right ventricular growth. A systemic-to-pulmonary shunt procedure is usually required as well. Critical pulmonic stenosis is usually associated with a more nearly normal right ventricle, and the response to percutaneous or surgical valvotomy is generally better. For both of these conditions, pulmonary resistance postoperatively must be kept as low as possible using oxygen, vasodilators, and optimal ventilatory management.

Transposition of the Great Arteries

Transposition of the great arteries is the commonest cause of cyanosis presenting in the neonatal period. As soon as the diagnosis is suspected, PGE_1 is begun to improve mixing across the ductus. Echocardiography is then performed to confirm the diagnosis and define anatomic detail, including the presence of concomitant lesions and left ventricular outflow tract obstruction, and to determine the coronary artery anatomy. An arterial switch operation is carried out within the first 2 weeks of life, unless some feature of the anatomy favors delay to an older age, at which time the type of correction is individualized.

Coarctation of the Aorta

Coarctation of the aorta varies in its presentation from profound congestive failure and peripheral hypoperfusion in neonates to asymptomatic hypertension in older children. In the critically ill newborn, PGE_1 may palliate severe coarctation until operation is performed, as it opens the ductus and restores distal aortic perfusion from the pulmonary artery. Echocardiography is usually adequate to detect the presence of the coarctation and any associated intracardiac defects. Surgical correction may be postponed for a few days in newborns if the PGE_1 is effective in restoring peripheral perfusion. This allows a semielective operation to be done on a stable patient. In older children, operation is done electively, usually to treat hypertension.

Patent Ductus Arteriosus

Patent ductus arteriosus is encountered commonly in premature infants with respiratory distress syndrome. Echocardiography establishes the diagnosis and excludes other significant intracardiac conditions such as an aortopulmonary window. In the newborn, indomethacin or ibuprofen may be used to attempt closure of the ductus without surgery. Operation is usually performed for difficulty in weaning from the ventilator or for severe congestive heart failure. In children, operation should be performed electively because of the long-term risk of endocarditis, as well as the risk of developing pulmonary vascular obstructive disease with a large patent ductus. In many instances, a patent ductus in an older infant or child may be closed percutaneously.

Aortic Stenosis

Aortic stenosis, depending on its severity, may cause symptoms at any age. Severe stenosis in infancy produces profound congestive failure and acidosis and requires emergency intervention. This extreme form is best managed with prompt echocardiographic diagnosis, followed by a brief period of medical stabilization with ventilation and vasopressor support before percutaneous or operative valvotomy. Milder forms of stenosis may be followed until symptoms occur or until the patient develops a sufficiently severe gradient that makes sudden death a risk.

Univentricular Heart

Univentricular heart encompasses a wide variety of anatomic configurations that share the common feature of having a single functional ventricular chamber. The associated defects and resultant physiology determine the clinical effects, degree of cyanosis, and approach to patient management. Usually, an initial palliative operation is required to increase or decrease pulmonary blood flow, with the aim of eventually carrying out a Fontan type of procedure to put the pulmonary and systemic circulations in series.

Tricuspid Atresia

Tricuspid atresia is a type of univentricular cardiac lesion characterized by the absence of the tricuspid valve and thus absence of the normal connection between the right atrium and right ventricle. The right ventricle is invariably hypoplastic. Associated defects determine the physiologic consequences of tricuspid atresia. Pulmonary blood flow may be increased, decreased, or normal depending on associated anatomic features, and the degree of cyanosis is similarly variable. Most patients have diminished pulmonary blood flow and require treatment with PGE_1 and systemic-to-pulmonary artery shunting in the neonatal period. Eventually, a Fontan operation is performed.

Hypoplastic Left Heart Syndrome

Hypoplastic left heart syndrome results in univentricular physiology based on an anatomic right ventricle associated with unimpeded pulmonary blood flow and systemic blood flow that is ductus dependent. Consequently, upon ductal closure, these infants can present with profound circulatory collapse and severe systemic acidosis. Initial management consists of intubation, PGE_1 to open the ductus arteriosus, inotropic support, bicarbonate administration to correct acidosis, and ventilatory management to limit pulmonary blood flow. With appropriate management, these very ill neonates can be stabilized to permit surgery under controlled and optimized conditions. They are usually treated by the Norwood procedure to produce balanced parallel circulations, followed by staged conversion to a Fontan procedure.

Truncus Arteriosus

Truncus arteriosus is an uncommon defect that presents in the neonatal period with congestive failure caused by excessive pulmonary blood flow. Total correction is generally performed in neonates and certainly by 2 or 3 months of age. If operation is delayed, pulmonary vascular obstructive disease is likely to develop, and in this setting, postoperative management may be challenging due to pulmonary hypertension.

Total Anomalous Pulmonary Venous Connection

Total anomalous pulmonary venous connection is another uncommon condition that usually presents in the first few weeks of life. The severity of the patient's symptoms is directly related to the degree of pulmonary venous obstruction, with severely obstructed pulmonary veins resulting in patient presentation in the newborn period. Operation is performed urgently in all cases, as there are few temporizing measures. PGE_1 is avoided, as restoration of ductal patency can worsen pulmonary congestion in the presence of obstructed pulmonary veins. The most critical element of postoperative care is management of the lungs, because of the effects of pulmonary venous obstruction and resulting pulmonary hypertension and lung injury. Invariably, several days of ventilation are required after surgery.

PREOPERATIVE PREPARATION

It is essential that all possible steps are taken to ensure that patients arrive in the operating room in optimal condition. The need for truly emergent operation has become rare because of improvements in diagnosis and management, especially the contributions of PGE_1 and effective resuscitation, which allow stabilization of most of the anomalies that cause severe collapse in newborns. Laboratory studies usually include blood gases, electrolytes, glucose, calcium, and hematocrit. A specimen for blood cross-matching is obtained as well. Typically, a chest radiograph, electrocardiogram, and echocardiogram are performed as part of the initial diagnostic investigation. Cardiac catheterization is required infrequently.

Critically ill neonates are likely to develop profound metabolic acidosis as an early indicator of poor cardiac output. This should be corrected with bicarbonate infusion as the ductus is being opened with PGE_1. Respiratory acidosis should be treated with mechanical ventilation to lower the patient's P_{CO_2}. Intubation may also be necessary if apnea develops as a side effect of PGE_1.

All babies, particularly premature infants, have difficulty with thermal autoregulation; thus, they are at risk for hypothermia. This can further aggravate hypoperfusion. Radiant warming devices with temperature control servomechanisms permit maintenance of normal body temperature without impeding access to the patient.

Catecholamine and milrinone support may be required along with transfusions if the patient is hypovolemic or cyanotic and anemic. With these techniques, it is rare for emergency operations to be performed, and the overall results have improved dramatically.

Ductus-Dependent Lesions

A considerable number of congenital heart defects that previously required urgent operative treatment in the neonatal period are now palliated by opening the ductus arteriosus and maintaining its patency with PGE_1 (Table 7-1) (2). This may be useful in patients with inadequate pulmonary blood flow (such as those with pulmonary or tricuspid atresia or tetralogy); inadequate systemic blood flow (such as those with coarctation, critical aortic stenosis, or hypoplastic left heart syndrome); or transposition of the great arteries as well as other less common conditions. PGE_1 permits time to improve the patient's hypoxia and acidosis. The patient may then come to the operating room with a lesser degree of urgency and in better condition to withstand a major operation. PGE_1 is administered intravenously at 0.01 to 0.1 μg/kg per minute. The lowest effective dose is used to prevent side effects, which include hypotension, seizures, fever, and apnea.

OPERATIVE CONSIDERATIONS

Monitoring Lines

Adequate intravenous access must be ensured to permit safe initiation of the operation; additional transthoracic lines for postoperative use are placed easily during the procedure. Conventional percutaneous catheterization of peripheral lines is usually possi-

Table 7-1. Lesions palliated by PGE_1 infusion

Lesions with inadequate pulmonary blood flow
Tetralogy of Fallot
Pulmonary atresia
Tricuspid atresia
Lesions with inadequate systemic blood flow
Coarctation
Interrupted aortic arch
Critical aortic stenosis
Hypoplastic left heart syndrome
Lesions with inadequate mixing
Transposition of the great arteries

PGE_1, prostaglandin E_1.

ble, but cutdowns may be required as well, particularly in neonates. Scalp vein catheters are precarious and should not be relied on for any critical medication or fluid infusion.

There are a number of commercially available products that facilitate insertion of central venous lines. We commonly employ a 5-Fr double- or triple-lumen catheter (Cook Critical Care, Bloomington, IN) inserted via the internal or external jugular vein after the patient is anesthetized. With use of the Seldinger technique, this catheter can be inserted easily by experienced users and has few complications.

Peripheral arterial cannulation is generally accomplished by percutaneous insertion into the radial artery, although cutdown is sometimes required, particularly in the neonate. A 22-gauge catheter is adequate for small children and most infants, and this can be maintained for several days with proper nursing care and continuous flushing (3). Although 24-gauge catheters may seem easier to insert, they are at higher risk for kinking and becoming nonfunctional; efforts should be made to insert at least a 22-gauge catheter. Percutaneous insertion may be facilitated by the use of a straight flexible guidewire (0.015 in). Alternatively, if this produces a poor arterial pressure tracing or if blood withdrawal is difficult, a short 22-gauge catheter may be exchanged over a guidewire to a 2.5-Fr catheter inserted up to 2 to 3 cm into the radial artery. This will usually yield better blood withdrawal and improve the phasic arterial pressure tracing. Femoral artery cannulation may be used as an alternative and likewise has few complications (4,5); meticulous attention must be directed to maintaining the sterility of the insertion site.

Patients undergoing uneventful operation for relatively simple defects generally require no additional catheters beyond those inserted preoperatively. At the conclusion of the more complex operative procedures, we often use a variety of transthoracic lines that permit more accurate hemodynamic monitoring and provide additional access for administration of volume and drugs. A right atrial catheter can be inserted easily via a pursestring suture in the right atrium, and it is brought out to the surface by a separate stab wound. Similarly, a left atrial catheter may be placed through a pursestring suture in the right superior pulmonary vein (Fig. 2-4). Meticulous line care is required to minimize the risk of air embolization from left atrial catheters, similar to adults. All transthoracic lines of this type must be removed before withdrawal of the patient's mediastinal drainage tubes, lest excessive bleeding from the heart lead to tamponade. This should not be done unless blood is available for transfusion, and coagulation values are adequate. The complication rate from these lines is far less than 1% (6) and justifies their use in appropriate patients.

Umbilical artery catheters are often helpful in the pre- and postoperative management of neonates (7). Often, the umbilical vessels can provide access for cardiac catheterization, and at the conclusion of catheterization, umbilical artery and vein catheters may be inserted for subsequent intra- and postoperative use (Fig. 7-1). Multiple-lumen catheters also may be used via umbilical access (8). Proper positioning of these lines, preferably below the level of the renal arteries, should be radiologically confirmed. It is desirable to remove umbilical artery lines as soon as possible,

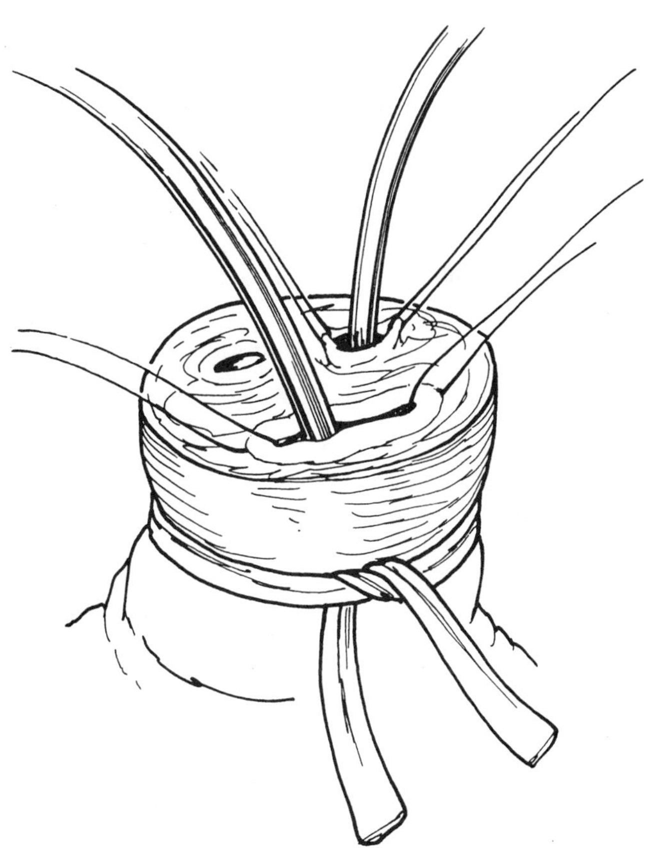

Fig. 7-1. Insertion of umbilical artery and vein catheters for neonatal monitoring and fluid and drug infusion. After a sterile prep and draping, the umbilicus is amputated to within 5–8 mm of the skin line. Two umbilical arteries and an umbilical vein (larger vessel) can be identified in the cross-section. Silk traction sutures (3-0 or 4-0) are placed through the edges of the cut vessels as shown, and gentle upward countertraction is exerted. An artery and the vein are then catheterized with a commercially available umbilical vessel catheter. The amount of each catheter one should insert to result in the catheter tip being at the level of the diaphragm can be estimated from the following formulas:

Artery: Inserted length (cm) = 8.5 + (1.6 × shoulder-umbilical length [cm])
Vein: Inserted length (cm) = 5.0 + (0.6 × shoulder-umbilical length [cm])

Shoulder-umbilical length is measured on a perpendicular line from the baby's shoulder to a transverse line drawn through the umbilicus. The traction sutures can be tied around each catheter to secure the insertion. To complete the procedure, umbilical tape is tied around the base of the umbilicus at the skin line to ensure a good seal around each catheter. (From Dunn P. Localization of the umbilical catheter by post-mortem measurement. *Arch Dis Child* 1966;41:69. Adapted from *The Harriet Lane Handbook*. Chicago: Year Book Medical Publishers, 1984.)

as they have been implicated in the development of necrotizing enterocolitis and arterial thrombosis (9), particularly in premature infants. We generally remove them after patients are extubated. Usually, patients are not fed until they are removed, although this practice varies from institution to institution. Similarly, umbilical venous lines may lead to portal vein thrombosis and should be removed within a few days after insertion, as the risk of this complication increases after 5 or 6 days of use, particularly if the line is used for transfusion (10). These lines are removed by first discontinuing heparinized saline infusion. Beginning with the umbilical venous line, these lines are slowly withdrawn until a small amount of bleeding is noted around each catheter. The catheter is then advanced back in 1 to 2 mm. After approximately 15 minutes, they may be completely withdrawn, as the umbilical vessels will have clotted.

POSTOPERATIVE CARE

Summarized in Appendix 4 are the usual doses of medications commonly used in infants and children.

Assessment of Cardiovascular Status

The evaluation of the small child or infant after cardiac surgery is a demanding task, requiring the utmost vigilance and attention to subtle changes.

Physical Examination

Because babies are capable of having major alterations in their clinical status in a short period of time and because cardiac output is usually not measured directly as in adult patients, the importance of the physical examination is clearly apparent.

One of the most important indicators of tissue perfusion in the infant is the distribution of skin temperature. Often, a distinct gradation in skin temperature from abdominal wall, to thigh, to calf, and to foot can be detected as the patient's cardiac output varies. The presence and volume of the peripheral pulses are a good index of cardiac output; inspection of the skin color and capillary refill of the nailbeds is also worthwhile. Particularly in neonates, central fever with a cool periphery is a sign of low cardiac output that requires prompt attention (11).

Examination of the chest and lung fields gives information regarding the adequacy of ventilation and can be an early warning of impending difficulty. When the patient is mechanically ventilated, chest excursion should be smooth and symmetric. Because the calculated ventilation tidal volume based on the patient's body weight may be misleading, we prefer to rely on a visual assessment of chest expansion to confirm the adequacy of the ventilatory volume. After extubation, the infant's breathing pattern should remain smooth, and there should be no nasal flaring, intercostal retraction, or use of accessory muscles.

Hepatomegaly is a common sign of congestive failure. The liver edge is easily palpated in most children, and it will rise and fall in response to treatment. Peripheral edema is common after cardiopulmonary bypass and does not always signify failure; however, it is an important indicator of total body fluid and generally signifies a need for diuresis. Children typically exhibit edema in the soft tissues of the upper back (the "flat back" sign) or the face, often to a degree not seen in the extremities. Palpating the tension of the cranial fontanelles, which are not fused in neonates, provides another method of assessing fluid status.

Auscultation of the heart in the young patient is difficult because of the rapid heart rate and respiratory rate. Nevertheless, it is important for surgeons caring for such patients to familiarize themselves with each patient's particular auscultatory findings to permit identification of changes in heart sounds that may indicate a physiologically important alteration. A new or changing murmur, presence or resolution of a gallop, and appearance of a friction rub should be noted and compared with previous examinations.

Mixed Venous Saturation

Mixed venous oxygen saturation (SVO_2) varies with the patient's oxygen consumption, hemoglobin concentration, arterial oxygen saturation, and cardiac output. If the first three factors are constant, changes in SVO_2 can be followed as an approximate indicator of cardiac output. In the setting of congenital heart surgery, this assumes that there are no new or residual left-to-right shunts that can falsely elevate mixed venous oxygen saturation. In appropriate patients, we use an indwelling pulmonary artery catheter that makes a colorimetric measurement of SVO_2 for continuous on-line determination of this variable. The catheter must be calibrated frequently by laboratory measurement of a carefully obtained pulmonary artery blood sample to ensure accuracy. We have found it most helpful to rely on fluctuations of SVO_2 over time rather than on an isolated value as the most valuable indicator of cardiac performance (12). In addition to its use to monitor fluctuations of SVO_2 over time, a sudden rise in saturation with diminution of peripheral perfusion can also signify opening of a left-to-right shunt, such as a residual VSD following VSD or tetralogy repair. In general, patients with good cardiac output and without residual shunts maintain an SVO_2 above 60%.

Treatment of Low Cardiac Output

Hypovolemia occurs commonly after operations for congenital heart defects; bleeding, blood sampling, vasodilation from rewarming, and diuresis all contribute to this. Appropriate infusions of blood, colloid, and crystalloid are administered to correct volume deficits and maintain approximate oxygen-carrying capacity. Left atrial and/or pulmonary artery catheters are useful in assessing the need for and results of volume replacement. Excessive volume loading can produce deleterious effects, however, and this adverse response to excessive fluid administration is most likely in infants and in more complex cardiac defects (13). As a general rule, infants and young children do not respond favorably to high levels of preload as do adults, and we rarely push the central venous pressure above 10 mm Hg or the left atrial pressure above 15 mm Hg, relying more heavily on catecholamine administration to improve cardiac output.

The general use of pharmacologic agents in the treatment of low cardiac output is discussed in Chapter 3. Dopamine and dobutamine are useful in stimulating the myocardium without causing vasoconstriction at moderate doses. Milrinone is especially useful in pediatric patients, as it reduces pulmonary vascular resistance, which is often a problem in these patients. Epinephrine is used in low doses when the above agents produce unsatisfactory results. Occasionally, nitroglycerin, nitroprusside, or PGE_1 is added for systemic afterload reduction. The target systolic arterial blood pressure, of course, is age related, ranging from 50 to 60 mm Hg in the neonate to 80 to 100 mm Hg in the young child.

Tamponade Physiology

Cardiac tamponade represents a life-threatening complication in children as it does in adults. The volume of fluid required to produce tamponade in children is, of course, much smaller; therefore, the surgeon must have a lower threshold for reopening the sternum when this occurs. The difficulty lies in making the diagnosis of tamponade, particularly in the absence of intracardiac pressure measurements, which often facilitate the diagnosis in adult patients. Tamponade must be suspected in any child who demonstrates diminished tissue perfusion and elevated venous pressure in the postoperative period without an identifiable cause. The index of suspicion must be particularly high when these findings occur in an otherwise stable child following removal of intracardiac monitoring lines. Tamponade may be heralded by mediastinal drainage tubes that suddenly stop draining or by temporary pacing wires that falter. Echocardiography may be unreliable in excluding the diagnosis in children. Sometimes a few chest compressions in an infant will initiate evacuation of a very recent ("fresh") tamponade. However, if this is not immediately successful, prompt sternal reopening is mandatory, either in the operating room or, if needed, in the intensive care unit. Sometimes, exploration is necessary to rule out this diagnosis even when the clinical signs are very "soft."

Infants are especially prone to develop tamponade physiology because of cardiac compression in the absence of mediastinal blood clots. A small amount of cardiac edema, swelling of the mediastinal tissues, or elevation of the diaphragm from ascites can produce this syndrome. Leaving the sternum open for a few days after surgery may prove lifesaving (14). Also, we sometimes leave a drain in the peritoneal cavity of infants to drain ascites fluid and help avoid elevation of the diaphragm. Some have advocated continuous fluid removal early after surgery in critically ill infants as a means of alleviating the consequences of edema. This may be achieved by continuous ultrafiltration (15,16) or early dialysis (15). Late tamponade due to pericardial effusion can occur following operations for congenital heart disease and, in some patients, can be life threatening (17,18). Prior to hospital discharge and at the first postoperative office visit, the neck veins should be examined and the patient should be checked for possible paradox. Aspirin (18) or steroids (19) may be useful for the treatment of postoperative pericardial effusions in this setting.

Residual Lesions

Residual lesions include those anatomic abnormalities that are not repaired at operation because of technical difficulty, unacceptable risk, or incomplete diagnosis and those that are deliberately left uncorrected for physiologic reasons. Typical examples include atrial or ventricular septal defects that are incompletely closed owing to technical error, resulting in excessive pulmonary blood flow. Other residua include a persistent gradient across a coarctation repair or persistent valvar stenosis after aortic or pulmonary valvotomy. Knowledge of residual lesions obtained by postoperative monitoring or echocardiography can guide the timing of late postoperative restudy (20).

Treatment of these conditions must be individualized according to the patient's symptoms, physical findings, and results of invasive and noninvasive studies. Residual lesions must be considered after operation if the patient has a worse-than-expected clinical course. If a patient is not progressing after surgery as expected, the adequacy of repair and the presence of residual lesions must be determined. Echocardiography is an essential first step in this process. If necessary, cardiac catheterization may be required. If a poor clinical course leads to restudy, and a significant unexpected residual lesion is found, immediate reoperation is often the best course to ensure a good short- and long-term outcome.

As mentioned above, sometimes defects are deliberately left unrepaired. An example is the atrial septal defect that is left open to allow right-to-left shunting when right ventricular function is impaired (21) or in patients after a Fontan procedure (22). Leaving residual right-to-left shunts in such situations has decreased the morbidity and mortality for right-sided failure sometimes observed following these types of operations.

Pulmonary Management

Pulmonary care in the young patient usually begins in the operating room with intubation. Although practices vary from institution to institution, if intubation is anticipated to be of short duration (intraoperative or early postoperative extubation), it may be done via the oral route, using an appropriately sized uncuffed tube (Table 7-2). The endotracheal tube is of the appropriate size if it maintains a good seal up to 25 to 30 cm H_2O airway pressure

Table 7-2. Endotracheal tube (ETT) size and intubation guidelines

Age	Internal Diameter (mm)[a]
Premature infant[b]	2.5–3.0[c]
Term infant[b]	3.0–3.5
3 mo–1 yr	4.0
1–2 yr	4.5
2–15 yr	$\frac{16 + \text{age (years)}}{4}$

[a]If no leak is present at airway pressures >30 cm H_2O, change to the next smaller tube.

[b]The head should not be extended for placement of the ETT in newborns due to anatomic differences compared to older patients.

[c]Most premature neonates can accept a 3.0 ETT. 2.5 ETTs have increased airway resistance and are difficult to suction adequately.

Source: Adapted from *The Harriet Lane Handbook*. Chicago: Year Book Medical Publishers, 1984.

but "leaks" at higher airway pressures. An uncuffed endotracheal tube that does not "leak" at higher airway pressures may be too large and should be changed. For most patients, who will require mechanical ventilation for at least 12 to 24 hours, we prefer to use a nasotracheal tube. Before intubation, 1 or 2 drops of 0.25% phenylephrine is placed into the selected nostril to produce mucosal vasoconstriction and, hence, reduce the risk of bleeding during heparinization. The nasal tube provides better opportunity for secure fixation and aids in oral hygiene. We obtain a postoperative chest film in the operating room prior to transfer of the patient to the intensive care unit. This confirms proper positioning of the tube in the trachea and proper positioning of intracardiac monitoring lines and may demonstrate a need for additional chest tubes. The connections between the endotracheal tube and the ventilator must be flexible enough to permit motion of the patient's head without moving the tube within the trachea. Failure to make provision for this may lead to unplanned tube removal or trauma to the airway. It is essential that patients requiring mechanical ventilation be provided with sufficient analgesia and sedation to prevent vigorous movements. Particularly in patients with postoperative pulmonary hypertension, high-dose sedation with narcotics such as fentanyl (at least 10 μg/kg per hour) or morphine (0.1 mg/kg per hour) combined with pharmacologic paralysis (vecuronium 0.1 mg/kg per hour) is usually necessary for the appropriate ventilatory control of the pulmonary circulation.

Maintenance of endotracheal tube patency is critical. In particular, small-caliber endotracheal tubes such as 3- or 3.5-mm tubes are prone to plugging at their distal tip with dried secretions. Particularly if surgery involved pulmonary artery branch mobilization, small amounts of blood may be present initially in the airway secretions and can contribute to plugging. Maintenance of tube patency requires saline irrigation and suctioning on a routine basis; if blood is present, irrigation with alkalinized saline may help mobilize secretions adherent to the endotracheal tube. Unexplained increases in P_{CO_2} in patients on pressure-cycled ventilators or unexplained increases in peak airway pressure in patients on volume-cycled ventilators should raise suspicion of partial endotracheal tube obstruction. Hand ventilation will sometimes help detect tube obstruction. If there is uncertainty, changing the endotracheal tube will resolve this important issue.

The postoperative care of children following cardiac surgery, particularly the care of the neonate, involves very close attention to respiratory care and ventilatory management (23,24). Atelectasis should be prevented by ensuring adequate tidal volume and providing appropriate chest physiotherapy. Endotracheal suctioning is important, but it must be used with great caution in the hemodynamically precarious patient. Particularly in the patient with pulmonary hypertension, vigorous airway suction can produce hypoxia, pulmonary vascular spasm, and cardiovascular collapse (25); premedication with additional narcotic plus manual hyperventilation with 100% oxygen may be needed before suctioning is performed. High ventilation pressures in well-relaxed patients without wheezing should quickly raise the suspicion of endotracheal tube plugging. Tubes that may be obstructed should be removed immediately and replaced; suctioning may not succeed in removing a mucous plug or clot that is acting as a "ball valve" on the tip of the tube.

Formerly, the only mechanical ventilators used for pediatric patients were of the pressure-cycled type. These ventilators deliver gas until a given pressure is reached, followed by an expiratory phase. In most neonates after cardiopulmonary bypass, inspiratory pressures of at least 20 to 25 cm H_2O are commonly required. Positive end-expiratory pressure (PEEP) of 3 to 5 cm H_2O is used to prevent alveolar collapse and improve functional residual capacity. The ventilatory rate typically is 15 to 20 per minute. We generally employ the intermittent mandatory ventilation mode because this allows the patient to establish his or her own breathing pattern and assists in weaning. The inspiratory/expiratory ratio (I/E) is usually 1:2.

Volume-cycled ventilators use a similar ventilatory rate, PEEP, and I/E ratio. The tidal volume is about 15 to 20 mL/kg, slightly more than that used in adults. The inspiratory pressures must be monitored and limits set to guard against barotrauma. High-frequency jet ventilation, although not in common use in postoperative cardiac infants, may be of value in selected cases of severe pulmonary failure, acute respiratory distress syndrome, refractory pulmonary hypertension, or after a Fontan procedure (26).

The F_iO_2 is reduced as rapidly as possible to prevent such complications as retrolental fibroplasia (Table 7-3). It is more important to individualize this in pediatric patients than in adults because of the unique physiologic requirements imposed by some of their cardiac anomalies.

Pulmonary Hypertension

Pulmonary hypertension is typically encountered in patients with large left-to-right shunts and those with left-sided obstructive lesions such as mitral stenosis, cor triatriatum, and obstructed total anomalous pulmonary venous return. If left untreated, the pulmonary vascular resistance may rise to systemic levels or higher and become irreversible (Eisenmenger syndrome); these patients are inoperable. One of the tasks of preoperative catheterization is to separate those patients with fixed elevation of pulmonary vascular resistance from those in whom the pulmonary vascular resistance falls to operable levels in response to oxygen and/or vasodilator drugs. Some of these latter borderline-operable patients will, thus, be operated on, and they demand great attention postoperatively.

The most important component of the treatment of postoperative pulmonary hypertension is proper ventilatory management. The fractional inspired oxygen (F_iO_2) is kept high, and hypercarbia and acidosis are avoided; a degree of respiratory alkalosis helps to lower

Table 7-3. Potential complications of ventilating neonates with high concentrations of oxygen

Retrolental fibroplasia
Excessive pulmonary blood flow in patients with left-to-right shunts
Increased pulmonary congestion in the presence of obstructed total anomalous pulmonary venous drainage

pulmonary artery pressure. The patient should receive adequate sedation and paralysis to prevent voluntary resistance to ventilation. These measures are often sufficient to maintain maximum pulmonary vasodilatation. Vigorous hand ventilation of the patient with 100% oxygen can alleviate episodes of pulmonary vascular spasm that appear periodically and may be lifesaving. Vasodilators such as nitroglycerin and nitroprusside or PGE_1 may be used. Milrinone is another valuable agent for lowering pulmonary artery resistance, and its positive inotropic effect may provide additional benefits. Dopamine may worsen the situation.

Inhaled *nitric oxide* has been used with good results to treat postoperative pulmonary hypertension as it appears to be a truly selective, potent pulmonary vasodilator (27). Since its approval for clinical use, nitric oxide has become a first-line treatment for significant pulmonary hypertension at many institutions. It is administered by a special ventilator apparatus in doses ranging from 1 to 80 parts per million (ppm). Recent data suggest that most patients respond to doses in the range of 5 to 40 ppm, and keeping the dose under 40 ppm minimizes potential complications such as alveolar injury, nitrogen dioxide generation, and methemoglobin formation (28). Withdrawal of nitric oxide therapy must be done gradually and with monitoring of clinical status because of the potential for rebound pulmonary hypertension (29).

Parallel Circulations and Control of the Pulmonary Circulation

One of the most challenging problems for postoperative management in congenital heart surgery is the care of patients with parallel circulations. Parallel circulations are encountered after palliation of any single-ventricle lesion, such as after the Norwood operation for hypoplastic left heart syndrome or after creation of a systemic-to-pulmonary shunt in complex lesions that include pulmonary atresia. In these patients, the systemic saturation achieved depends on the relative amounts of pulmonary and systemic blood flow, which is expressed as the ratio $\dot{Q}_P/\dot{Q}_S$. Figure 7-2 shows an example of the systemic saturation achieved as a function of $\dot{Q}_P/\dot{Q}_S$, assuming a completely mixed circulation such as that encountered in single ventricle physiology and, for the purpose of illustration, assuming a systemic saturation of 50%. Note that 100% saturation is approached asymptotically so that very high ratios of $\dot{Q}_P/\dot{Q}_S$ are required to achieve high levels of systemic saturation. It is important to note that increasing systemic saturation is obtained not only by increasing pulmonary blood flow but also by decreasing systemic flow. This has particularly important implications in the management of the neonate. *In utero,* there is relatively little pulmonary blood flow. As a result, a fetus with single-ventricle physiology needs only to pump to the systemic circulation plus the blood flow to the placenta. The neonatal single ventricle has therefore not accommodated to pumping large volume loads such as may be the case in parallel circulations. Furthermore, there is evidence to suggest that single ventricles with right ventricular morphology may be less efficient than single ventricles with left ventricular morphology, the former situation encountered in the hypoplastic left heart syndrome. In these neonates, a higher

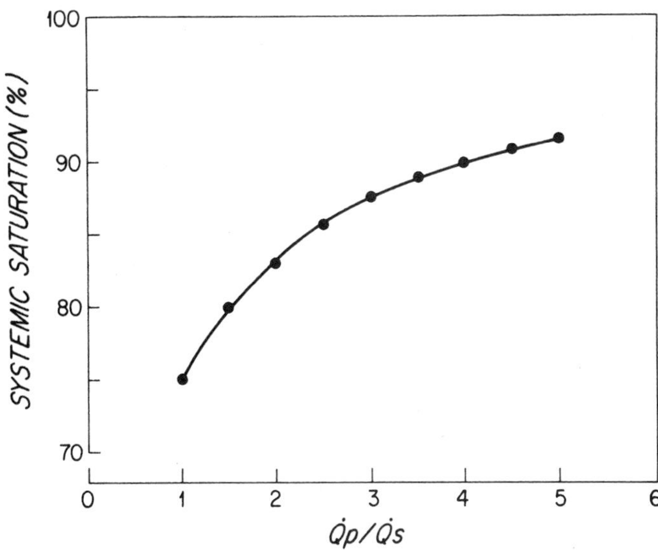

Fig. 7-2. Illustration of systemic saturation achieved as a function of the pulmonary-to-systemic flow ratio ($\dot{Q}_P/\dot{Q}_S$). Note that 100% saturation is approached asymptotically.

systemic saturation may signify not only increasing $\dot{Q}_P$ but also decreasing $\dot{Q}_S$. Thus, neonates with single-ventricle physiology are capable of being well saturated but having a consequent low output state and acidosis. In essence, whatever blood flow goes through the lungs does not go through the systemic circulation and vice versa.

The essence of managing such neonates is the control of pulmonary blood flow so as to maintain adequate systemic perfusion while having adequate saturation for oxygen transport. With time, the neonatal single ventricle adapts to increasing volume load and meets the demands of the systemic circulation, while providing substantial amounts of pulmonary blood flow. However, early after such operations as the Norwood procedure for hypoplastic left heart syndrome, it may be particularly challenging to maintain adequate systemic perfusion. This issue is further complicated by the fact that early after creation of a surgically placed systemic-to-pulmonary shunt, it is desirable to maintain systemic output and pressure to help maintain shunt patency.

To date, no single intravenous pharmacologic agent has been found that provides either highly selective vasoconstriction or highly selective vasodilation of only the pulmonary or only the systemic circulation. Rather, the systemic and pulmonary circulations must be "balanced" in these neonates by careful postoperative ventilatory management, usually aimed initially at decreasing pulmonary blood.

Table 7-4. Control of pulmonary blood flow

Factors That increase $\dot{Q}_p$	Factors That Decrease $\dot{Q}_p$
↑ F_iO_2	↓ F_iO_2
Alkalosis; Hypocarbia	Acidosis; Normo- or mild hypercarbia
Mean airway pressure	Mean airway pressure
↓ PEEP	↑ PEEP
↓ I:E ratio	↑ I:E ratio
↓ tidal volume	↑ tidal volume

$\dot{Q}_p$, pulmonary blood flow; F_iO_2, fractional inspired oxygen; PEEP, positive end-expiratory pressure; I:E ratio, inspiratory:expiratory ratio.

There are three key ventilatory parameters that have important effects on the pulmonary circulation (see Table 7-4):

1. *F_iO_2*. Particularly in the neonate, the pulmonary circulation will respond to increasing concentrations of inspired oxygen by vasodilation; conversely, decreasing inspired oxygen concentrations down to room air will result in some pulmonary vasoconstriction. In extreme circumstances, F_iO_2 may be decreased to 0.17% to 0.18% to achieve control of excessive pulmonary blood flow.
2. *pH and carbon dioxide.* Respiratory alkalosis and hypocarbia may produce pulmonary vasodilation (30), and conversely, normocarbia and normal pH may produce some increase in pulmonary vascular resistance.
3. *Airway pressure.* By direct mechanical effect, increasing airway pressure also opposes pulmonary blood flow. The airway pressure can be varied in two ways. PEEP can be added or removed to increase or decrease correspondingly the mean airway pressure. Pulmonary blood flow may also be decreased by increasing the relative amount of time the ventilator spends in inspiration versus expiration (I/E ratio). A similar effect to increase the mean airway pressure (and hence decrease pulmonary blood flow) can be achieved by using very large tidal volumes (20 to 25 mL/kg); however, inspired CO_2 (1% to 4%) must be added to normalize P_{CO_2} (31).

To illustrate, after the Norwood procedure for first-stage palliation of hypoplastic left heart syndrome, it is sometimes necessary to limit pulmonary blood flow. The single ventricle with right ventricular morphology requires time to accommodate pumping to parallel circulations, and in these neonates, excessive systemic saturation is common and is usually accompanied by poor systemic perfusion and acidosis. Thus, these infants are frequently ventilated immediately after surgery with room air. The ventilatory rate and total volume are adjusted, so that normocarbia results and hyperventilation is avoided. PEEP may be added up to 5 to 7 cm H_2O, and a relatively long inspiratory time is selected, so that the I/E ratio is 1:2 to 1:3. Cardiac performance is then maximized by ensuring optimal filling pressures and by the use of inotropic agents. In general, achieving precise control of ventilatory parameters early after surgery usually requires continuous narcotic sedation and pharmacologic paralysis. Oxygen-carrying capacity is optimized by raising the hematocrit to about 40%.

In contrast, patients who have undergone a Fontan procedure must have pulmonary vascular resistance minimized (32). These patients are ventilated after surgery with little or no PEEP and with short inspiratory times; atelectasis may be minimized by the use of intermittent ventilatory sighs or by intermittent hand ventilation. Hypoxia is assiduously avoided. In-series circulations after a Fontan procedure function best with spontaneous ventilation (33), and accordingly, efforts should be made to extubate these patients as early as possible after operation.

Extubation of the postoperative patient requires hemodynamic stability, freedom from severe edema, smooth respiratory motion of the chest wall with spontaneous breathing, and acceptable blood gases. Most patients are extubated after a short period of time with an intermittent mandatory ventilation rate of 5 per minute. We do not think infants should have the additional stress of a continuous positive airway pressure trial, because this requires a great deal of effort as the baby attempts to overcome the combined resistance of continuous positive airway pressure and a small-caliber endotracheal tube. The intravenous administration of dexamethasone (0.5 mg/kg) several hours before and after tube removal in infants assists in reducing airway edema and may help to prevent reintubation. Racemic epinephrine inhalation (2.25%, 1 mL in 5 mL of saline) also helps control postextubation stridor due to upper airway edema. Airway edema and consequent obstruction may be more of a problem following prolonged intubation or in babies who have been very active prior to extubation and more likely to have tube-related airway trauma. In addition to airway edema, intraoperative phrenic nerve injury and the resulting diaphragmatic paralysis may also result in acute respiratory failure following extubation.

Tracheostomy may be required in the care of some infants who cannot be separated from the ventilator after several weeks. It often seems that tracheostomy, by providing a shorter airway pathway and permitting easier suctioning for removal of secretions, permits weaning from the ventilator in a short time. Meticulous surgical technique is required for this procedure: Injury to the cricoid cartilage must be avoided to prevent subglottic stenosis, the proper-size tube should be inserted, and the device must be secured in place to avoid trauma to the skin and trachea. No one except the responsible surgical team should attempt removal or repositioning of the tube for the first 5 to 7 days; after that time, the tube can be removed easily for cleaning and reinserted.

Cardiac Rhythm Management

Arrhythmias can occur frequently following correction of congenital cardiac defects in children and include a wide range of brady- and tachyarrhythmias, with an overall incidence approaching 50% (34). Some arrhythmias may be related anatomically to surgery, such as heart block following VSD closure or tachyarrhythmias following procedures involving extensive suture lines in the atria, like Fontan procedures or atrial switch procedures for transposition.

As in the case of adult patients, bradyarrhythmias are managed by pacing. Pacing electrodes may be placed on the atria and ventricles, and smaller-caliber electrodes are available for use in pediatric patients. Despite smaller cardiac dimensions, efforts should be made to avoid unipolar pacing because of higher thresholds and lower reliability. In particular, atrial pacing electrodes should be sufficiently far apart to yield an adequate signal for atrial sensing to permit DDD pacing. The right atrial free wall near the atrioventricular groove and the cephalic atrial wall between the atrial appendages produce optimum temporary pacing wire properties in pediatric patients (35).

Among the tachyarrhythmias occurring after pediatric cardiac surgery, junctional ectopic tachycardia (JET) can produce substantial morbidity because of its effect on overall cardiac performance. It should be aggressively treated. This tachyarrhythmia appears as a regular rhythm at a rate that can vary between 150 and 250 per minute. Although P-wave activity may be difficult to recognize during JET, this rhythm is characterized by atrioventricular dissociation (36). JET is managed by first ensuring that sympathetic tone is minimized. Adequate sedation should be ensured, and doses of catecholamine inotropic agents should be minimized. Pancuronium exerts a vagolytic action, and if it is being used for muscle relaxation, it should be switched to another agent. Systemic cooling to approximately 34°C may be of value in small infants, and if topical cooling is used, adequate muscle relaxation should be used to block shivering.

Increasingly, amiodarone is being used to control JET, as well as other tachyarrhythmias that may be poorly tolerated. In the postoperative setting, if simple measures such as cooling and minimizing drug infusions are ineffective in controlling JET, intravenous amiodarone loading and maintenance infusion should be instituted if the arrhythmia is poorly tolerated, as manifested by evidence of low cardiac output (37,38).

Fluids, Electrolytes, and Nutrition

Routine Fluid and Electrolyte Management

Postoperatively, intelligent fluid administration requires careful consideration of the patient's cardiac output, systemic and pulmonary pressures, filling pressures, urine output, and blood loss. In the immediate postoperative period, our initial plan of volume replacement dictates infusion of red blood cells and/or plasma equal in volume to that lost via mediastinal drainage and blood sampling on an hour-by-hour basis. The volume expander chosen is dictated by the desired hematocrit: normal in acyanotic patients and elevated in cyanotic patients.

Usual full maintenance fluid requirements in a child are 100 mL/kg per day for the first 10 kg of body weight, plus 50 mL/kg per day for the second 10 kg, plus 20 mL/kg per day for weight over 20 kg. In patients after cardiopulmonary bypass, this calculated volume is reduced by half because of the tendency for these patients to retain large volumes of excess water. Dextrose, 5% in water (±0.2 N saline), with 20 mEq/L of potassium chloride added on day 2, is generally used for maintenance fluids.

Further alterations in volume and composition of intravenously administered fluids depend on the clinical situation and measurements of hematocrit, electrolytes, and blood gases. It must be recalled that hyponatremia is almost always dilutional and requires fluid restriction, although small infants may require some sodium administration. Fluid restriction may be difficult because of the large number of intravenous lines that are at risk of occlusion if flow rates are low. Syringe infusion pumps with digital control are the most reliable devices for precise administration of small volumes of fluid as well as critical medications. For most arterial and central venous lines, at least 1.5 to 2.0 mL per hour is required to maintain patency (3). Arterial lines should receive saline or 0.5 N saline without dextrose; other lines should receive 5% or 10% dextrose. Heparin should be added (1 U/mL).

Nutritional Management

The typical child who undergoes an uneventful open-heart operation should be able to begin clear liquids by mouth a short time (6 hours) after the endotracheal tube is removed. If liquids are well tolerated, a regular diet for age may be resumed later that day. Postoperative ileus is unusual in most cardiac patients, and there is no reason to withhold nourishment. One exception to this rule is the patient undergoing repair of coarctation (below). Most neonates may similarly begin sugar solution after extubation, with a rapid progression to breast milk or formula.

The more critically ill infant poses a more difficult problem in nutritional management, and a need for prolonged ventilation makes normal feeding impossible. Whenever possible, we prefer to use the patient's gastrointestinal tract as a route for alimentation. Feedings are started via an orogastric tube with 5% dextrose or balanced electrolyte solution (e.g., Pedialyte) with frequent residuals measured to guard against gastric dilatation. Formula may then be initiated at increasing volumes and concentrations until the infant is receiving 120 to 180 kcal/kg per day. If additional volume must be administered to reach this nutritional intake, diuretics may be needed. Diarrhea or stools positive for reducing substances require discontinuation of the feedings, followed by resumption at a slightly lower rate or concentration. Intolerances to formula mandate formula changes.

Intravenous hyperalimentation may be needed if the gastrointestinal tract is not usable. Central administration is preferable, as higher solute concentrations can be given with less volume. Lipids are added to increase the calorie intake.

Glucose

Glucose homeostasis is frequently deranged in infants with severe congenital heart defects. This derangement may be most severe when circulatory arrest is employed (39). Hyperglycemia is particularly common in the postoperative period, and this may lead to osmotic diuresis, dehydration, and increase in serum osmolarity, which may lead to cerebral hemorrhage. Plasma glucose values below 200 mg/dL need not be treated beyond reducing the rate or concentration of dextrose-containing intravenous solutions. Glucose levels above 300 mg/dL require the intravenous administration of regular insulin, 0.1 to 0.2 U/kg, every 6 to 12 hours until glucose levels stabilize. Standing orders for "sliding scale" insulin should never be used in infants because of the risk of dangerous hypoglycemia. Hypoglycemia must be prevented by frequent monitoring of glucose levels in patients receiving insulin, and dextrose infusions should be administered if the levels fall below 100 mg/dL (40). The small glycogen stores in neonates and limited capacity for gluconeogenesis make hypoglycemia the greater danger. Neonates may not manifest any clinical evidence of hypoglycemia until serum glucose levels fall below 30 mg/dL, at which point the patient is at risk for cerebral insult. This is completely preventable in most cases by using maintenance solutions containing 10% dextrose, estimating blood glucose frequently using bedside test strips, and confirming test strip values with measurements of blood glucose levels by the laboratory. When plasma glucose levels fall below 50 mg/dL despite these precautions, the patient should receive small dextrose-containing fluid boluses through a secure central venous catheter, and the concentration of dextrose in the maintenance solutions should be increased to ≥10% (40).

Calcium

Hypocalcemia most commonly occurs in neonates and may cause irritability, seizures, and abnormalities of cardiac rhythm. Measurement of ionized, not total, calcium is easily accomplished and is the best guide to calcium replacement (normal ionized calcium level, 1 to 2 mmol/L). Replacement may be particularly necessary when blood products have been administered. Calcium supplementation should be provided as a 10% calcium gluconate infusion and should be infused slowly 1 to 2 mL/kg at a time through a central venous line exclusively (41). Particularly in neonates, hypocalcemia may be recurrent, especially if the DeGeorge syndrome is present; in this circumstance, it can be added to the maintenance solutions (calcium gluconate, 2 g/L).

Hypomagnesemia may coexist very rarely with hypocalcemia, and it should be suspected when symptomatic hypocalcemia does not respond to calcium infusion alone (42). Although laboratory measurements of serum magnesium levels are, at best, an uncertain indicator of total body magnesium, levels below 1.4 mEq/L are abnormal. Tetany unresponsive to calcium is treated with 0.2 mL of 50% magnesium sulfate administrated intramuscularly every 4 hours.

Potassium

Hypokalemia is most commonly due to urinary losses and administration of bicarbonate ion. Unlike adult cardiac patients, who are often very sensitive to hypokalemia, children rarely develop ventricular irritability because of moderately low serum potassium levels. Unless the potassium falls below 3.0 mEq/L, additional potassium supplementation is usually unnecessary. Enteral administration of potassium is preferred to intravenous administration if the gastrointestinal route is available and the deficit is modest. Intravenously administered potassium chloride requires a central venous catheter and should be given slowly at a dose of 0.1 to 0.2 mEq/kg over 20 to 30 minutes, followed by redetermination of the potassium level.

More dangerous is significant hyperkalemia, which most commonly occurs because of renal failure and metabolic acidosis. Elevated serum potassium levels lead to progressive electrical instability of the heart and eventually to cardiac arrest. Hyperkalemia may be palliated temporarily by the administration of calcium, bicarbonate, and/or glucose and insulin. These measures, however, only shift the potassium to the intracellular compartment. Removal of potassium is best accomplished with vigorous diuresis, if possible, or the use of ion exchange resins (Kayexalate) as enemas. Kayexalate is prepared as a slurry (1 g/mL of sorbitol solution), and it is administered through an indwelling rectal tube. Dialysis is not an efficient method of rapid potassium removal but may be used to stabilize the serum concentration while other measures take effect.

Special Problems

Coagulation Disorders and Transfusion

Younger patients are at greater risk than adults for excessive peripheral edema after cardiopulmonary bypass. As extreme anemia and dilution of serum oncotic pressure encourage edema formation, we usually use a blood prime in our bypass circuit in infants and small children.

Patients with congenital heart defects are more likely than most individuals to have abnormal preoperative coagulation tests (43). This is particularly evident in cyanotic patients. In most respects, replacement of blood products in the pediatric patient undergoing cardiac operation follows the same principles used for adults. Some cardiac surgeons believe that there is a beneficial effect of transfusing fresh whole blood in achieving hemostasis immediately after open heart operations and that this benefit surpasses that of component therapy. There is some objective evidence to support this belief (44), but it is often impractical in practice owing to the time required to perform screening serologic tests. It is useful to remove as much free water as possible by hemofiltration while on bypass to "make room" for fresh frozen plasma and platelet transfusions in these patients.

Paradoxical Hypertension After Coarctation Repair

Despite technically adequate surgical correction of aortic coarctation, severe hypertension in the early postoperative period occurs in 37% to 63% of patients (45,46). Proposed mechanisms of this hypertension include elevated sympathetic activity (47,48) and elevated renin (49). It is interesting to note that paradoxical hypertension does not occur after balloon dilatation of the coarctation (50). Postoperative hypertension is less of a problem in neonatal coarctation repair.

Preoperative treatment with β-blockers effectively prevents this paradoxical hypertension (51). The patient begins atenolol (1 mg/kg per day) orally, starting 2 weeks before operation. When hypertension does occur after coarctation repair, we prefer to treat it as we would other forms of systemic hypertension, with nitroprusside infusion beginning at 0.5 µg/kg per minute and increasing as needed in addition to intravenous β-blockade. Alternatively, if hypertension is not easily controlled, intravenous esmolol (52) or labetalol (53) can be used. We restart atenolol when oral intake has begun for additional pressure control and to assist in weaning nitroprusside. Particularly in older patients, persistent hypertension may be a significant problem. In these patients, high-dose β-blockade combined with potent antihypertensives such as angiotensin-converting enzyme inhibitors or calcium channel blocking agents may be needed.

Blood pressure control in these patients is important to prevent the complication of mesenteric arteritis, which commonly followed coarctation repair in past years. In these patients, who were generally older than the patients operated on now, hypertension occurred "paradoxically" after several days. Mesenteric arteritis may result in intestinal necrosis. For this reason, we do not permit oral intake after coarctation repair until the abdomen is soft and bowel sounds are vigorous.

Temperature Regulation

Neonates cannot regulate their body temperature because of their relatively large surface area, limited subcutaneous fat, and inability to generate heat by shivering. Use of radiant warming devices prevents hypothermia in these patients while permitting access for necessary care. Automatic radiant heaters incorporate skin temperature probes to regulate warming by using skin temperature in a servomechanism feedback system. Either elevation or depression of body temperature may be a sign of infection.

Neurologic Complications of Cardiac Surgery in Children

Effects of Profound Hypothermia and Circulatory Arrest

Neurologic issues in pediatric cardiac surgery are the most devastating and most feared complications. Although the neurologic risk of surgery to correct relatively simple defects is very low, studies have shown that operations for very complex lesions, particularly single-ventricle lesions, and operations done using prolonged circulatory arrest are associated with greater decrements in neurocognitive function (54). In the extreme, operations for complex congenital cardiac defects, particularly those requiring prolonged hypothermic circulatory arrest, can produce devastating neurologic complications, including choreoathetosis that can be manifest even up to 1 week following surgery (55).

Infants under 5 kg in weight may benefit from operation using profound hypothermia and circulatory arrest. This technique has been applied in a wide variety of congenital heart defects and permits operating in a bloodless field without the obstruction that perfusion cannulas may create in the smaller patient. Some surgeons are concerned that this technique may lead to cerebral injury and developmental delay, perhaps to a very subtle degree (54), and more frequently, strategies are being utilized to avoid this technique, even when complex aortic arch surgery is required.

Because neurologic complications can be devastating, this area has been the subject of considerable investigation. Some studies suggested that subtle changes in cognitive function occur with use of circulatory arrest and that this may be related to excessively short periods of core cooling on bypass before circulatory arrest is effected (56); more recent studies have suggested that use of circulatory arrest is associated primarily with long-term issues of motor coordination (57). Recent studies have shown that neurologic function may be improved early following hypothermic circulatory arrest if pH–stat blood gas management is used during cardiopulmonary bypass (58). Control of blood glucose levels and pH during reperfusion may also be of particular importance in avoiding cerebral injury (59). Together, all of these measures have helped improve neurologic outcome following surgery for congenital heart defects, so that recent studies have suggested a declining incidence of these dreaded complications (60).

Seizure Activity

Infants are at high risk for seizures after cardiac operations because of electrolyte imbalance, osmotic shifts, anoxic cerebral insult, or air or thrombotic emboli through persistent shunts. These most commonly occur after the use of deep hypothermic arrest. Seizure activity in babies may vary from obvious tonic-clonic motions to subtle eye, tongue, or mouth movements. In the neonate or infant who is mechanically ventilated and with adjunct pharmacologic paralysis, seizures may be masked and may be manifested only by tachycardia, hypertension, mydriasis, or bronchorrhea; the sudden appearance of any of these signs should raise suspicion of seizure activity in the paralyzed patient. In all cases, vigorous treatment is indicated to prevent the cerebral consequences of unchecked seizures. Initial control may be obtained with intravenously administered diazepam (0.1 mg/kg). Phenobarbital, the preferred maintenance agent, should be given intravenously in two loading doses of 10 mg/kg each, followed by a maintenance dose of 5 mg/kg per day divided into b.i.d. doses. Phenytoin (20-mg/kg i.v. loading dose and 5 mg/kg per day divided b.i.d.) is an alternative maintenance agent (61).

Computed tomography scanning or ultrasound examination of the brain in neonates may be needed to exclude the possibility of intraventricular hemorrhage. Sudden changes in serum osmolarity may predispose the infant to this problem. Therefore, no more than 5 to 6 mOsm/kg per hour should be given in any 1 hour to neonates. Hyperventilation and steroids are used for treatment of this condition.

Renal Failure

We generally strive to maintain a urine output of approximately 1 mL/kg per hour in children after cardiac operations. Oliguria combined with rising blood urea nitrogen and creatinine levels indicates renal failure. Renal failure in the neonatal period usually results from prerenal causes: low cardiac output, sepsis, and hypovolemia. Postrenal factors such as obstructive uropathy must also be considered and excluded with ultrasound. Correction of the underlying cause will correct the renal dysfunction in most cases. Peritoneal dialysis is indicated for severe volume overload or persistent metabolic acidosis. Some surgeons advocate early aggressive dialysis in infants to prevent the edema formation and fluid and electrolyte problems common in these patients (15).

Sepsis

Bacterial sepsis is unfortunately common in the newborn period and may further complicate the care of the patient with congenital heart defects. *Streptococcus* sp. are probably the most common cause of neonatal sepsis, followed by the common hospital-acquired pathogens such as *Staphylococcus* and *Pseudomonas*. Rising or falling temperature, lethargy, pallor, mottling, decreasing platelet count, hemodynamic instability, and poor feeding are typical manifestations of sepsis. The nonspecificity of these signs and the frequency with which they occur in cardiac patients without sepsis are testimony to the difficulty in prompt diagnosis of sepsis. Laboratory studies may reveal elevated or depressed white count, thrombocytopenia, hyperglycemia, and acidosis (62).

The surgeon must maintain a high index of suspicion regarding the presence of infection, even during the first postoperative night and particularly in the postoperative patient with multiple indwelling lines and foreign material within the heart. Avoidance of septic complications is achieved by minimizing the number of invasive devices and the length of time they are used, meticulous nursing procedures, and prophylactic change of lines that must be in place for a prolonged time. When infection is suspected, vigorous attempts should be made to identify the source with blood, urine, and sputum cultures, chest radiographs, and possibly computed tomography scans. Meningitis must also be considered, and cerebrospinal fluid cultures should be obtained.

After cultures have been obtained, the routine antibiotic regimen is changed, and broad-spectrum antibiotics may be instituted, usually vancomycin and an aminoglycoside. More specific coverage may be determined by the culture results. Doses of antibiotics used may require modification according to the patient's renal function. This may be abnormal because of the immaturity of the kidneys, as well as renal injury related to the underlying illness or operative complications.

Prosthetic Valves in Children

Most surgeons make great efforts to avoid implantation of prosthetic heart valves in children with congenital defects. Poor valve longevity in pediatric patients often requires accepting a less-than-ideal reconstructive operation in preference to valve replacement. Longer-term follow-up with homograft valves and pulmonary autograft valves in the aortic position is now available, and the results appear promising (63).

The accelerated calcification of bioprostheses is well known (64), and few such valves are used today. Mechanical valves are occasionally required despite the need for anticoagulation, which may be difficult to manage in growing children. Although some surgeons have reported early success in utilizing mechanical valves in pediatric patients without warfarin, longer follow-up revealed an excessive rate of thromboembolic complications (65). It is well established that warfarin must be used in children who have mechanical prosthetic valves, despite the potential problems of noncompliance or bleeding complications (66). With meticulous follow-up, late mortality due to anticoagulation in this patient population is low (67). Therefore, we have continued to use warfarin anticoagulation as we would for adult patients with mechanical valves.

Postoperative Investigations

Postoperative Echocardiography

Echocardiography, because of the detailed anatomic information it can provide and its noninvasive nature, is a nearly ideal technique for postoperative investigation of patients with congenital heart defects. We have found echocardiography to be most useful in assessing ventricular function and determining the presence of significant blood and fluid collections. Injections of saline containing microbubbles provide an echocardiographic contrast medium to demonstrate the presence of transseptal shunts. Color flow Doppler facilitates shunt detection and the estimation of valve regurgitation and stenosis. If the presence of mediastinal drainage tubes obscures the echocardiographic windows needed for a postoperative study, transesophageal echocardiography is a useful alternative. Caution must be exercised, particularly in infants, to make sure that inadvertent endotracheal tube dislodgement does not occur during echo probe manipulation. Transthoracic echo, with or without transesophageal echo, has made early postoperative cardiac catheterization of critically ill infants virtually unnecessary.

REFERENCES

1. Pfammatter JP, Berdat P, Hammerli M, et al. Pediatric cardiac surgery after exclusively echocardiography-based work-up. *Int J Cardiol* 2000;74:185–190.
2. Freed MD, Heymann MA, Lewis AB, et al. Prostaglandin E_1 in infants with ductus arteriosus-dependent congenital heart disease. *Circulation* 1981;64:899–905.
3. Sellden H, Nilsson K, Larsson L, et al. Radial arterial catheter in children and neonates: a prospective study. *Crit Care Med* 1987;15: 1106–1109.
4. Graves PW, Davis AL, Maggi JC, et al. Femoral artery cannulation for monitoring in critically ill children: prospective study. *Crit Care Med* 1990;18:1363–1366.
5. Glenski JA, Beynen FM, Brady J. A prospective evaluation of femoral artery monitoring in pediatric patients. *Anesthesiology* 1987;66:227–229.
6. Gold JP, Jonas RA, Lang P, et al. Transthoracic intracardiac monitoring lines in pediatric surgical patients: a ten-year experience. *Ann Thorac Surg* 1986;42:185–191.
7. Butt WW, Whyte H. Blood pressure monitoring in neonates: comparison of umbilical and peripheral artery catheter measurements. *J Pediatr* 1984;105:630–632.
8. Pinheiro JM, Fisher MA. Use of a triple-lumen catheter for umbilical venous access in the neonate. *J Pediatr* 1992;120:624–626.
9. Marsh JL, King W, Barrett C, et al. Serious complications after umbilical artery catheterization for neonatal monitoring. *Arch Surg* 1975;110:1203–1208.
10. Kim JH, Lee YS, Kim SH, et al. Does umbilical vein catheterization lead to portal venous thrombosis? Prospective US evaluation in 100 neonates. *Radiology* 2001;219:645–650.
11. Kirklin JK, Blackstone EH, Kirklin JW, et al. Intracardiac surgery in infants under age 3 months: predictors of postoperative in-hospital cardiac death. *Am J Cardiol* 1981;48:507–512.
12. Schranz D, Schmitt S, Oelert H, et al. Continuous monitoring of mixed venous oxygen saturation in infants after cardiac surgery. *Intensive Care Med* 1989;15:228–232.
13. Burrows FA, Williams WG, Teoh KH, et al. Myocardial performance after repair of congenital cardiac defects in infants and children. Response to volume loading. *J Thorac Cardiovasc Surg* 1988;96:548–556.
14. Tabbutt S, Duncan BW, McLaughlin D, et al. Delayed sternal closure after cardiac operations in a pediatric population. *J Thorac Cardiovasc Surg* 1997;113:886–893.

15. Zobel G, Stein JI, Kuttnig M, et al. Continuous extracorporeal fluid removal in children with low cardiac output after cardiac operations. *J Thorac Cardiovasc Surg* 1991;101:593–597.
16. Thompson LD, McElhinney DB, Findlay P, et al. A prospective randomized study comparing volume-standardized modified and conventional ultrafiltration in pediatric cardiac surgery. *J Thorac Cardiovasc Surg* 2001;122:220–228.
17. Kron IL, Rheuban K, Nolan SP. Late cardiac tamponade in children. A lethal complication. *Ann Surg* 1984;199:173–175.
18. Beland MJ, Paquet M, Gibbons JE, et al. Pericardial effusion after cardiac surgery in children and effects of aspirin for prevention. *Am J Cardiol* 1990;65:1238–1241.
19. Wilson NJ, Webber SA, Patterson MW, et al. Double-blind placebo-controlled trial of corticosteroids in children with postpericardiotomy syndrome. *Pediatr Cardiol* 1994;15:62–65.
20. Lang P, Chipman CW, Siden H, et al. Early assessment of hemodynamic status after repair of tetralogy of Fallot: a comparison of 24 hour (intensive care unit) and 1 year postoperative data in 98 patients. *Am J Cardiol* 1982;50:795–799.
21. DiDonato RM, Jonas RA, Lang P, et al. Neonatal repair of tetralogy of Fallot with and without pulmonary atresia. *J Thorac Cardiovasc Surg* 1991;101:126–137.
22. Bridges ND, Mayer JE Jr, Lock JE, et al. Effect of baffle fenestration on outcome of the modified Fontan operation. *Circulation* 1992;86:1762–1769.
23. Meliones J, Kern F, Schulman S. Pathophysiologic approach to respiratory support for patients with congenital heart disease: pediatric cardiovascular intensive care. *Prog Pediatr Cardiol* 1995;4.
24. Kocis KC, Dekeon MK, Rosen HK, et al. Pressure-regulated volume control vs. volume control ventilation in infants after surgery for congenital heart disease. *Pediatr Cardiol* 2001;22:233–237.
25. Hopkins RA, Bull C, Haworth SG, et al. Pulmonary hypertensive crises following surgery for congenital heart defects in young children. *Eur J Cardiothorac Surg* 1991;5:628–634.
26. Kocis KC, Meliones JN, Dekeon MK, et al. High-frequency jet ventilation for respiratory failure after congenital heart surgery. *Circulation* 1992;86(suppl III):III27–III32.
27. Frostell C, Fratacci M-D, Wain JC, et al. Inhaled nitric oxide. A selective pulmonary vasodilator reversing hypoxic pulmonary vasoconstriction. *Circulation* 1991;83:2038–2047.
28. Atz AM, Wessel DL. Delivery and monitoring of inhaled nitric oxide. *Curr Opin Crit Care* 1997;3:243–249.
29. Atz AM, Adatia I, Wessel DL. Rebound pulmonary hypertension after inhalation of nitric oxide. *Ann Thorac Surg* 1996;62:1759–1764.
30. Morray JP, Lynn AM, Mansfield PB. Effect of pH and pCO_2 on pulmonary and systemic hemodynamics after surgery in children with congestive heart disease and pulmonary hypertension. *J Pediatr* 1988;113:474–479.
31. Jobes DR, Nicolson SC, Steven JM, et al. Carbon dioxide prevents pulmonary overcirculation in hypoplastic left heart syndrome. *Ann Thorac Surg* 1992;54:150–151.
32. O'Brien P, Elixson EM. The child following the Fontan procedure: nursing strategies. *AACN Clin Issue Crit Care Nurs* 1990; 1:46–58.

33. Lofland GK. The enhancement of hemodynamic performance in Fontan circulation using pain free spontaneous ventilation. *Eur J Cardiothorac Surg* 2001;20:114–118.
34. Valsangiacomo E, Schmid ER, Schüpbach RW, et al. Early postoperative arrhythmias after cardiac operation in children. *Ann Thorac Surg* 2002;74:792–796.
35. Kashima I, Aeba R, Katogi T, et al. Optimal position to atrial epicardial leads for temporary pacing in infants after cardiac surgery. *Ann Thorac Surg* 2001;71:1945–1948.
36. Gillette PC. Diagnosis and management of postoperative junctional ectopic tachycardia. *Am Heart J* 1989;118:192–194.
37. Figa FH, Gow RM, Hamilton RM, et al. Clinical efficacy and safety of intravenous amiodarone in infants and children. *Am J Cardiol* 1994;74:573–577.
38. Perry J, Fenrich AL, Hulse JE, et al. Pediatric use of intravenous amiodarone: efficacy and safety in critically ill patients from a multicenter protocol. *J Am Coll Cardiol* 1996;27:1246–1250.
39. Benzing G III, Francis PD, Kaplan S, et al. Glucose and insulin changes in infants and children undergoing hypothermic open-heart surgery. *Am J Cardiol* 1983;52:133–136.
40. LaFranchi S. Hypoglycemia of infancy and childhood. *Pediatr Clin North Am* 1987;34:961–982.
41. Tsang RC, Steichen JJ, Chan GM. Neonatal hypocalcemia. Mechanism of occurrence and management. *Crit Care Med* 1977;5: 56–61.
42. Satur C, Stubington S, Jennings A, et al. Magnesium flux during and after open heart operations in children. *Ann Thorac Surg* 1995;59:921–927.
43. Colon-Otero G, Gilchrist GS, Holcomb GR, et al. Preoperative evaluation of hemostasis in patients with congenital heart disease. *Mayo Clin Proc* 1987;62:379–385.
44. Mohr R, Martinowitz U, Lavee J, et al. The hemostatic effect of transfusing fresh whole blood versus platelet concentrates after cardiac operations. *J Thorac Cardiovasc Surg* 1988;96: 530–534.
45. Fox S, Pierce WS, Waldhausen JA. Pathogenesis of paradoxical hypertension after coarctation repair. *Ann Thorac Surg* 1980;29: 135–141.
46. Stansel HC, Tabry IF, Poirier RA, et al. One hundred consecutive coarctation resections followed from one to thirteen years. *J Pediatr Surg* 1977;12:279–286.
47. Benedict CR, Grahame-Smith DG, Fisher A. Changes in plasma catecholamines and dopamine beta-hydroxylase after corrective surgery for coarctation of the aorta. *Circulation* 1978;57:598–602.
48. Sealy WC. Paradoxical hypertension after repair of coarctation of the aorta: a review of its causes. *Ann Thorac Surg* 1990;50:323–329.
49. Rocchini AP, Rosenthal A, Barger AC, et al. Pathogenesis of paradoxical hypertension after coarctation resection. *Circulation* 1976;54:382–387.
50. Choy M, Rocchini AP, Beekman RH, et al. Paradoxical hypertension after repair of coarctation of the aorta in children: balloon angioplasty versus surgical repair. *Circulation* 1987;75:1186–1191.
51. Gidding SS, Rocchini AP, Beekman R, et al. Therapeutic effect of propranolol on paradoxical hypertension after repair of coarctation of the aorta. *N Engl J Med* 1985;312:1224–1228.

52. Smerling A, Gerson WM. Esmolol for severe hypertension following repair of aortic coarctation. *Crit Care Med* 1990;18:1288–1290.
53. Bojar RM, Weiner B, Cleveland RJ. Intravenous labetalol for control of hypertension following repair of coarctation of the aorta. *Clin Cardiol* 1988;11:639–641.
54. Forbess JM, Visconti KJ, Hancock-Friesen C, et al. Neurodevelopmental outcome after congenital heart surgery: results from an institutional registry. *Circulation* 2002;106(suppl I):I95–I102.
55. DeLeon G, Ilbawi M, Arcilla R, et al. Choreoathetosis after deep hypothermia without circulatory arrest. *Ann Thorac Surg* 1990; 50:714–719.
56. Bellinger DC, Wernovsky G, Rappaport LA, et al. Cognitive development of children following early repair of transposition of the great arteries using deep hypothermic circulatory arrest. *Pediatrics* 1991;87:701–707.
57. Bellinger DC, Wypij D, Kuban KC, et al. Developmental and neurologic status of children 4 years of age after heart surgery with hypothermic circulatory arrest or low-flow cardiopulmonary bypass. *Circulation* 1999;100:526–532.
58. duPlessis AJ, Jonas RA, Wypij D, et al. Perioperative effects of alpha-stat versus pH-stat strategies for deep hypothermic cardiopulmonary bypass infants. *J Thorac Cardiovasc Surg* 1997;114: 991–1001.
59. Ekroth R, Thompson RJ, Lincoln C, et al. Elective deep hypothermia with total circulatory arrest: changes in plasma creatine kinase BB, blood glucose, and clinical variables. *J Thorac Cardiovasc Surg* 1989;97:30–35.
60. Menache CC, duPlessis AJ, Wessel DL, et al. Current incidence of acute neurologic complications after open-heart operations in children. *Ann Thorac Surg* 2002;73:1752–1758.
61. Painter MJ, Bergman I, Crumrine P. Neonatal seizures. *Pediatr Clin North Am* 1986;33:91–109.
62. Donovan EF. Perioperative care of the surgical neonate. *Surg Clin North Am* 1985;65:1061–1081.
63. Elkins RC, Lane MM, McCue C. Ross operation in children: late results. *J Heart Valve Dis* 2001;10:736–741.
64. Dunn JM. Porcine valve durability in children. *Ann Thorac Surg* 1981;32:357–368.
65. Sade RM, Crawford FA Jr, Fyfe DA, et al. Valve prostheses in children: a reassessment of anticoagulation. *J Thorac Cardiovasc Surg* 1988;95:553–561.
66. Stewart S, Cianciotta D, Alexson C, et al. The long-term risk of warfarin sodium therapy and the incidence of thromboembolism in children after prosthetic cardiac valve replacement. *J Thorac Cardiovasc Surg* 1987;93:551–554.
67. Calderone CA, Raghuveer G, Hills CB, et al. Long-term survival after mitral valve replacement in children <5 years: a multi-institutional study. *Circulation* 2001;104(suppl I):I143–I147.

Mechanical Cardiac Support and Transplantation

Despite all best surgical and medical efforts, patients may suffer heart conditions or perioperative complications that require more than the usual surgical therapy and postoperative management. For these patients, mechanical device support of the failing heart may be lifesaving, and, when required, replacement of the heart may be the only potentially successful form of therapy.

INTRAAORTIC BALLOON COUNTERPULSATION

The most commonly used method of mechanical circulatory support is, by far, intraaortic balloon counterpulsation, which is erroneously called the *intraaortic balloon pump* (IABP). In most patients, the IABP is inserted percutaneously via the femoral artery (Fig. 8-1). The sausage-shaped balloon is advanced to the thoracic aorta, with the tip being placed just distal to the takeoff of the left subclavian artery. Balloon inflation and deflation are timed to the cardiac cycle: either the electrocardiogram or the arterial pressure wave. Deflation of the balloon during early systole provides afterload reduction (decreased impedance to ventricular emptying), with a resultant increase in cardiac output of up to approximately 20%. Inflation of the balloon during diastole results in increased coronary artery perfusion pressure and flow. In contrast to most inotropic drugs, the appropriately timed IABP provides a reduction in both left ventricular work and myocardial oxygen consumption. Because of these properties, the IABP is frequently used in patients with low cardiac output. Patients with ongoing myocardial ischemia such as unstable angina or complicated myocardial infarction are also potential candidates for IABP support. Balloon pump support is particularly advantageous in patients with severe mitral valve regurgitation or postinfarction ventricular septal defect as it improves the forward ejection of left ventricular blood into a lowered resistance circuit, thus reducing the severity of the regurgitation or left-to-right shunting. Although IABP assist is usually for 1 to a few days to allow for recovery of the myocardium, support for long periods (even weeks) is possible, although rarely indicated. IABP support in children has been reported but is generally not the support method of choice as other methods such as extracorporeal membrane oxygenation are usually preferred (1,2).

An IABP is typically inserted when the patient's cardiac index is <1.8 to 2.0 L/min/m^2 despite moderate doses of inotropic drugs (such as epinephrine at 0.075 µg/kg per minute or dobutamine at 10 µg/kg per minute) in the absence of hypovolemia or reversible conditions such as tamponade. Because of the augmentation of coronary blood flow, it may also be indicated in patients with ongoing myocardial ischemia even if the cardiac output is not severely reduced. It should not, however, be placed in patients with aortic valve insufficiency, aortic dissection, or thoracic aortic aneurysm.

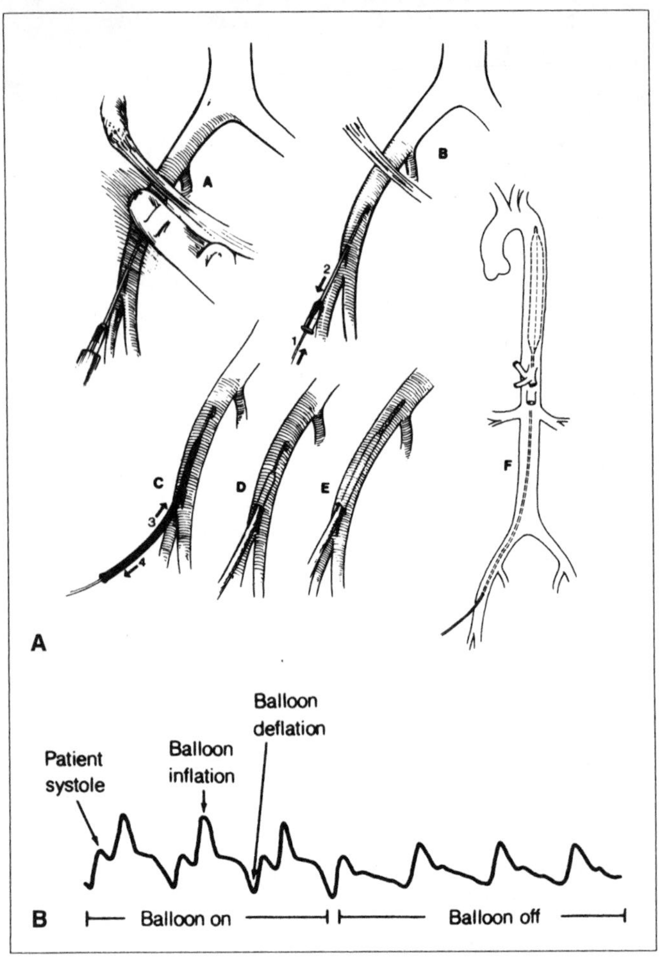

Fig. 8-1. Percutaneous insertion of an intraaortic balloon pump via the femoral artery. A: Insertion technique. If a femoral arterial line is not already present, the femoral artery is localized with a needle and syringe. Ideally, the artery should be entered immediately below the inguinal ligament (*A*). A guidewire is introduced via the needle (or femoral arterial line, if present) and into the iliofemoral tree (*B*). The needle is withdrawn over the guidewire, using gentle pressure to prevent bleeding around the insertion site, and dilators are serially introduced over the guidewire to dilate the femoral puncture site (*C*). An intraaortic balloon pump insertion sheath is then inserted over the final dilator (*D, E*). The dilator is removed, and the balloon is inserted into the sheath. The balloon is then directed into the descending aorta (*F*). Passage of the balloon can be facilitated if a long guidewire is used (150 cm) to help negotiate the balloon through the iliofemoral arterial system. B: Proper balloon timing is shown in this tracing of arterial blood pressure. Balloon inflation occurs during patient diastole, and balloon deflation occurs as the patient's heart ejects so as to produce mechanical afterload reduction.

Severe atherosclerosis of the descending aorta (which can be visualized by transesophageal echocardiography) may also be a relative contraindication due to the risk of peripheral embolization of dislodged plaque.

Balloon pump support may be initiated prior to surgery in high-risk patients for whom there is a significant likelihood of postoperative IABP requirement. In this situation, the IABP is often inserted in the cardiac catheterization laboratory using fluoroscopy to guide placement, often en route to the operating room. This is particularly useful for patients with severe peripheral vascular disease in whom insertion may be more difficult due to femoral artery involvement. Candidates for preoperative IABP insertion include those with poor left ventricular function (ejection fraction <25% to 30%), unstable angina, or acute myocardial infarction and those undergoing an anticipated difficult repeat coronary bypass procedure. IABP utilization in such situations has proven to improve patient outcome and to be cost-effective (3–5).

Patients with increased risk for intraoperative complications (such as a repeat operation in the patient with patent but diseased old vein grafts) or with moderately impaired left ventricular function may not require a preoperative IABP but are still at increased risk for the need for support to wean from cardiopulmonary bypass (CPB). In these patients, it is useful to place a small catheter in the femoral artery after the induction of anesthesia but prior to beginning the procedure. This is placed to a transducer to confirm the intraarterial location. If an IABP is needed for CPB separation, it can then be advanced over a wire. For patients with severe aortoiliac occlusive disease or other conditions preventing femoral artery insertion, it is possible to place the IABP through the ascending aorta (Fig. 8-2) (2,6). Removal usually requires reoperation, depending on the technique employed.

Complications related to IABP occur in at least 10% of patients, with the most common being leg ischemia (2,7). Patients with peripheral vascular occlusive disease and poor preoperative left ventricular are at increased risk, with other conditions such as hypertension, diabetes, and female gender being potential contributors. For the ischemic limb, surgical intervention is usually required. Early IABP removal with thromboendarterectomy and femoral artery repair is usually required. If the leg is ischemic but the patient is IABP dependent, revascularization may be accomplished by construction of a femoral artery-to-femoral artery crossover graft. Other IABP complications include iliac or aortic dissection, bleeding, infection, and paraplegia. A rare problem is balloon entrapment. This occurs after the balloon develops a leak and blood enters the balloon, clots, and then prevents easy removal. If this occurs, open surgical removal and arterial repair are usually indicated, although management by clot lysis (via thrombolytic drug injection into the drive lumen of the catheter) has also been reported (8).

MECHANICAL CARDIAC SUPPORT

A patient who remains in a low output state despite inotropic and IABP support may be a candidate for mechanical circulatory support. This is most often provided with a blood pump termed a ventricular assist device (VAD). Most commonly, this occurs in one of

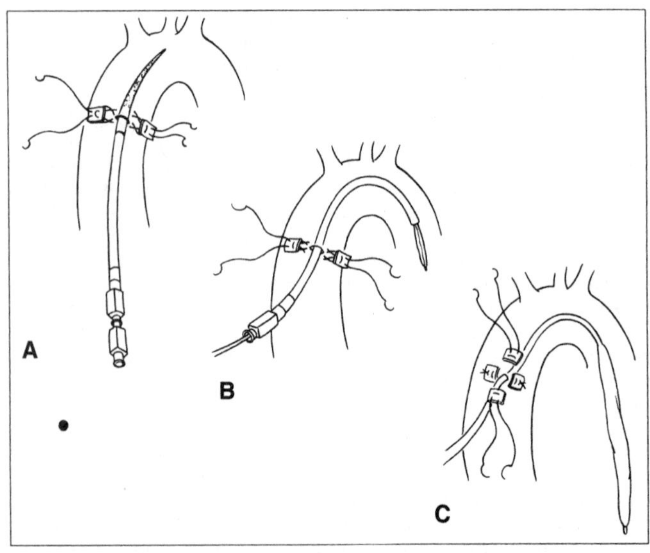

Fig. 8-2. Technique for transthoracic intraaortic balloon placement. With use of two concentric pursestring sutures, a guidewire and dilators are introduced into the ascending aorta and passed around the aortic arch into the descending aorta. An insertion sheath is placed over the guidewire and dilators and directed beyond the brachiocephalic vessels (*A*). The intraaortic balloon pump catheter and balloon are then introduced over the guidewire, via the sheath, into the descending aorta (*B*). The position must be estimated visually by the surgeon, so that the proximal extent of the balloon is beyond the left subclavian artery (*C*). The sheath is then withdrawn from the aorta, and the pursestring sutures are tightened using short tourniquets. The balloon may be subsequently removed by withdrawing the balloon catheter out the aortotomy, achieving digital control of the aortotomy site, and tightening and tying down the pursestring sutures.

three situations: (a) in the patient who cannot be weaned from CPB during a cardiac surgical procedure (*postcardiotomy cardiogenic shock*), (b) in the patient with chronic heart failure who is awaiting transplantation but who deteriorates hemodynamically (*bridge to transplantation*), and (c) in the patient with end-stage heart failure who is not eligible for a heart transplant (*destination therapy*). In the patient with postcardiotomy cardiogenic shock, the decline in myocardial performance is related to perioperative myocardial stunning, and recovery of ventricular function is anticipated (although not certain). Short-term VAD support will allow time for ventricular recovery. The bridge-to-transplant patient is an approved cardiac transplant candidate who suffers from chronic congestive heart failure. If the patient experiences a life-threatening decline, most often manifest by a deterioration in end-organ function related to hypoperfusion, long-term VAD support may allow the patient to survive until a donor heart is available. In the fall of 2002, the Food and Drug Administration (FDA) approved permanent use of an intracorporeal VAD in patients with end-stage heart failure who are not candidates for cardiac transplantation (9). In this instance, the VAD remains *in situ* for the remainder of the patient's life.

Occasionally, a patient who presents with acute myocarditis and cardiogenic shock, or a patient who suffers an acute decompensation of chronic heart failure, may *recover* ventricular function following weeks or months of VAD support (10–12). Active areas of investigation include identifying patients who might benefit from interim circulatory support and the mechanism(s) by which recovery occurs (13). Whether or not myocardial recovery is sustained in these patients following device removal remains to be determined.

The mechanical blood pump utilized most frequently is the VAD. Depending upon the cannulation scheme employed, the single-ventricle VAD is designed to function either in series or parallel with the native heart. Two VADs may be employed to provide biventricular support. The total artificial heart is implanted orthotopically, much like a donor heart. The recipient heart is removed when an artificial heart is inserted. Although there has been a resurgence of interest in the artificial heart in the recent past, its current use is limited to a few academic centers as part of an FDA-approved clinical trial (14).

Postcardiotomy Cardiogenic Shock

The patient who has undergone a technically complete operation but who cannot be weaned from CPB, despite use of an IABP, may be supported with a mechanical blood pump (15,16). The device is used to maintain the systemic (and/or pulmonary) circulation, with the endpoint being the recovery of ventricular function. When the ventricle has recovered, the mechanical blood pump is removed. For many years, it was estimated that 0.5% to 1% of patients who undergo an open heart operation will not be able to be weaned from CPB following completion of the procedure despite the use of inotropic agents and an IABP. More recently, the need for VAD support in the postcardiotomy cardiogenic shock situation has declined, perhaps due to better myocardial protection or the introduction of more potent inotropic agents. Regardless, when needed, patient survival following VAD implantation for this purpose remains suboptimal, with only about 25% of the patients surviving to be discharged from the hospital. This is often due to complications related to organ systems other than the heart.

Patient Selection

An effort should be made preoperatively to identify patients who might be at risk for profound postoperative ventricular dysfunction. One such patient group at high risk for postoperative left heart failure comprises those who enter the operating room with a low ejection fraction (<20% to 25%). If a patient has underlying left ventricular dysfunction in association with critical aortic stenosis or occlusive coronary artery disease in combination with viable myocardium, improved left ventricular function following either aortic valve replacement or coronary revascularization is anticipated (17). Should such a patient fail to be weaned from

CPB, blood pump support is a reasonable undertaking, with the expectation that myocardial recovery will occur. For patients with a low ejection fraction who have marginal potential for recovery of myocardial function following operative intervention, it is prudent to perform a cursory pretransplant evaluation. If the patient requires VAD support upon completion of the operation, the endpoint changes from recovery of ventricular function to the bridge-to-transplant application.

Unfortunately, the inability to wean a patient from CPB is usually unanticipated. Thus, the decision regarding the use of a VAD in this situation is made urgently in the operating room. When the operation is completed and the patient has been converted to a functional cardiac rhythm but still cannot be weaned from CPB, echocardiography or visual inspection will demonstrate poor left ventricular wall motion. In rapid sequence, the patient should be placed on appropriate inotropic support and an IABP. If the patient cannot be weaned from CPB despite these interventions, consideration should be given to the use of a VAD. To be considered a candidate for VAD use, the patient should have undergone a complete and technically successful open-heart procedure with the expectation that ventricular recovery is a possibility. Furthermore, the patient should have a reasonable expectation for operative survival. Preoperative conditions that may negatively impact the potential for survival include renal failure, irreversible pulmonary hypertension, severe peripheral vascular disease, and advanced age (older than 75 years). Operative events that may adversely impact the potential for patient recovery include a low flow state or prolonged hypotension, either of which might precipitate a neurologic event or renal failure. If the patient is considered a reasonable candidate for recovery and a return of ventricular function, it is imperative to proceed rapidly with VAD implantation to avoid the adverse effects of prolonged CPB.

Device Selection and Implantation Technique

Although not approved by the FDA for this clinical application, centrifugal pumps have been widely used successfully for interim support of either the left or the right heart (18,19). The centrifugal pump is an extracorporeal device that requires systemic anticoagulation. The pump and console are located at the patient's bedside. Use of a centrifugal pump generally requires a perfusionist to be in attendance for pump management.

Two air-driven pulsatile devices are approved by the FDA for the use as either a left or a right ventricular assist device (LVAD, RVAD). The Abiomed BVS 5000 Biventricular Support System (Abiomed, Danvers, MA) is an extracorporeal device connected by percutaneous cannulas to the patient, with the blood pump and drive console being located at the patient's bedside (Table 8-1) (20,21). This device is particularly useful for postcardiotomy support as it is easily implanted and removed. Full-time attendance by a perfusionist is not required as the device may be managed by appropriately trained nursing staff. Continuous anticoagulation, however, is required (activated clotting time 180 to 200 seconds or activated partial thromboplastin time 1.5 to 2.0 times control). The Thoratec VAD System (Thoratec Corp., Pleasanton, CA, U.S.A.) offers greater patient mobility in that the blood pump is paracorporeal in location, being positioned on the pa-

Table 8-1. Ventricular assist devices

Indication	Device	Left, Right, or Biventricular Support
PCCS	Abiomed BVS 5000	Biventricular
PCCS, bridge	Thoratec VAD system	Biventricular
Bridge	Thoratec HeartMate IP LVAS	Left
Bridge, DT	Thoratec HeartMate VE LVAS	Left
Bridge	Novacor LVAS	Left

Bridge, bridge to cardiac transplantation; DT, destination therapy; PCCS, postcardiotomy cardiogenic shock.

tient's anterior abdominal wall (22). The blood pump is connected to a bedside console.

Patients who cannot be weaned from CPB usually suffer from left heart failure (Table 8-2). Thus, left ventricular support is provided first. The usual configuration for short-term left heart support is VAD inflow from the patient's left atrium with VAD outflow to the patient's ascending aorta (23,24). Whereas left atrial inflow does not provide as efficient uptake as left ventricular apex cannulation, it avoids injury to the apical myocardium that may be viable and will participate in ventricular recovery, so that eventual removal of the LVAD will be possible. With left atrial cannulation, LVAD explantation can usually be accomplished without the use of CPB.

If the patient cannot be weaned from CPB despite inotropic support and the IABP, the patient remains on CPB as preparations are made for LVAD implantation (25). A left atrial pressure line is

Table 8-2. Definition of ventricular failure

Left ventricle	
Profound left ventricular wall motion abnormalities by transesophageal echocardiography	
Left atrial pressure	≥15–20 mm Hg
Peak systolic aortic pressure	≤90 mm Hg
Cardiac index	≤2.0 L/min/m^2
Despite: Functional cardiac rhythm	
Inotrope administration	
Intraaortic balloon counterpulsation	
Right ventricle	
Cardiac index	≤2.0 L/min/m^2
Right atrial pressure	≥20 mm Hg
Left atrial pressure	≤10 mm Hg
Distended right ventricle	
Hypocontractile right ventricular free wall	
Inability to volume load the left ventricle	

inserted via the right superior pulmonary vein. The presence of the left atrial line facilitates decision making when weaning from CPB on the LVAD. For left atrial cannulation, the interatrial groove is developed, and the left atrial cannula is inserted via the right lateral wall of the left atrium. The outlet graft is anastomosed in an end-to-side fashion to the ascending aorta. If a centrifugal pump is used as an LVAD, a standard arterial CPB cannula is employed for VAD outflow. For left heart support utilizing a left atrial inflow cannula, the inflow and outflow cannulas exit the pericardium in the right subcostal region. The cannulas are completely de-aired and connected to the VAD circuit.

Right heart performance is maximized using temporary pacing and selective inotrope infusion. Agents that are particularly effective for right heart support include isoproterenol and milrinone. Inhaled nitric oxide (10 to 20 parts per million) effectively unloads a failing right heart by reducing pulmonary vascular resistance (26). Left and right heart preload are monitored simultaneously. LVAD flow is initiated as CPB flow is decreased. The goal is a systemic systolic blood pressure in excess of 90 mm Hg with a cardiac index well above 2.0 L/min/m^2. If the right heart is functioning satisfactorily, the central venous pressure (CVP) should remain below 10 to 15 mm Hg (Table 8-3). If LVAD filling is satisfactory, the left atrial pressure will be below 10 mm Hg.

Following termination of CPB, transesophageal echocardiography is performed. Ideally, the left heart should be well decompressed. As the left atrial cannula often does not completely decompress the left heart, the native aortic valve will often open intermittently (as the volume-loaded, albeit failing, left heart ejects). A bubble study is performed to evaluate for a patent foramen ovale. If a foramen ovale is present, this must be closed due to the potential for systemic desaturation. The latter scenario is possible due to the reduction of left atrial pressure in association with mild right ventricular dysfunction. The increase in right atrial pressure relative to the low left atrial pressure results in a right-to-left shunt at the atrial level. The resultant systemic desaturation can be profound and lead to central nervous system sequelae. If a patent

Table 8-3. Hemodynamic status during left ventricular assistance

CVP (mm Hg)	LAP (mm Hg)	Systolic AoP (mm Hg)	CI (L/min/m^2)	Diagnosis
<20	<10	>90	>2.0	Satisfactory pumping
<15	<10	<90	<2.0	Hypovolemia
<20	>20	<90	<2.0	Inlet cannula obstruction
>20	<10	<90	<2.0	Right ventricular failure

AoP, aortic pressure; CI, cardiac index; CVP, central venous pressure; LAP, left atrial pressure.

foramen ovale is present, the patient is converted to bicaval venous cannulation, CPB is reinstituted, and the defect is closed through a small right atriotomy.

Persistent right heart dysfunction results in a low left atrial pressure with inadequate left-sided filling. LVAD flow is suboptimal, and the CVP is elevated. Visual inspection of the right heart demonstrates right ventricular distention. If inotrope administration and the use of nitric oxide do not correct the right ventricular dysfunction, RVAD implantation is indicated (27). The usual configuration for RVAD implantation is right atrial inflow with pulmonary artery outflow. The Abiomed BVS 5000, Thoratec paracorporeal pump, or any centrifugal pump can be configured for right heart support. Inflow and outflow cannulas exit the chest via the left subcostal region. Figure 8-3 shows RVAD and LVAD cannulation.

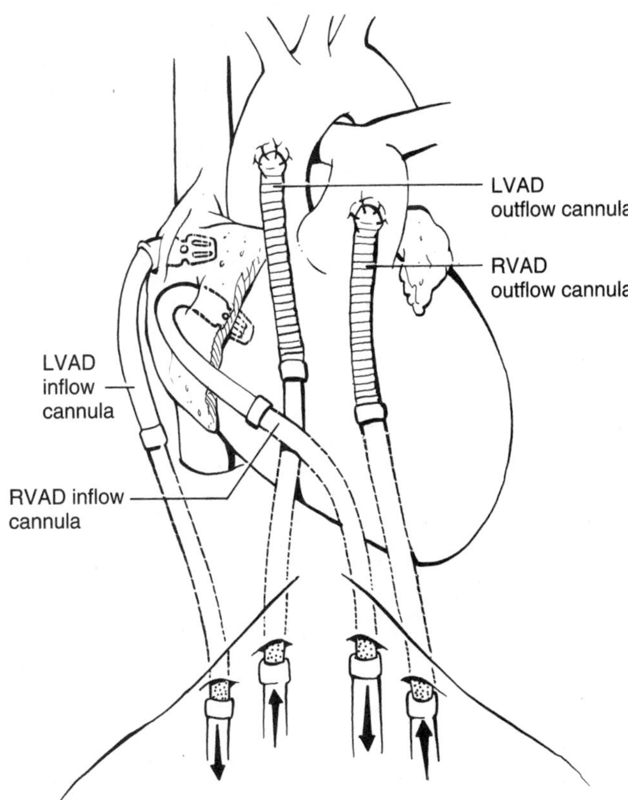

Fig. 8-3. Cannulation scheme for biventricular assistance for postcardiotomy cardiogenic shock. Left ventricular assistance employs left atrial inflow and aortic outflow cannulas. Right ventricular assistance utilizes right atrial inflow and main pulmonary artery outflow cannulas. LVAD, left ventricular assist device; RVAD, right ventricular assist device.

Occasionally, a patient will develop isolated right ventricular dysfunction while left ventricular contractility is preserved. This most commonly occurs following an inferior wall myocardial infarction or secondary to acute right ventricular distention associated with a sizable pulmonary embolism. In this situation, the patient's left heart will be decompressed and contracting vigorously. The right heart will be distended and hypocontractile. The CVP will exceed 20 mm Hg, while pulmonary artery pressures will be low. If tailored inotropic therapy does not result in improved left ventricular preload and right heart decompression, RVAD implantation should follow. The RVAD uptake is via the right atrium with return to the main pulmonary artery. Pulmonary artery or the left atrial pressure should be monitored, as it may be necessary to limit RVAD flow to avoid pulmonary congestion.

Following termination of CPB, protamine sulfate is slowly administered to reverse the heparin effect and return the activated clotting time to baseline. Nonsurgical bleeding is often the norm following an extended CPB time. If a patient is considered to be a potential VAD candidate preoperatively, aprotinin is employed (see Chapter 5). If aprotinin has not been utilized, ϵ-aminocaproic acid (5 g i.v. before CPB, 5 g i.v. on CPB, 1 to 2 g per hour i.v. thereafter for up to 8 hours) may be administered following decannulation. The two drugs are not, however, administered together. Specific coagulation deficits are corrected with the administration of blood component therapy. Chest closure can be problematic due to the presence of VAD cannulas and coronary bypass conduits, but is attempted because reapproximation of the sternal edges and soft tissues reduces postoperative bleeding. If it is not possible to close the chest primarily, the sternum is stented open. As myocardial edema resolves over the ensuing days, delayed chest closure is often possible.

Postoperative Care

The primary postoperative consideration following LVAD implantation is to ensure adequate systemic perfusion. This is based in part upon the ability of the right heart to move blood through the pulmonary vasculature to the left heart and thus, in turn, to the LVAD. For this, the right heart must be adequately supported. This ensures satisfactory left heart filling and reduces systemic venous congestion, thereby facilitating end-organ perfusion. Assuming the patient has an effective cardiac rhythm, the right heart is supported with tailored inotropic administration and inhaled nitric oxide as described in *Cardiac Transplantation.* Failing these treatment modalities, an RVAD is used to replace the function of the native right heart.

The postcardiotomy cardiogenic shock patient is at risk for postoperative hemorrhage. The etiology of this bleeding is multifactorial (28). Platelet dysfunction, due to CPB and the IABP (if present), is a prime causative factor. A reduction in serum clotting factors, excessive fibrinolysis, and the presence of multiple suture lines and cannula access sites also contribute. When this occurs, coagulation studies are obtained, and the coagulopathy is corrected with appropriate blood product and clotting factor administration. If the patient is considered to be a candidate for heart transplantation, leukodepleted blood products are used to help avoid antibody development.

In the first 24 hours following VAD insertion, the patient is allowed to awaken for neurologic assessment. Early extubation helps to avoid nosocomial pneumonia. Because a prolonged CPB time results in a capillary leak syndrome with an increase in extravascular lung water, a diuretic is administered. This is often in the form of a continuous furosemide infusion, the goal being an output that exceeds intake over the first 24 hours. Within 12 to 24 hours of surgery, all noncritical tubes and lines are removed in order to avoid infectious complications. All of the extracorporeal blood pumps require systemic anticoagulation, but systemic anticoagulation is not begun until the patient's coagulation studies have returned to normal and mediastinal tube drainage has fallen below 50 mL per hour for 2 to 3 hours. Following this, heparin (800 to 1,000 U per hour i.v., goal partial thromboplastin time 1.5 to 2.0 times control) is used as the systemic anticoagulant. The usual intensive care unit precautions are employed, including stress ulcer prophylaxis, nutritional support, and infection control.

Weaning from Mechanical Circulatory Support

Following VAD implantation, ventricular recovery usually occurs in a few days. The simplest way to assess ventricular recovery is using pulmonary arterial and left atrial pressure lines. For the LVAD-only patient, device flow is slowly reduced over a number of hours while monitoring the filling pressures and cardiac output. If the left ventricle has recovered, these hemodynamic parameters will be maintained despite a mild to modest reduction in LVAD flow. If the reduced LVAD flow results in an elevation in left atrial or pulmonary artery pressures, LVAD flow should again be increased to decompress the left heart, which facilitates left ventricular recovery.

If LVAD support is required for more than a few days, the monitoring catheters are often withdrawn. In this case, echocardiography can be used to monitor left ventricular contractility while reducing LVAD flow (29). If ventricular recovery has occurred, a reduction in LVAD flow is associated with improved left-sided wall motion, and the native aortic valve opens with each cardiac contraction.

The natural inclination is to rapidly wean the patient from the mechanical blood pump for fear of a complication related to the presence of the device. Weaning attempts should be delayed, however, to allow time for ventricular recovery and to make sure that end organs have recovered from the acute insult of the initial operation. Weaning should be performed slowly to avoid volume overloading of the left ventricle. Furthermore, it is best to wean the patient from left heart support without the use of additional inotropic drugs, which cause increased oxygen consumption by the recovering ventricle. In addition, if a patient is weaned from the LVAD without the use of inotropic support, these agents can be employed judiciously following device removal should that be necessary. LVAD flow is reduced to a minimum of 1.5 to 2 L per minute, with flow maintained at that minimal rate for an extended period of time to ensure patient stability prior to device removal. We prefer that the patient be hemodynamically stable on a minimum of 2 L of LVAD flow for at least 12 to 24 hours prior to device explantation. During this time, it is imperative that the patient's anticoagulation be therapeutic to avoid VAD thrombosis.

If ventricular function is recovered, the patient is returned to the operating room for VAD removal. CPB is not usually required for explantation. If echocardiographic and visual inspection of the heart suggests that there is unequivocal recovery of ventricular function, the device is simply withdrawn. To be certain that the patient has recovered ventricular function, in the operating room, we usually administer heparin and discontinue VAD support for a number of minutes prior to device explantation (Table 8-4). By so doing, we ensure that the patient is hemodynamically stable without LVAD support. The left atrial cannula is then withdrawn, the outlet graft is transected adjacent to the aorta, and the stump of the graft is oversewn. Chest closure and patient care are conventional thereafter.

Bridge to Cardiac Transplant

Mechanical circulatory support as a bridge to cardiac transplant is a frequent indication for mechanical blood pump use (30). In this situation, a patient who is a candidate for heart transplantation but who deteriorates hemodynamically prior to the availability of a donor heart is offered interim use of a mechanical blood pump. The endpoint in this clinical situation is device removal at the time of cardiac transplantation. As a result, the focus in patient care is different from that in the postcardiotomy cardiogenic shock situation, as the heart is not expected to recover. Rather, the goal is to improve systemic perfusion and end organ function. Furthermore, the patient is rehabilitated, physically and nutritionally, in preparation for the subsequent heart transplant. Excellent pretransplant and posttransplant survival is possible.

Four different devices are available for use as a bridge to cardiac transplantation (Table 8-1). The Thoratec VAD is the same device approved for use in the postcardiotomy cardiogenic shock patient

Table 8-4. Indicators of ventricular recovery

Left ventricle	
In the absence of left ventricular assistance:	
Peak systolic arterial pressure	≥90 mm Hg
Cardiac index	>2.0 L/min/m^2
Pulmonary artery pressures do not rise	
Concentric contraction of left ventricular free wall and septum by TEE	
No more than one inotropic drug required	
Right ventricle	
In the absence of right ventricular assistance:	
Peak systolic arterial pressure	≥90 mm Hg
Central venous pressure	<10–15 mm Hg
Cardiac index	>2.0 L/min/m^2
Pulmonary artery pressures are maintained	
If an LVAD is in place, LVAD flow is maintained	
Brisk contraction of right ventricular free wall	
No more than one inotropic or pulmonary vasodilator drug required	

LVAD, left ventricular assist device; TEE, transesophageal echocardiography.

population (31). This paracorporeal blood pump is capable of providing either right or left heart support. Intracorporeal devices include the HeartMate IP LVAS, the HeartMate VE LVAS (both manufactured by Thoratec Corp.), and the Novacor LVAS (World-Heart, Oakland, CA) (32–34). The HeartMate IP LVAS is an implantable pneumatically powered device, whereas the HeartMate VE LVAS and Novacor LVAS are electric blood pumps. These pumps are implanted in the patient's anterior abdominal wall or left upper quadrant of the abdomen proper. The electric blood pumps permit improved patient mobility as the VADs are powered by a lightweight external battery pack and control system. All of these devices allow months or even a year or two of trouble-free support; patients who receive an electric implantable blood pump may be discharged from the hospital (35). As the donor organ shortage has resulted in prolonged waiting times prior to cardiac transplantation, quality-of-life issues in patients receiving mechanical circulatory support become increasingly important.

Patient Selection

The patient must fulfill all cardiac transplant inclusion and exclusion criteria and be on the active transplant waiting list (36). Typically, the approved cardiac transplant recipient who deteriorates hemodynamically is hospitalized in an intensive care unit with invasive hemodynamic monitoring lines, inotropic drugs maximized, and, often, an IABP. However, as results with mechanical circulatory support in this patient population have improved and the duration of waiting times prior to transplantation has increased, the use of an IABP is not always necessary prior to VAD implantation. When a potential transplant recipient is admitted to the hospital with hemodynamic deterioration, preliminary contact with the patient by the mechanical blood pump team ensures that the patient and family understand the concept of mechanical circulatory support and have adequate social support to permit use of this therapeutic modality. Financial concerns and insurance issues are best addressed prior to blood pump insertion.

A preoperative checklist is utilized to evaluate LVAD candidates (Table 8-5). The patient should be infection-free. Systemic anticoagulation is discontinued if possible or is converted to heparin infusion if continued thromboprophylaxis is required. An echocardiogram is performed to rule out left ventricular thrombus (which would complicate placement of the VAD inflow cannula in the left ventricular apex) and to assess aortic valve competency (severe aortic insufficiency needs to be corrected at the time of LVAD implantation) and the presence of a patent foramen ovale (37). The patient's abdomen is examined as previous intra-abdominal operations may provide technical hurdles for implantable LVAD insertion. A prior incision in the subcostal region may affect preperitoneal placement of an implantable blood pump. Patients who have received an implantable defibrillator in the distant past may have a generator in the left upper abdominal quadrant that may need to be removed or repositioned when the LVAD is implanted.

If a patient is a candidate for mechanical circulatory support as a bridge to cardiac transplantation, the operation is usually performed on an urgent, but not emergency, basis. A blood type and

Table 8-5. Preoperative checklist for the ventricular assist device patient

Baseline laboratory studies
Complete blood count
Renal panel
Liver function tests
Coagulation studies
Serum prealbumin
Type and cross (leukodepleted blood products)
Urinalysis

Right heart catheterization
Determine reversibility of pulmonary hypertension

Echocardiography—evaluate for:
Left ventricular thrombus
Aortic insufficiency
Patent foramen ovale

Baseline neurologic examination

Review old operative notes and catheterization data

New intravenous and hemodynamic monitoring lines the night prior to surgery

Informed consent

Preoperative antibiotics and skin preparation

cross-match are performed. All intravenous catheters and lines are moved to new sites before LVAD insertion to reduce the infection risk. The antibiotic regimen is complex and specifically designed to provide prophylaxis against a broad spectrum of organisms associated with mechanical blood pumps (Table 8-6).

Operative Management

The first decision in managing the bridge-to-transplant patient is device selection. The advantage of the *paracorporeal* Thoratec VAD is that it can be configured for either left or right heart support

Table 8-6. Perioperative antibiotics for the ventricular assist device patient

Drug	Route	Preoperative Dose	Postoperative Dose
Vancomycin hydrochloride	i.v.	1 g	1 g q 12 h for 48 h
Levofloxacin	i.v.	500 mg	500 mg q 24 h for 48 h
Rifampin	p.o.	600 mg	600 mg q 24 h for 48 h
Fluconazole	i.v.	200 mg	200 mg q 24 h for 48 h

(Fig. 8-4). However, this pneumatically powered blood pump lacks portability due to the presence of the external drive unit. The electric *implantable* blood pumps are more portable, and patients supported with these devices are eligible for hospital discharge. In addition, the HeartMate VADs have a unique blood-contacting surface that does not require systemic anticoagulation. For patients supported with these VADs, aspirin therapy alone suffices. The implantable blood pumps are technically more difficult to implant and explant because a preperitoneal pocket is required (38). In general, we prefer to use an implantable blood pump for the bridge-to-transplant patient as the patient has increased mobility and the potential for hospital discharge. Patients who are small (body surface area $\leq 1.5\ m^2$) and those in whom there is a high likelihood of biventricular failure are usually implanted with a paracorporeal device. That way, an identical VAD can be used for right and left heart support should biventricular assistance be required.

Patients receive aprotinin intraoperatively to reduce both cytokine release and the need for postoperative blood transfusion. LVAD configuration for the bridge-to-transplant application usually involves placement of a cannula through the left ventricular apex for device inflow and a graft to the aorta for outflow. A

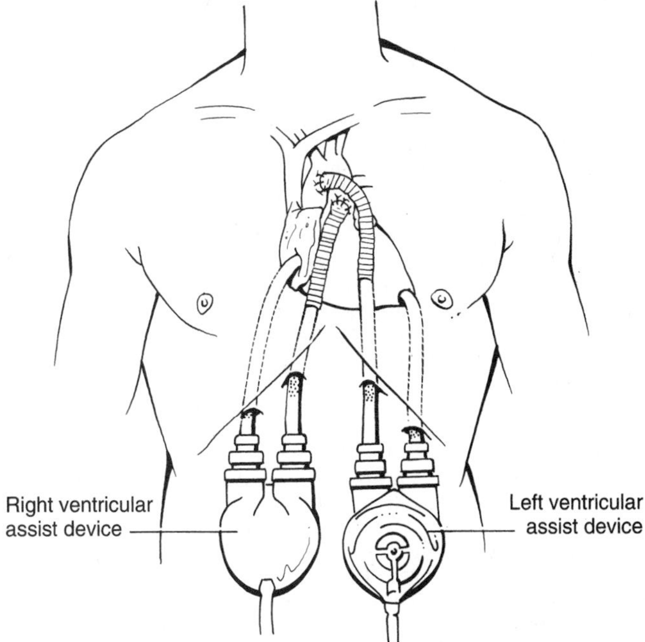

Fig. 8-4. Cannulation scheme for Thoratec biventricular assistance. The left ventricular assist device withdraws blood from the left ventricular apex and returns it to the ascending aorta. The right ventricular assist device withdraws blood from the right atrium and returns it to the pulmonary artery.

standard sternotomy incision is employed (39). CPB is used with an aortic and a single venous cannula unless a patent foramen ovale is present, in which case bicaval cannulation is necessary. The outlet graft-to-aortic anastomosis is usually performed prior to the initiation of CPB, and it is performed as low on the ascending aorta as possible to permit complete removal of the outlet graft at the time of cardiac transplantation. We prefer cardioplegic arrest for left ventricular cannulation. This allows a thorough inspection of the inner aspect of the left ventricle and facilitates placement of sutures about the apex cannula exit site. The heart and mechanical blood pump circuit are compulsively de-aired. The patient is weaned from CPB as LVAD flow is initiated.

If the extracorporeal VAD is employed, the heart is approached through a standard median sternotomy, and the inflow and outflow cannulas traverse the skin in the left subcostal region. The remaining operative considerations are identical to those described above.

Patients who are listed as candidates for cardiac transplantation have been previously screened for the presence of irreversible pulmonary hypertension. Thus, right ventricular failure is usually not an issue in the bridge-to-transplant patient population. Low pulmonary vascular resistance allows passive blood flow through the right heart, even in the presence of mild right ventricular dysfunction. Even so, left and right ventricular preload should be carefully monitored as left heart support is initiated. Left ventricular decompression can unmask right ventricular failure, and if it occurs, it is managed as described previously. Transesophageal echocardiography is used to evaluate the effectiveness of left ventricular decompression. With left ventricular apex cannulation, the entire output of the left heart should be via the VAD, and the left heart will be well decompressed. The native aortic valve should not open at all. A bubble study is performed to identify a patent foramen ovale; if present, it should be closed.

Chest closure details include placement of mediastinal and VAD pocket drains, positioning of the outlet graft to the right of the midline to avoid injury on reentry, and pericardial closure, using a prosthetic pericardial membrane, if necessary (40). These measures will facilitate reentry at the time of subsequent sternotomy for the transplantation operation.

Postoperative Care

Following VAD implantation, the goal is to avoid development of a complication that would prevent subsequent cardiac transplantation. Initially, the VAD patient is removed from the cardiac transplant waiting list. The patient is placed back on the list when recovery, wound healing, and relatively normal kidney, lung, and liver function are achieved. The patient is usually extubated, and the majority of tubes and lines are removed within 24 hours of VAD implantation. Perioperative antibiotics are continued for 48 hours, during which time all invasive monitoring lines are usually withdrawn. A coagulopathy, if any, is corrected and anticoagulation begun within the first 24 hours following VAD implantation. Patients receiving the HeartMate device receive aspirin, whereas warfarin is provided for all other patients. The therapeutic international normalized ratio is 2.5 to 3.5. Enteral feedings are initiated with a small-diameter feeding tube. Smaller-sized patients who receive an implantable blood pump may develop early satiety due to compression of the stomach by the left upper quadrant VAD. Patients are mobilized early and aggressive cardiac rehabilitation initiated. Range-of-motion exercises are initiated within 12 to 24 hours. Ambulation begins as soon as invasive hemodynamic monitoring lines are withdrawn (41).

Patients who receive an implantable blood pump have drains placed in the blood pump pocket to avoid a pocket hematoma or seroma that might spontaneously drain through the driveline exit site. Drainage from the driveline exit site interferes with tissue ingrowth at the driveline–skin exit site interface and may increase the potential for driveline bacterial colonization. The drains are left in place until the drainage is <50 mL for 24 hours.

The patient who is a candidate for home discharge and the family receive preoperative teaching regarding the concept of mechanical circulatory support (42). This may include a visit by a patient who is currently receiving VAD support. Thereafter, a staged training program is initiated. Following surgery, the patient learns to manage the power source and battery changes. The patient or family member performs driveline exit site care, and both are taught to deal with emergency troubleshooting and management of the mechanical blood pump. At discharge, community members who might come in contact with the patient also receive specialized training. This list of community members might include local health care providers, community cardiac rehabilitation specialists, as well as family members or friends.

Long-Term Issues

Avoidance of infection is of paramount importance in the VAD patient who is to subsequently undergo cardiac transplantation with inherent immunosuppression (43). Standard endocarditis prophylaxis is employed when the patient visits the dentist or undergoes any procedure that carries a risk of bacteremia. Superficial driveline or cannula exit site colonization is usually treated with local wound care. If exit site colonization is associated with fever or an elevation in white blood count, we initiate antistaphylococcal antibiotic therapy. The coverage continues for the duration of VAD support. Blood-borne sepsis can lead to VAD endocarditis that carries with it the risk of embolism. If endocarditis develops, consideration should be given to VAD replacement.

Heart transplant candidates with an implanted VAD undergo weekly measurement of panel-reactive antibody (PRA) titers (44). In this test, the recipient's serum is mixed with a panel of randomly selected white blood cells. The purpose of this test is to identify preformed antibodies in the recipient's serum that may place the recipient at risk for hyperacute rejection or decreased long-term survival following cardiac transplantation (45). Recipients who are at increased risk for the formation of preformed antibodies include those who have had previous blood transfusions or women who have been pregnant.

Ventricular Assist Device Explantation and Cardiac Transplantation

If all has gone well during the period of VAD support, the patient is at home when a donor heart becomes available. The patient immediately returns to the hospital, and the prothrombin time is corrected if the patient has been receiving warfarin. If a prospective cross-match is required, we bring two potential recipients to the hospital. The second patient serves as a backup recipient should the primary recipient's prospective cross-match result be positive.

Blood product requirements can be excessive, and thus the blood bank is notified of the pending VAD explant and transplant to ensure that adequate blood products are available. Timing of the cardiac transplant can be complex. This is particularly true in the patient who has been supported with an implantable blood pump. These patients require a complex redo sternotomy that can require 2 or even 3 hours of dissection prior to implantation of the donor heart (46). Frequent communication between donor and recipient surgical teams is imperative. Standard antibiotic prophylaxis is employed. The patient is prepped and draped in a routine fashion, with the exception that cannula skin exit sites are excluded from the operative field to avoid mediastinal contamination. Femoral artery and vein cannulation is routine due to the potential for injuring mediastinal structures at the time of sternal re-entry and to maximize aortic length. Every effort is made to divide the aorta distal to the outlet graft-to-aortic anastomosis to eliminate the volume of foreign material retained in the mediastinum following cardiac transplant.

On sternal entry, the inlet side of the pump is not exposed until CPB is initiated to avoid the potential for air embolism. As CPB is initiated, VAD pumping is discontinued and the outlet graft clamped. The recipient cardiectomy and donor implant are performed in an identical fashion to that described in *Cardiac Transplantation.* Following the cardiac transplant and chest closure, the skin exit sites are exposed. These are debrided, irrigated, and closed primarily. Patient management is conventional thereafter.

Destination Therapy

Patients who suffer end-stage heart failure but who are not eligible for heart transplantation may be candidates for permanent LVAD support. Patients considered for *destination therapy* have New York Heart Association (NYHA) Class IV heart failure despite optimal medical therapy, left ventricular ejection fraction of <25%, and a life expectancy of <2 years. For this purpose, the implantable electrically driven device, specifically the HeartMate VE LVAS, has been used (9). Such patients with terminal heart failure experience considerable improvement in heart failure class, length of survival, and quality of life. In general, surgical and management considerations are the same as when the device is used for bridging to transplantation.

CARDIAC TRANSPLANTATION

Patients with advanced heart failure are initially treated with conventional medical therapy including diuretics, afterload-reducing agents, antiarrhythmics, if indicated, and, in selected patients, biventricular pacing. Patients with ischemic cardiomyopathy, with viable myocardium in the distribution of a stenotic coronary artery, may be treated with high-risk coronary revascularization. Nevertheless, the mainstay in surgical therapy for patients with advanced inoperable heart failure remains cardiac transplantation.

Cardiac Recipient Selection

Cardiac transplant recipient selection criteria are listed in Table 8-7 (47,48). The typical candidate has NYHA functional Class 4 heart failure and has an ejection fraction of <20%. A patient with NYHA Class 3 heart failure can be considered a candidate for transplantation if his or her measured exercise maximal oxygen consumption (Vo_2 max) is <14 mL/kg per minute. In general, the patient's prognosis with medical management alone is poor, with a 1-year life expectancy of <50%. Occasionally, a patient with intractable angina and non-bypass-able occlusive coronary artery disease or a patient with refractory life-threatening ventricular arrhythmias may be considered a candidate for cardiac transplantation despite not suffering from NYHA functional Class 3 or 4 symptomatology. Advanced age is a relative contraindication to cardiac transplantation. Although patients older than 65 to 70 years have successfully undergone transplantation, usual selection criteria limit this therapy to patients 65 years or younger (49). The majority of adults who undergo cardiac transplantation suffer from ischemic cardiomyopathy or idiopathic dilated cardiomyopathy, with most being between the ages of 35 and 64 years (50). Occasional older patients are placed on an "alternate waiting list" and may be offered only a donor heart that has been deemed unsuitable for use in patients on the standard waiting list (51).

As the patient is being screened, operative reports from previous cardiac operations should be reviewed, especially in patients with congenital heart disease (52,53). Details of previous operations permit a better estimate of operative risk and may lead to modifications in the donor cardiectomy (54). For example, additional length of either the aorta, the systemic veins, or the pulmonary artery may be required to allow reconstruction of

Table 8-7. Cardiac transplant recipient selection and exclusion criteria

Selection criteria
NYHA Class 4 not amenable to surgical treatment
Estimated 1-y mortality >50%
Chronologic age ≤65 y
No systemic illness (other than abnormalities related to heart failure)
Normal pulmonary artery pressures or reversible pulmonary hypertension
Emotional stability, with strong family support system
Exclusion criteria
Fixed pulmonary hypertension
Irreversible hepatic, renal, or pulmonary disease
Active systemic or pulmonary infection
Uncorrected systemic or cerebrovascular disease
Active peptic ulcer disease
Active history of substance abuse
Active malignancy
Diabetes mellitus with end-organ damage

NYHA, New York Heart Association.

congenital cardiac anomalies. If the patient has had previous coronary revascularization, knowledge of the presence and location of bypass grafts, and whether or not they are patent, facilitates risk assessment and operative planning.

Once a patient is deemed a suitable candidate for cardiac transplantation, the patient is placed on the cardiac transplant waiting list. The patient is listed with the United Network for Organ Sharing (UNOS) and is assigned a recipient status level. The status level determines the urgency with which the recipient is offered a donor heart. UNOS status levels are listed in Table 8-8 (55). The patient provides the listing center with a 24-hour telephone number and carries a pager to allow the transplant center to contact him or her immediately following a donor heart offer. Transplant waiting list times vary by recipient blood type and body weight, but can measure months to even a year or two (56,57). During that time, the patient is closely monitored and managed medically to preserve end-organ function. If end-organ dysfunction appears, consideration must be given to supporting the patient with a mechanical blood pump. Any change in the patient's clinical condition would be reflected in the UNOS listing. Up to three-quarters of patients are hospitalized or on life support at the time of cardiac transplant. Due to the shortage of donor hearts, up to one-third of patients will die while awaiting cardiac transplantation.

Cardiac Donation

Cardiac Donor Selection Criteria

The majority of cardiac donors have suffered a traumatic injury or intracranial hemorrhage (Table 8-9) (58). When a patient fulfills

Table 8-8. UNOS cardiac transplant recipient status

Status 1A	The patient is admitted to the listing transplant center hospital and has at least one of the following: Mechanical circulatory support (VAD ≤30 d),[a] artificial heart, IABP Mechanical circulatory support >30 d, with device-related complication Mechanical ventilation High-dose inotropes, continuous hemodynamic monitoring Life expectancy <7 d
Status 1B	At least one of the following: VAD >30 d without complication Continuous i.v. infusion of inotropes
Status 2	All other actively listed patients
Status 7	Patient temporarily removed from the transplant waiting list

IABP, intraaortic balloon pump; UNOS, United Network for Organ Sharing; VAD, ventricular assist device.

[a] VAD patients are permitted to accumulate 30 d of Status 1A time, following VAD implantation, regardless of whether or not they are hospitalized.

Table 8-9. Cardiac donor selection and exclusion criteria

Selection criteria
Pronounced brain dead
Age <46 y (advanced age warrants further cardiac work-up)
No history of cardiac disease
Minimal vasopressor support
Normal hemodynamics
Normal echocardiographic wall motion
No untreated bacterial infection
Exclusion criteria
Closed-chest injury resulting in myocardial contusion
Known history of cardiac disease (previous cardiac operation or history of ischemic or valvular heart disease)
Systemic infection including hepatitis B or C positivity
Unwitnessed cardiac arrest or prolonged cardiac resuscitation
HIV positivity or history of high-risk behavior
Systemic malignancy (primary brain tumor excluded)

HIV, human immunodeficiency virus.

brain death criteria, the regional Organ Procurement Organization (OPO) is notified of the presence of a potential organ donor. Informed consent for specific organ donation is obtained from the donor's nearest relative, and at that point, the OPO personnel assumes both medical and financial responsibility for the donor's care. OPO personnel access the UNOS transplant waiting list, and the heart is offered to a recipient based upon blood type, body weight, status, and time spent on the waiting list.

When the transplant center receives a heart offer, the recipient surgeon should request details concerning the donor's demise, including the cause of death, resuscitative efforts, if any, and events of note during the donor's hospitalization. The heart offer is directed to a specific recipient on the transplant waiting list. The blood types of both donor and recipient are confirmed, and the donor weight is requested to ensure that the size match between donor and recipient is appropriate. When a recipient is listed for transplantation, the cardiac transplant center is asked to select a minimum acceptable weight for a cardiac donor. In general, the minimum acceptable weight for the cardiac donor is 80% of the recipient's body weight (59). Any donor at, or above, that weight will be considered a suitable match for a recipient of the same blood type. There can be a substantial size mismatch, with the donor body weight far exceeding the recipient body weight, as cardiomegaly in the recipient will allow insertion of an oversized donor heart into a recipient with a smaller body. Undersized donor hearts are less well tolerated. When a small donor heart is implanted into a large recipient, right ventricular performance can be a problem even in the presence of normal pulmonary artery pressures. Right ventricular failure may occur. Preexisting pulmonary hypertension may exacerbate right ventricular dysfunction. The obese donor may have a heart that is smaller than predicted by body weight. Likewise, the donor should be oversized with respect to the recipient's body weight if the recipient suffers from pulmonary hypertension or the donor heart ischemic time is expected to be prolonged.

If the potential donor has suffered from a blunt chest injury, the electrocardiogram and cardiac enzymes are carefully reviewed. The electrocardiogram should be normal, although global ST-segment abnormalities and T-wave changes can occur in association with head trauma, unrelated to myocardial injury. The creatine phosphokinase determination is often difficult to interpret in the multiply injured patient due to skeletal muscle injury. Creatine phosphokinase isoenzymes or troponin allow identification of a myocardial source. The donor with a significant myocardial contusion is excluded from consideration for cardiac donation.

Potential cardiac donors undergo an echocardiogram to assess global ventricular function (60). Segmental wall motion abnormalities are located, valvular function is assessed, and valvular vegetations, if present, are identified. Cardiac catheterization is used selectively (61). As a general rule, coronary angiography is performed in male donors over 40 years of age, female donors over 45 years of age, and in younger ones with a history of smoking, hyperlipidemia, or familial coronary artery disease.

As part of the cardiac recipient screening process, a PRA screen is performed. If the PRA is >10% (and at some centers, if the PRA is anything other than 0), a lymphocytotoxic cross-match is performed. For this, lymph node tissue from the prospective donor is mixed with the prospective recipient's serum. If the recipient serum contains preformed antibodies to the donor lymph node tissue, the test is positive and identifies the recipient as being at increased risk for hyperacute rejection if the donor heart is utilized. This usually precludes the use of this heart in this recipient.

Donor Management

Although the OPO is responsible for donor management, the recipient surgeon may be called upon to provide input (62,63). Appropriate management of the potential donor will serve to maximize the use of organs (64). Patients with a neurologic injury have often been fluid restricted. In addition, donors frequently suffer from diabetes insipidus. As a result, there is usually a volume deficit that must be corrected. The donor should receive appropriate volume resuscitation and vasopressor drug administration. Vasopressin (0.25 to 1 U per minute i.v.) may also be used to treat diabetes insipidus. Central hemodynamic monitoring is utilized with the goal of a CVP of 5 to 10 mm Hg. With volume administration, inotropic drug doses can usually be decreased. Although the efficacy of thyroid hormone replacement is uncertain, if thyroid hormone replacement is utilized, triiodothyronine (maximal dose 0.6 μg/kg i.v.) is administered over 30 minutes (65). If a multiorgan retrieval is planned, the donor is cross-matched for packed red blood cells. A prophylactic antibiotic is administered prior to organ retrieval.

Donor Cardiectomy

The heart is usually retrieved as part of a multiorgan harvest. Timing of donor cardiectomy is determined by the number of organs being retrieved, the transportation time between the donor and recipient hospitals, and the complexity of mediastinal dissection in the recipient. The issue of timing between donor and recipient operations is critical to minimize the donor heart ischemic time.

A midline incision is created from the suprasternal notch to the symphysis pubis. The heart is inspected to ensure that there are no signs of cardiac trauma. Dyskinetic wall motion in the right or left ventricle may be identified by visual inspection or transesophageal echocardiography if that modality is utilized in the operating room. The surface of the heart should be gently palpated to identify occult coronary artery plaques, although care is taken in palpating the heart, as the donor heart tends to be prone to arrhythmias.

Following cardiac inspection, the abdominal team completes their dissection prior to cardiac removal. When the chest and abdominal dissections are complete, the donor is fully heparinized. A cardioplegia needle is inserted into the ascending aorta (Fig. 8-5),

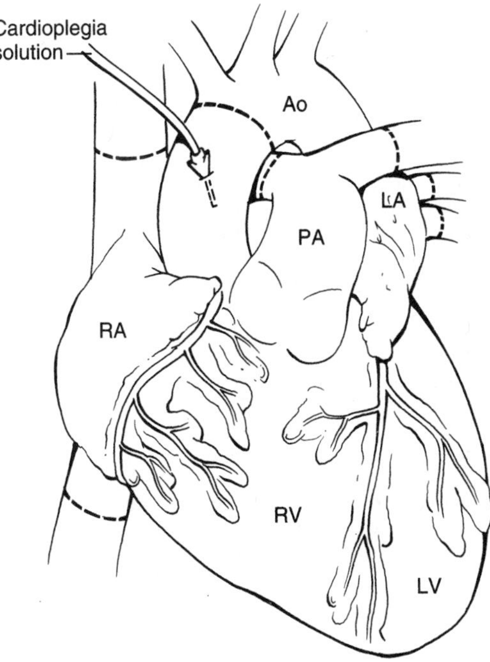

Fig. 8-5. Schematic of donor cardiectomy. Cold cardioplegia is administered into the aortic root after an aortic cross-clamp is applied. The heart is vented by transecting the inferior vena cava and left inferior pulmonary vein. If there is a simultaneous lung donation, the left heart is vented by opening the left atrial appendage. Once the heart is arrested, the donor cardiectomy is completed by dividing the superior vena cava and remaining pulmonary veins and transecting the great vessels along the dotted lines shown in the figure. RA, right atrium; RV, right ventricle; PA, pulmonary artery; LA, left atrium; LV, left ventricle; Ao, aorta.

and then the superior and inferior venae cavae are divided. Warm blood is evacuated from the chest to facilitate myocardial cooling. The aorta is cross-clamped and cold hyperkalemic cardioplegia administered into the aortic root (66). Although a variety of cardioplegic solutions have been employed, we find a simple, readily available cardioplegic solution to consist of 1 L of 5% dextrose in half-normal saline to which potassium chloride (20 mEq) and sodium bicarbonate (10 mEq) are added. Ice is applied to the surface of the heart to provide topical cooling.

Following cardioplegia administration, the heart is excised. The superior vena cava is divided well above the cavoatrial junction to avoid injuring the sinoatrial node, higher if the bicaval implant technique is used. The pulmonary veins are divided individually. The aorta is divided at the level of the innominate artery, and either the distal main pulmonary artery or the right and left main pulmonary arteries are divided. The donor cardiectomy is modified in the face of a simultaneous lung retrieval. If the lungs are being retrieved from the same donor, the donor cardiectomy can proceed in one of two ways. The donor heart can be removed first with the lungs to follow. Alternatively, the heart–lung bloc can be excised and moved to a back table where the three organs are separated (67). Regardless of technique employed, if the lungs are being harvested, the pulmonary veins must accompany the lungs. The donor heart is briefly inspected to ensure that a foramen ovale, if present, is identified and closed. The valves are inspected to ensure that there is no evidence of occult endocarditis or valve abnormality, particularly if there was an indwelling central line. The heart is packaged in layered plastic bags filled with ice-cold saline solution, and the packaged heart is placed in an ice-filled cooler for transportation to the recipient hospital.

Cardiac Recipient Management

Cardiac Recipient Preparation

When the recipient hospital is contacted by the OPO with a cardiac offer, the heart is accepted for a specific patient on the cardiac transplant waiting list. That recipient is immediately contacted and questioned with regard to the presence of any new conditions that might be a contraindication to transplantation, such as an acute infection. The potential recipient is asked to take nothing further by mouth and to travel to the hospital immediately. On arrival, a history and physical examination are performed to confirm that the potential recipient remains a suitable candidate. If the recipient has a high PRA, blood is immediately obtained for performance of the lymphocytotoxic cross-match. Frequently, recipient serum will be banked at the transplant center to facilitate performance of the cross-match.

The recipient's anterior chest, abdomen, and both anterior thighs are clipped, and the patient subsequently showers with chlorhexidine. If the patient has been receiving warfarin, the prothrombin time may be corrected with vitamin K and fresh frozen plasma as indicated. Monitoring lines include a radial arterial line, one or two large-bore peripheral intravenous catheters, and a central venous catheter. We employ a pulmonary artery catheter routinely in all cardiac transplant recipients. This catheter is inserted via the left internal jugular vein, thereby preserving the right internal jugular vein for subsequent cardiac biopsies. It is important that all catheters and lines be inserted with meticulous sterile technique.

Preoperative immunosuppressive agents are administered according to the schedules described below. The patients receive gram-positive and gram-negative antibiotic coverage (vancomycin and ceftriaxone). Perioperative antibiotic coverage continues for 48 hours following cardiac transplantation.

Timing of the Donor and Recipient Operations

Perhaps the most challenging portion of the cardiac transplant procedure is the timing of both the donor and the recipient cardiectomy. The primary focus of this portion of the operation is to minimize the period of time between application of the aortic cross-clamp in the donor and removal of the aortic cross-clamp in the recipient. Myocardial preservation is always important, but this is particularly true in cardiac transplantation, when the donor heart is frequently undersized and is expected to perform in a setting of pulmonary hypertension following a period of prolonged ischemia. The donor heart should arrive as the recipient cardiectomy is being completed. Close communication between the cardiac and abdominal organ retrieval teams is paramount as abdominal organ retrieval time can vary dramatically depending upon organs to be retrieved as well as anatomic hurdles encountered during the abdominal organ dissection.

Implant team considerations can have a profound impact upon the speed with which the cardiac recipient is taken to the operating room. It may take several hours for the patient simply to arrive at the hospital. Preformed antibodies in the recipient's blood and the requisite lymphocytotoxic cross-match may require several additional hours prior to determining that the potential recipient is suitable. In this instance, we often bring a second back-up recipient to the hospital to minimize any potential delay should the lymphocytotoxic cross-match be positive in the primary recipient. Additionally, a patient who has had previous cardiac surgery may require multiple hours of additional dissection prior to reaching the point in the operation when donor heart implantation can occur.

The recipient is moved to the operating room well in advance of the anticipated anesthetic induction time. We prefer that the recipient not be anesthetized until the donor team has actually visualized the donor heart and has communicated that it is functioning satisfactorily. At that time, the recipient operation begins.

Recipient Operative Management

The beginning of anesthesia is dictated by the progress of the donor operation. Because the recipient has advanced heart failure, anesthetic induction and maintenance require careful monitoring and pharmacologic management. A narcotic-based anesthetic is employed to minimize myocardial depression. Volume administration is minimized, and filling pressures are monitored with invasive hemodynamic monitoring lines. The recipient cardiectomy is performed through a median sternotomy. CPB employs bicaval venous cannulation and aortic cannulation. If the recipient has had previous cardiac surgery or if a VAD is in place, the femoral vessels may be accessed for arterial cannulation and inferior vena caval return. A superior vena caval cannula will need to be connected to the CPB circuit once the mediastinal dissection is complete. Heparin is administered, and the activated clotting time is measured to ensure that the anticoagulation level is therapeutic. If the patient is grossly fluid overloaded, we employ continuous ultrafiltration during CPB for volume removal. The patient is cooled to a core temperature of 27°C. The aorta is cross-clamped, and caval snares are applied to isolate the heart from the blood path. The recipient cardiectomy is accomplished by dividing the atria along the atrioventricular grooves (Fig. 8-6) (68). The great vessels are divided just distal to the semilunar valves. The recipient left atrial appendage is excised to eliminate a potential source for intracardiac thrombus formation. The tips of the commissures are maintained on the pulmonary artery to facilitate orientation of the pulmonary artery as the donor heart is implanted. This avoids pulmonary artery torsion, a potential cause of right heart failure in the donor heart. Although the in-

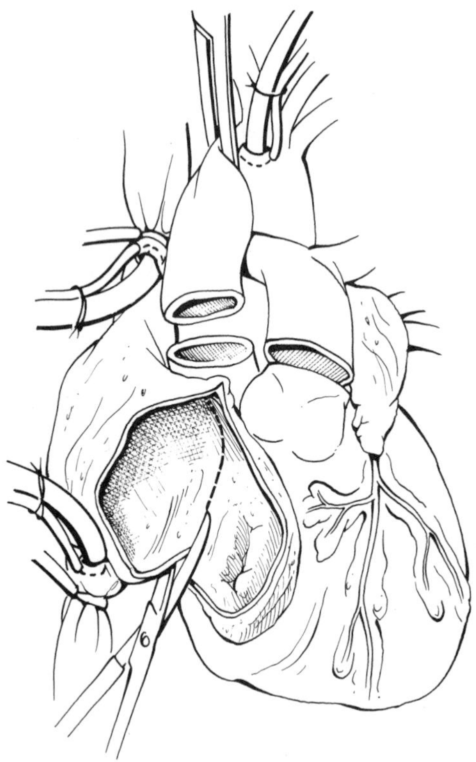

Fig. 8-6. The recipient cardiectomy. The patient is placed on cardiopulmonary bypass using bicaval venous cannulation and aortic arterial cannulation. The heart is isolated from the blood path with caval snares and the aortic cross-clamp. The great vessels are divided at the level of the semilunar valves. The ventricles are removed by dividing the atria along the atrioventricular groove.

trapericardial dissection is performed prior to the arrival of the donor heart, the recipient cardiectomy is not usually completed until the donor heart has safely arrived in the hospital.

The donor implant is accomplished by anastomosing the left followed by the right atrial cuffs to the recipient counterparts (Fig. 8-7). The pulmonary artery anastomosis follows. Care is taken to trim the pulmonary artery to the appropriate length to avoid redundancy of this vessel that can result in kinking and increased afterload to the right heart. Rewarming is completed as the aortic anastomosis is performed. Prior to completing the aortic anastomosis, the caval snares are removed, and the heart is permitted to fill with blood. The heart is de-aired and the aortic anastomosis completed.

Some centers have converted from the standard biatrial implant technique to a bicaval implant technique (Fig. 8-8) (69,70). In the latter procedure, the recipient right atrium is excised in its entirety, and the recipient superior and inferior venae cavae are divided at the point at which they would normally have entered the

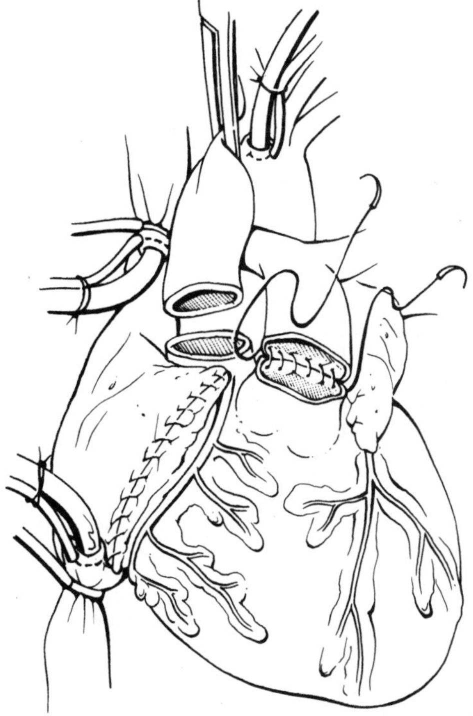

Fig. 8-7. The cardiac implant is accomplished by anastomosing the donor atrial cuffs to their recipient counterparts. The great vessel anastomoses follow. Care is taken to avoid injuring the donor sinoatrial node.

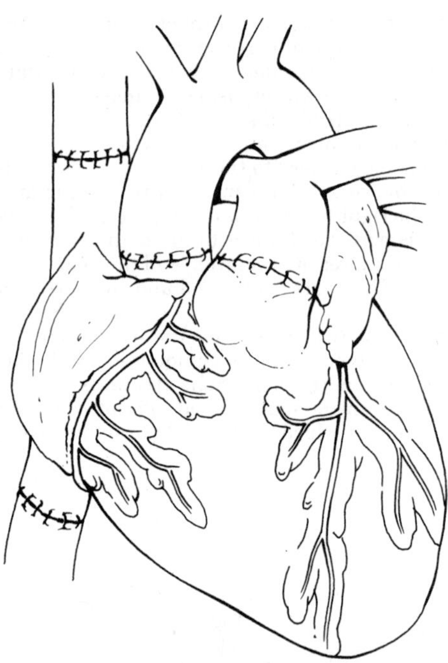

Fig. 8-8. The bicaval cardiac implant utilizes the standard left atrial cuff anastomosis. However, the donor right atrium is not opened. The donor superior and inferior venae cavae are anastomosed directly to the recipient cavae.

recipient right atrium, leaving a small cuff of right atrial tissue attached to the cavae. The implant technique is modified such that a caval-to-caval anastomosis is performed on both the superior and the inferior venae cavae. This eliminates the redundant right atrium associated with the standard biatrial technique. Proponents of this procedure note improved right ventricular performance and reduction in the incidence of tricuspid regurgitation.

The patient usually converts to sinus rhythm upon release of the aortic cross-clamp. Because the donor heart is denervated, the recipient will require chronotropic support. Although we place temporary pacing wires on both the donor atrium and the ventricle, chronotropic support is usually achieved with isoproterenol (1 to 4 μg per minute i.v.). The goal is a heart rate of approximately 100 beats per minute, recognizing that younger hearts are much more responsive to this intravenous medication. If the donor heart does not respond to isoproterenol administration, temporary pacing can be employed. Atrial pacing or atrioventricular sequential pacing are the most physiologically effective pacing modes.

Patients with chronic heart failure frequently have elevated pulmonary artery pressures and pulmonary vascular resistance. The donor heart is particularly susceptible to right ventricular failure, as it is not accustomed to the increased afterload (71). Thus, it is important that the right heart be supported following release of the aortic cross-clamp and that the CVP be carefully monitored as CPB is discontinued. Once again, isoproterenol is the drug of choice for support of right ventricular function as it increases the donor heart rate, has a positive inotropic effect, and reduces pulmonary vascular resistance. Right ventricular contractility is evaluated visually, and if it is impaired, milrinone, epinephrine, or dobutamine can be added to the drug regimen. If pulmonary artery pressures remain elevated, inhaled nitric oxide (10 to 20 parts per million) may be administered (72). If right ventricular function is a problem, a left atrial pressure line is inserted to monitor left ventricular preload.

Many heart transplant recipients have received preoperative warfarin, and the warfarin effect may be reversed preoperatively, although time may not always allow for this and it may not be necessary (73). Aprotinin is often administered during CPB, especially in patients undergoing repeat sternotomy (74). If the associated coagulopathy has not been corrected preoperatively, up to 8 U of fresh frozen plasma can be added to the CPB circuit during terminal rewarming. Excess water is removed with hemofiltration during CPB. Postoperatively, the patient will often require transfusion with either blood or blood products. This is particularly true in patients who have had a previous sternotomy or who have been supported with a mechanical blood pump. Packed red blood cells and platelets are administered through a leukodepletion filter to avoid an antigen load. Clotting factor administration contributes to increased pulmonary vascular resistance (and, thus, right ventricular dysfunction). Intraoperative blood loss is minimized and transfusions given only as required.

Postoperative Management

Hemodynamics

In the absence of hyperacute rejection or a problem with donor heart preservation, the left ventricle usually contracts satisfactorily following cardiac transplant (75). Right ventricular dysfunction, however, can result in central venous hypertension and inadequate left ventricular preload. The CVP is carefully monitored, and right ventricular distention is avoided. Within 24 to 48 hours, the pulmonary vascular resistance usually falls, and medications used for right heart support can be weaned. Tricuspid regurgitation, if present, usually improves as the pulmonary artery pressures fall. Chronotropic support with isoproterenol is often required for 4 to 7 days depending upon the patient's heart rate. Isoproterenol can be administered peripherally and does not require intensive care unit monitoring. Thus, this drug can be slowly withdrawn over a number of days using the heart rate as the endpoint. Early in the postoperative course, we attempt to maintain a heart rate above 90 beats per minute. Toward the end of the first postoperative week, we accept a heart rate above 70 to 80 beats per minute.

Infection

Patients undergoing heart transplantation receive perioperative antibiotic prophylaxis for both gram-positive and gram-negative organisms that is continued postoperatively until the mediastinal tubes and lines are removed, usually 48 hours following the heart transplant. Patient isolation and reverse precautions are not employed; however, traffic is minimized in the patient room. More importantly, all personnel who enter the patient room utilize good hand-washing technique.

Cytomegalovirus (CMV) and *Toxoplasmosis gondii* can be transmitted from a seropositive donor into a seronegative recipient. CMV, in particular, can produce a flu-like syndrome with pneumonitis, enteritis, and hepatitis (76). Patients infected with CMV appear to be at increased risk for accelerated allograft coronary artery disease. Recipients who are seronegative preoperatively that receive a heart from a CMV-seropositive donor are treated with intravenous ganciclovir for 21 days, followed by oral ganciclovir for 3 months, followed by oral acyclovir for 1 year. CMV-seropositive recipients who receive a seropositive donor heart are treated prophylactically with intravenous ganciclovir until hospital discharge. This is followed by oral acyclovir. Seronegative recipients who receive a seronegative donor heart receive oral acyclovir starting immediately following extubation. CMV titers are checked every 6 months. If seroconversion occurs, oral ganciclovir is administered for 3 months, followed by oral acyclovir for 3 months. In all of these scenarios, low-dose oral acyclovir is continued for a minimum of 1 year following transplantation. Acyclovir is discontinued thereafter, provided the prednisone dose is <10 mg per day. Seronegative recipients for *T. gondii* who receive a seropositive donor heart are prophylactically treated with pyrimethamine and folinic acid for 6 weeks (77). Oral candidiasis ("thrush") is prevalent in the immunosuppressed patient population. To avoid this infectious complication, the recipients receive nystatin oral suspension (100,000 U/mL, 5-mL p.o. swish and swallow after meals and at bedtime) for 4 to 6 weeks. Prophylaxis against *Pneumocystis carinii* consists of trimethoprim and sulfamethoxazole.

Immunosuppression

The drug protocols used for immune suppression therapy of cardiac transplant recipients vary from institution to institution and are constantly changing. The purpose of this discussion is to provide general patient care guidelines and examples of commonly used therapeutic regimens. Immunosuppression begins prior to the cardiac transplant (78–80). The mainstay of immunosuppressive protocols is *triple-drug therapy,* utilizing cyclosporine, azathioprine, and steroids. Currently, the triple-medication protocol is reserved primarily for patients who have received mechanical circulatory support prior to cardiac transplant as these recipients enter the operating room with normal renal function.

The majority of our patients are managed with a *cytolytic induction* protocol (81,82). This protocol avoids the renal dysfunction associated with the triple-medication protocol, delays the first episode of rejection, and decreases the risk of rejection during the first 6 months following transplantation. However, the use of monoclonal antibodies is associated with significant systemic side effects, may be associated with a higher early incidence of infection, and can result in sensitization to these agents. At the University of Iowa, patients managed with the cytolytic induction protocol receive azathioprine prior to transplant. Intraoperatively, the patients receive methylprednisolone and muromonab-CD3 (OKT3).

The OKT3 is usually administered late in the implant procedure (as the pulmonary artery anastomosis is completed) to avoid a systemic response to OKT3 as CPB is discontinued. Postoperatively, the patients receive OKT3. T-Lymphocytic cell lysis and resultant cytokine release can lead to a systemic reaction characterized by fever and low systemic vascular resistance. Thus, the OKT3 dose is preceded by the following medications: diphenhydramine hydrochloride (50 mg i.v.), cimetidine (300 mg i.v.), and acetaminophen (650 mg p.o./p.r.). All of these medications are administered 30 minutes to 1 hour before OKT3 administration on postoperative days 1 through 3. OKT3 postmedications (diphenhydramine hydrochloride, cimetidine, and acetaminophen) are administered 6, 12, and 18 hours after OKT3 on postoperative days 1 through 3. The postoperative cytolytic induction protocol also includes azathioprine and methylprednisolone followed by prednisone when taking orally. Cyclosporine is instituted on postoperative days 4 to 6 as determined by the patient's renal function.

An alternative immunosuppressive protocol for adult cardiac transplant recipients employs a *monoclonal antibody* specific for the activated T-cell interleukin-2 receptor (83). This protocol provides the benefit of induction therapy without the associated risk of OKT3 and the inconvenience of OKT3 pre- and postmedications. Patients managed with this regimen receive preoperative cyclosporine and mycophenolate mofetil and intraoperative methylprednisolone. Postoperatively, the patient receives cyclosporine, mycophenolate mofetil, steroids, and daclizumab (84).

Other Management Issues

If the cardiac transplant has been performed uneventfully and the implanted heart functions satisfactorily, the patient is weaned from mechanical ventilation and rapidly extubated. Chronic left ventricular dysfunction is frequently associated with preoperative pulmonary congestion. Postoperatively, the patient receives diuretic drug treatment to eliminate excess pulmonary extravascular lung water. In order to avoid a precipitous decline in preload, this diuresis is most effectively accomplished with a continuous furosemide infusion (adult dose 5 to 40 mg per hour i.v.) to maintain a urine output of 50 to 100 mL more than the total intravenous fluid intake each hour. Rapid extubation reduces the potential for hospital-acquired pneumonia. The incidence of infectious complications is further reduced by early withdrawal of percutaneous lines and tubes, including the urinary drainage catheter. Patients with chronic heart failure frequently suffer cardiac cachexia. Enteral nutritional via a feeding tube is instituted if the patient is unable to meet his or her caloric need in the first 48 hours following cardiac transplant. Cardiac transplant recipients, with the exclusion of those supported with a mechanical blood pump, are usually deconditioned by their chronic heart failure. Therefore, physical therapy is begun in the intensive care unit following extubation (85).

Chronically ill heart failure patients who have a protracted hospitalization related to cardiac transplantation are at risk for the development of stress ulcers and thus are treated prophylactically with cimetidine or lansoprazole. Postoperative anemia is treated, in part, with iron sulfate (325 mg p.o. t.i.d., before meals), beginning on postoperative day 7, for 6 weeks. Aspirin (81 mg p.o. every day) is administered beginning on postoperative day 7. Patients who receive chronic steroid therapy are at risk for the development of osteoporosis (86). All patients receive calcium carbonate (500 mg p.o. t.i.d.) beginning on postoperative day 3 and a daily multivitamin that contains 400 IU of vitamin D beginning on day 7. Because patients who receive cyclosporine frequently develop hyperlipidemia, pravastatin (10 mg p.o. every day) is administered beginning on postoperative day 7 (87).

Long-Term Problems

Rejection

The risk of acute rejection is highest in the first 3 months following cardiac transplant. Thereafter, the risk of rejection decreases but remains constant (88). Risk factors for rejection during the first year following cardiac transplantation include a recipient of younger age, a donor or recipient of female gender, CMV positivity, or a recipient who has had a significant prior infection. After 1 year following cardiac transplantation, the risk of recurrent rejection is more common in patients who have a CMV infection or who experienced multiple rejection episodes during the first post-transplant year. Cardiac rejection is often presaged by unexplained weight gain, unexplained arrhythmia, decrease in blood pressure, or increase in heart rate. Rejection surveillance is accomplished using endomyocardial biopsies. The first biopsy is performed 7 days following transplant and is followed by weekly or biweekly biopsies for the next 2 months. Thereafter, the biopsy schedule is individualized according to the occurrence of rejection. At the minimum, an endomyocardial biopsy is performed on an annual basis. The biopsy tissue is histologically graded according to the International Society for Heart and Lung Transplantation (ISHLT) criteria (Table 8-10) (89).

Patients who develop mild cellular rejection (ISHLT grade 1B, 2, or 3A) are treated with a prednisone pulse (50 mg p.o. b.i.d. for

Table 8-10. International Society for Heart and Lung Transplantation Standardized Cardiac Biopsy Grading Scale

Grade	Histologic Findings
No rejection	—
1A	Focal (perivascular or interstitial) infiltrate without necrosis
1B	Diffuse but sparse infiltrate without necrosis; one focus only with aggressive infiltration and/or focal myocyte damage
3A	Multifocal aggressive infiltrates and/or myocyte damage
3B	Diffuse inflammatory process with necrosis; diffuse aggressive polymorphous infiltrate, ± edema, ± hemorrhage, ± vasculitis, with necrosis

5 days) followed by a taper in the dose back to the maintenance schedule. Methotrexate may be administered depending upon the patient's white blood count (90). The cyclosporine dose is increased to maintain therapeutic levels. A pulse dose of cyclophosphamide is given with the dose dictated by the white blood count. Azathioprine is discontinued, and cyclophosphamide is subsequently used for the long-term therapy. The patient is observed and undergoes a repeat biopsy in 7 to 14 days.

Moderate cellular rejection (ISHLT grade 3A, 3B, or 4) is treated in a manner dictated by the presence or absence of hemodynamic compromise. If the patient has no hemodynamic instability, pulse steroid coverage is provided using methylprednisolone followed by oral prednisone. If the patient demonstrates hemodynamic compromise as defined by the presence of relative hypotension (systolic blood pressure 20 mm Hg less than baseline), a new third heart sound, increase in jugulovenous pressure, or a decrease in left ventricular systolic function as evidenced by echocardiography, the patient receives antithymocyte globulin, methylprednisolone, and then oral prednisone.

Infection

The patient experiences the greatest risk for infection in the immediate postoperative period and during periods of augmented immunosuppression used for the treatment of rejection (91). Infection is more common in older patients, those who have required mechanical ventilation or mechanical circulatory support prior to transplantation, and those for whom monoclonal antibody therapy was used for immunosuppression induction. Viral and bacterial infections predominate in this patient population. Any patient who demonstrates a fever or rise in white blood count should be aggressively evaluated, recognizing that a leukocytosis may accompany steroid treatment. The evaluation and management of a patient with suspected sepsis include wound and catheter site examination, urinalysis, sputum and blood cultures, and chest radiograph. Should the patient develop a fever or evidence of peripheral thrombophlebitis, the intravenous catheter should be moved to a new site. In general, antibiotic therapy is reserved for treatment of a known infection.

Malignancy

Malignancies are the second most common cause of late death in patients who undergo a cardiac transplant, occurring in up to 15% of patients (92). The most common tumors are cutaneous neoplasms, non-Hodgkin's lymphoma, and lung cancer. Lymphoproliferative disorders occur more commonly in patients who received high-dose immunosuppressive therapy or induction therapy with OKT3. Lymphoproliferative malignancies, in particular B-cell lymphomas, are more common in recipients who were seronegative for the Epstein–Barr virus prior to transplant. When suspected, the cancers are diagnosed using standard techniques. Treatment is tumor specific and includes a reduction in the immunosuppressive dose.

Allograft Coronary Artery Disease

The etiology of allograft coronary artery disease is multifactorial (93,94). Because the donor heart is denervated, cardiac transplant recipients rarely present with angina. Shortness of breath, diaphoresis, nausea, edema, and a new cardiac murmur are suggestive of myocardial ischemia. Allograft coronary artery disease is the most common cause of late death following transplantation. Thus, vigilance must be maintained throughout the life of the transplant patient. Two months following cardiac transplantation, the patient undergoes right and left heart catheterization, including coronary angiography to provide a baseline evaluation with which subsequent coronary angiograms can be compared. Thereafter, patients undergo an annual assessment of left ventricular ejection fraction, echocardiogram, and cardiac catheterization to assess hemodynamics and coronary anatomy. If occlusive coronary artery disease or ventricular dysfunction develops, the frequency of follow-up is increased to every 6 months. Allograft coronary artery disease does not present as typical native coronary artery disease with segmental stenoses. Rather, the coronary arteries taper throughout their length, providing an angiographic appearance of a "pruned tree." These findings can sometimes be subtle, making it important to compare the current angiogram with the angiogram obtained previously. The only effective treatment for allograft coronary artery disease is repeat cardiac transplantation (95).

REFERENCES

1. Duncan BW. Mechanical support for infants and children with cardiac disease. *Ann Thorac Surg* 2002;73:1670–1677.
2. Baskett RJF, Ghali WA, Maitland A, et al. The intraaortic balloon pump in cardiac surgery (Review). *Ann Thorac Surg* 2002;74: 1276–1287.
3. Dietl CA, Berkheimer MD, Woods EL, et al. Efficacy and cost-effectiveness of preoperative IABP in patients with ejection fraction of 0.25 or less. *Ann Thorac Surg* 1996;62:401–409.
4. Christenson JT, Simonet F, Badel P, et al. Optimal timing of preoperative intraaortic balloon pump support in high-risk coronary patients. *Ann Thorac Surg* 1999;68:934–939.
5. Kang N, Edwards M, Larbalestier R. Preoperative intraaortic balloon pumps in high-risk patients undergoing open heart surgery. *Ann Thorac Surg* 2001;72:54–57.
6. Burack JH, Uceda P, Cunningham JN. Transthoracic intraaortic balloon pump: a simplified technique. *Ann Thorac Surg* 1996;62: 299–301.
7. Arafa OE, Pedersen TH, Svennevig JL, et al. Vascular complications of the intraaortic balloon pump in patients undergoing open heart operations: a 15-year experience. *Ann Thorac Surg* 1999;67: 645–651.
8. Fukushima Y, Yoshioka M, Hirayama N, et al. Management of intraaortic balloon entrapment. *Ann Thorac Surg* 1995;60: 1109–1111.
9. Rose EA, Gelijns AC, Moskowitz AJ, et al. Long-term mechanical left ventricular assistance for end-stage heart failure. *N Engl J Med* 2001;345:1435–1443.
10. Chen JM, Spanier TB, Gonzalez JJ, et al. Improved survival in patients with acute myocarditis using external pulsatile mechanical ventricular assistance. *J Heart Lung Transplant* 1999;18:351–357.

11. Frazier OH, Benedict CR, Radovancevic B, et al. Improved left ventricular function after chronic left ventricular unloading. *Ann Thorac Surg* 1996;62:675–682.
12. Loebe M, Müller J, Hetzer R. Ventricular assistance for recovery of cardiac failure. *Curr Opin Cardiol* 1999;14:234–248.
13. Young JB. Healing the heart with ventricular assist device therapy: mechanisms of cardiac recovery. *Ann Thorac Surg* 2001;71: S210–S219.
14. Dowling R, Etoch SW, Stevens K, et al. Initial experience with the AbioCor implantable replacement heart at the University of Louisville. *ASAIO J* 2000;46:579–581.
15. Goldstein DJ, Oz MC. Mechanical support for postcardiotomy cardiogenic shock. *Semin Thorac Cardiovasc Surg* 2000;12:220–228.
16. Richenbacher WE. Ventricular assistance for postcardiotomy cardiogenic shock. In: Richenbacher WE, ed. *Mechanical circulatory support.* Austin, TX: Landes BioScience, 1999:78–105.
17. Mickleborough LL, Carson S, Tamariz M, et al. Results of revascularization in patients with severe left ventricular dysfunction. *J Thorac Cardiovasc Surg* 2000;119:550–557.
18. Hoy FBY, Mueller DK, Geiss DM, et al. Bridge to recovery for postcardiotomy failure: is there still a role for centrifugal pumps? *Ann Thorac Surg* 2000;70:1259–1263.
19. Curtis JJ, Walls JT, Wagner-Mann CC, et al. Centrifugal pumps: description of devices and surgical techniques. *Ann Thorac Surg* 1999;68:666–671.
20. Sezai A, Minami K, El-Banayosy A, et al. Mechanical circulatory support with Abiomed BVS 5000 and BioMedicus BP-80 for postcardiotomy cardiogenic shock. *J Congest Heart Failure Circ Support* 2001;1:445–448.
21. Samuels LE, Holmes EC, Thomas MP, et al. Management of acute cardiac failure with mechanical assist: experience with the Abiomed BVS 5000. *Ann Thorac Surg* 2001;71:S67–S72.
22. Farrar DJ. The Thoratec ventricular assist device: a paracorporeal pump for treating acute and chronic heart failure. *Semin Thorac Cardiovasc Surg* 2000;12:243–250.
23. DiCorte CJ, Van Meter CH Jr. Abiomed RVAD and LVAD implantation. *Oper Tech Thorac Cardiovasc Surg* 1999;4:301–317.
24. Pae WE Jr, Lundblad O. Thoratec paracorporeal pneumatic ventricular assist device. *Oper Tech Thorac Cardiovasc Surg* 1999;4: 352–368.
25. Samuels LE, Kaufman MS, Thomas MP, et al. Pharmacological criteria for ventricular assist device insertion following postcardiotomy shock: experience with the Abiomed BVS system. *J Cardiac Surg* 1999;14:288–293.
26. Argenziano M, Choudhri AF, Moazami N, et al. Randomized, double-blind trial of inhaled nitric oxide in LVAD recipients with pulmonary hypertension. *Ann Thorac Surg* 1998;65:340–345.
27. Fukamachi K, McCarthy PM, Smedira NG, et al. Preoperative risk factors for right ventricular failure after implantable left ventricular assist device insertion. *Ann Thorac Surg* 1999;68:2181–2184.
28. Pavie A, Szefner J, Leger P, et al. Preventing, minimizing, and managing postoperative bleeding. *Ann Thorac Surg* 1999;68:705–710.
29. Barzilai B, Dávila-Román VG, Eaton MH, et al. Transesophageal echocardiography predicts successful withdrawal of ventricular assist devices. *J Thorac Cardiovasc Surg* 1992;104:1410–1416.

30. Richenbacher WE. Ventricular assistance as a bridge to cardiac transplantation. In: Richenbacher WE, ed. *Mechanical circulatory support.* Austin, TX: Landes BioScience, 1999:106–137.
31. Körfer R, El-Banayosy A, Arusoglu L, et al. Single-center experience with the Thoratec ventricular assist device. *J Thorac Cardiovasc Surg* 2000;119:596–600.
32. Sun BC, Catanese KA, Spanier TB, et al. 100 long-term implantable left ventricular assist devices: the Columbia Presbyterian interim experience. *Ann Thorac Surg* 1999;68:688–694.
33. Maher TR, Butler KC, Poirier VL, et al. HeartMate left ventricular assist devices: a multigeneration of implanted blood pumps. *Artif Organs* 2001;25:422–426.
34. Ramasamy N, Vargo RL, Kormos RL, et al. Intracorporeal support: the Novacor left ventricular assist system. In: Goldstein DJ, Oz MC, eds. *Cardiac assist devices.* Armonk, NY: Futura, 2000: 323–339.
35. Richenbacher WE, Seemuth SC. Hospital discharge for the ventricular assist device patient: historical perspective and description of a successful program. *ASAIO J* 2001;47:590–595.
36. Williams MR, Oz MC. Indications and patient selection for mechanical ventricular assistance. *Ann Thorac Surg* 2001;71: S86–S91.
37. Rao V, Slater JP, Edwards NM, et al. Surgical management of valvular disease in patients requiring left ventricular assist device support. *Ann Thorac Surg* 2001;71:1448–1453.
38. McCarthy PM. Implantable left ventricular assist device insertion techniques. *Oper Tech Thorac Cardiovasc Surg* 1999;4:277–300.
39. Slater JP, Williams M, Oz MC. Implantation techniques for the TCI HeartMate left ventricular assist systems. *Oper Tech Thorac Cardiovasc Surg* 1999;4:330–344.
40. Vitali E, Russo C, Tiziano C, et al. Modified pericardial closure technique in patients with ventricular assist device. *Ann Thorac Surg* 2000;69:1278–1279.
41. Jaski BE, Lingle RJ, Kim J, et al. Comparison of functional capacity in patients with end-stage heart failure following implantation of a left ventricular assist device versus heart transplantation: results of the experience with left ventricular assist device with exercise trial. *J Heart Lung Transplant* 1999;18:1031–1040.
42. Seemuth SC, Richenbacher WE. Education of the ventricular assist device patient's community services. *ASAIO J* 2001;47:596–601.
43. Gordon SM, Schmitt SK, Jacobs M, et al. Nosocomial bloodstream infections in patients with implantable left ventricular assist devices. *Ann Thorac Surg* 2001;72:725–730.
44. Tsau PH, Arabía FA, Toporoff B, et al. Positive panel reactive antibody titers in patients bridged to transplantation with a mechanical assist device. Risk factors and treatment. *ASAIO J* 1998;44: M634–M637.
45. Loh E, Bergin JD, Couper GS, et al. Role of panel-reactive antibody cross-reactivity in predicting survival after orthotopic heart transplantation. *J Heart Lung Transplant* 1994;13:194–201.
46. Oz MC, Levin HR, Rose EA. Technique for removal of left ventricular assist devices. *Ann Thorac Surg* 1994;58:257–258.
47. Cupples SA, Spruill LC. Evaluation criteria for the pretransplant patient. *Crit Care Nurs Clin North Am* 2000;12:35–47.

47. Cimato TR, Jessup M. Recipient selection in cardiac transplantation: contraindications and risk factors for mortality. *J Heart Lung Transplant* 2002;21:1161–1173.
49. Blanche C, Blanche DA, Kearney B, et al. Heart transplantation in patients seventy years of age and older: a comparative analysis of outcome. *J Thorac Cardiovasc Surg* 2001;121:532–541.
50. Hosenpud JD, Bennett LE, Keck BM, et al. The Registry of the International Society for Heart and Lung Transplantation: eighteenth official report—2001. *J Heart Lung Transplant* 2001;20: 805–815.
51. Laks H, Scholl FG, Drinkwater DC, et al. The alternate recipient list for heart transplantation: does it work? *J Heart Lung Transplant* 1997;16:735–742.
52. Carrel T, Neth J, Mohacsi P, et al. Perioperative risk and long-term results of heart transplantation after previous cardiac operations. *Ann Thorac Surg* 1997;63:1133–1137.
53. Uthoff K, Wahlers T, Cremer J, et al. Previous open heart operation: a contribution to impaired outcome after cardiac transplantation? *Ann Thorac Surg* 1997;63:117–123.
54. Vouhé PR, Tamisier D, Le Bidois J, et al. Pediatric cardiac transplantation for congenital heart defects: surgical considerations and results. *Ann Thorac Surg* 1993;56:1239–1247.
55. Renlund DG, Taylor DO, Kfoury A, et al. New UNOS rules: historical background and implications for transplantation management. *J Heart Lung Transplant* 1999;18:1065–1070.
56. Chen JM, Weinberg AD, Rose EA, et al. Multivariate analysis of factors affecting waiting time to heart transplantation. *Ann Thorac Surg* 1996;61:570–575.
57. Kauffman HM, McBride MA, Shield CF, et al. Determinants of waiting time for heart transplants in the United States. *J Heart Lung Transplant* 1999;18:414–419.
58. Brock MV, Salazar JD, Cameron DE, et al. The changing profile of the cardiac donor. *J Heart Lung Transplant* 2001;20:1005–1009.
59. Morley D, Boigon M, Fesniak H, et al. Posttransplantation hemodynamics and exercise function are not affected by body-size matching of donor and recipient. *J Heart Lung Transplant* 1993; 12:770–778.
60. Gilbert EM, Krueger SK, Murray JL. Echocardiographic evaluation of potential cardiac transplant donors. *J Thorac Cardiovasc Surg* 1988;95:1003–1007.
61. Hauptman PJ, O'Connor KJ, Wolf RE, et al. Angiography of potential cardiac donors. *J Am Coll Cardiol* 2001;37:1252–1258.
62. Wheeldon DR, Potter CDO, Oduro A, et al. Transforming the "unacceptable" donor: outcomes from the adoption of a standardized donor management technique. *J Heart Lung Transplant* 1995;14: 734–742.
63. Holmquist M, Chabalewski F, Blount T, et al. A critical pathway: guiding care for organ donors. *Crit Care Nurse* 1999;19:84–98.
64. Zaroff JG, Rosengard BR, Armstrong WF, et al. Consensus conference report: maximizing use of organs recovered from the cadaver donor: cardiac recommendations. *Circulation* 2002;106:836–841.
65. Jeevanandam V, Todd B, Regillo T, et al. Reversal of donor myocardial dysfunction by triiodothyronine replacement therapy. *J Heart Lung Transplant* 1994;13:681–687.

66. Jahania MS, Sanchez JA, Narayan P, et al. Heart preservation for transplantation: principles and strategies. *Ann Thorac Surg* 1999;68:1983–1987.
67. Hinkamp TJ, Montoya A, Bakhos M, et al. Heart and lung grafts harvested en bloc: operative technique, utilization, and results. *Ann Thorac Surg* 1993;56:1381–1385.
68. Bolman RM III. Heart transplantation technique. *Oper Tech Thorac Cardiovasc Surg* 1999;4:98–113.
69. Brandt M, Harringer W, Hirt SW, et al. Influence of bicaval anastomoses on late occurrence of atrial arrhythmia after heart transplantation. *Ann Thorac Surg* 1997;64:70–72.
70. Aziz TM, Burgess MI, El-Gamel A, et al. Orthotopic cardiac transplantation technique: a survey of current practice. *Ann Thorac Surg* 1999;68:1242–1246.
71. Bittner HB, Chen EP, Biswas SS, et al. Right ventricular dysfunction after cardiac transplantation: primarily related to status of donor heart. *Ann Thorac Surg* 1999;69:1605—1611.
72. Carrier M, Blaise G, Bélisle S, et al. Nitric oxide inhalation in the treatment of primary graft failure following heart transplantation. *J Heart Lung Transplant* 1999;18:664–667.
73. Morris CD, Vega JD, Levy JH, et al. Warfarin therapy does not increase bleeding in patients undergoing heart transplantation. *Ann Thorac Surg* 2001;72:714–718.
74. Prendergast TW, Furukawa S, Beyer J III, et al. Defining the role of aprotinin in heart transplantation. *Ann Thorac Surg* 1996;62:670–674.
75. Jahania MS, Mullett TW, Sanchez JA, et al. Acute allograft failure in thoracic organ transplantation. *J Cardiac Surg* 2000;15:122–128.
76. Rubin RH. Prevention and treatment of cytomegalovirus disease in heart transplant patients. *J Heart Lung Transplant* 2000;19:731–735.
77. Holliman RE, Johnson JD, Adams S, et al. Toxoplasmosis and heart transplantation. *J Heart Transplant* 1991;10:608–610.
78. McGoon MD, Frantz RP. Techniques of immunosuppression after cardiac transplantation. *Mayo Clin Proc* 1992;67:586–595.
79. Taylor DO, Olsen SL, Renlund DG. State of the art immunosuppressive regimens: routine and rescue. *Coronary Artery Dis* 1992;3:806–816.
80. Almenar L, Rueda J, Osa A, et al. Incidence of side effects of immunosuppressants commonly used in heart transplantation. *Transplant Proc* 1999;31:2519–2521.
81. Bristow MR, Gilbert EM, Renlund DG, et al. Use of OKT3 monoclonal antibody in heart transplantation: review of the initial experience. *J Heart Transplant* 1998;7:1–11.
82. Rodriguez JA, Crespo-Leiro MG, Paniagua MJ, et al. Induction of immunosuppression with OKT3 following heart transplantation: kidney function as a criterion for control of protocol duration. *Transplant Proc* 1999;31:2517–2518.
83. John R, Rajasinghe HA, Chen JM, et al. Long-term outcomes after cardiac transplantation: an experience based on different eras of immunosuppressive therapy. *Ann Thorac Surg* 2001;72:440–449.
84. Beniaminovitz A, Itescu S, Lietz K, et al. Prevention of rejection in cardiac transplantation by blockade of the interleukin-2 receptor with a monoclonal antibody. *N Engl J Med* 2000;342:613–619.

85. Braith RW, Edwards DG. Exercise following heart transplantation. *Sports Med* 2000;30:171–192.
86. Cremer J, Strüber M, Wagenbreth I, et al. Progression of steroid-associated osteoporosis after heart transplantation. *Ann Thorac Surg* 1999;67:130–133.
87. Fellström B. Impact and management of hyperlipidemia post-transplantation. *Transplantation* 2000;70:SS51–SS57.
88. Kubo SH, Naftel DC, Mills RM Jr, et al. Risk factors for late recurrent rejection after heart transplantation: a multiinstitutional, multivariable analysis. *J Heart Lung Transplant* 1995;14: 409–418.
89. Billingham ME, Cary NRB, Hammond ME, et al. A working formulation for the standardization of nomenclature in the diagnosis of heart and lung rejection: Heart Rejection Study Group. *J Heart Transplant* 1990;9:587–593.
90. Bourge RC, Kirklin JK, White-Williams C, et al. Methotrexate pulse therapy in the treatment of recurrent acute heart rejection. *J Heart Lung Transplant* 1992;11:1116–1124.
91. Fishman JA, Rubin RH. Infection in organ-transplant recipients. *N Engl J Med* 1998;338:1741–1751.
92. Kwok BW, Hunt SA. Neoplasia after heart transplantation. *Cardiol Rev* 2000;8:256–259.
93. Weis M, von Scheidt W. Coronary artery disease in the transplanted heart. *Annu Rev Med* 2000;51:81–100.
94. McGiffin DC, Savunen T, Kirklin JK, et al. Cardiac transplant coronary artery disease. A multivariable analysis of pretransplantation risk factors for disease development and morbid events. *J Thorac Cardiovasc Surg* 1995;109:1081–1089.
95. Srivastava R, Keck BM, Bennett LE, et al. The results of cardiac retransplantation: an analysis of the Joint International Society for Heart and Lung Transplantation/United Network for Organ Sharing Thoracic Registry. *Transplantation* 2000;70:606–612.

Appendices

Appendix 1

Nomogram for Determining Body Surface Area from Height and Weight

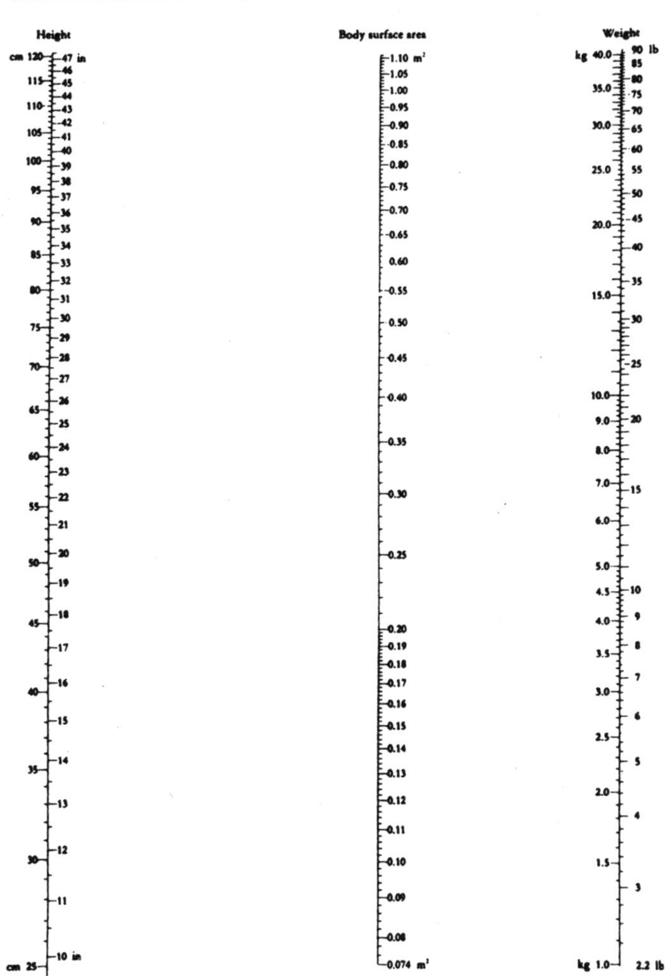

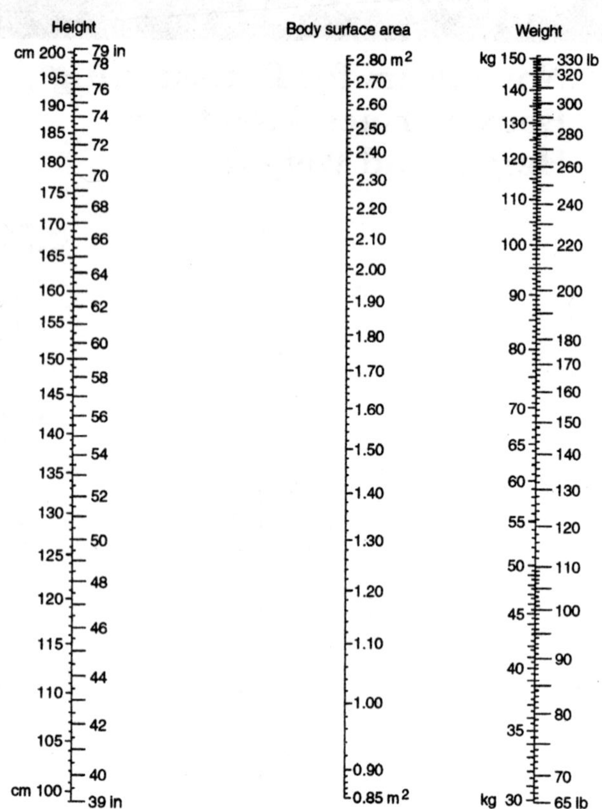
Height
Body surface area
Weight
cm 200
79 in
78
195
76
190
74
185
72
180
70
175
68
170
66
165
64
160
62
155
60
150
58
145
56
140
54
135
52
130
50
125
48
120
46
115
44
110
42
105
40
cm 100
39 in
2.80 m2
2.70
2.60
2.50
2.40
2.30
2.20
2.10
2.00
1.90
1.80
1.70
1.60
1.50
1.40
1.30
1.20
1.10
1.00
0.90
0.85 m2
kg 150
330 lb
320
140
300
130
280
120
260
110
240
100
220
90
200
80
180
170
160
70
150
65
140
60
130
55
120
50
110
45
100
40
90
80
35
70
kg 30
65 lb

Appendix 2

Recommendations for Preventing Bacterial Endocarditis

Patients at risk for bacterial endocarditis

High-Risk Group	Moderate-Risk Group	Low-Risk Group
Prosthetic valves (including mechanical, bioprosthetic, and allografts)	Acquired valvular dysfunction	Previous coronary artery bypass procedure
Previous bacterial endocarditis	Hypertrophic cardiomyopathy	Cardiac pacemakers and implanted defibrillators
Complex cyanotic congenital heart disease (e.g., single-ventricle states, transposition of great arteries, tetralogy of Fallot)	Most other congenital cardiac malformations (uncorrected ASD, VSD, PDA, aortic coarctation, bicuspid aortic valve)	Previously repaired ASD, VSD, or PDA (without residua beyond 6 mo)
Surgically constructed systemic pulmonary shunts or conduits	Mitral valve prolapse with valvular regurgitation and/or thickened leaflets	Isolated secundum ASD; mitral valve prolapse without regurgitation; physiologic, functional, or innocent heart murmurs

ASD, atrial septal defect; PDA, patent ductus arteriosus; VSD, ventricular septal defect.
Patients in the high-risk and low-risk groups should receive antibiotic prophylaxis for invasive procedures that may cause bacteremia (e.g., dental extractions, prophylactic cleaning of teeth, tonsillectomy, lung surgery, intestinal or biliary tract, prostate surgery, urethral dilatation, cystoscopy, or drainage of an abscess). Patients in the low-risk group do not appear to require any antibiotic prophylaxis. For details, see Dajani AS, Taubert KA, Wilson W, et al. Prevention of bacterial endocarditis. Recommendations by the American Heart Association. *Circulation* 1997;96:358–366.

Antibiotic prophylaxis regimens for dental, oral, respiratory tract, or esophageal procedures

Situation	Drug	Dose
Standard prophylaxis	Amoxicillin	Adult: 2.0 g; child: 50 mg/kg p.o. 1 h before procedure
Unable to take oral medications	Ampicillin	Adult: 2.0 g i.m. or i.v.; child: 50 mg/kg i.m. or i.v. within 30 min before procedure
Allergic to penicillin	Clindamycin ***or***	Adult: 600 mg; child: 20 mg/kg p.o. 1 h before procedure
	Cephalexin[a] or cefadroxil[a] ***or***	Adult: 2.0 g; child: 50 mg/kg p.o. 1 h before procedure
	Azithromycin or clarithromycin	Adult: 500 mg; child: 15 mg/kg p.o. 1 h before procedure
Allergic to penicillin and unable to take oral medications	Clindamycin ***or***	Adult: 600 mg; child: 20 mg/kg i.m. or i.v. within 30 min before procedure
	Cefazolin[a]	Adult: 1.0 g; child: 25 mg/kg i.m. or i.v. within 30 min before procedure

[a] Cephalosporins should not be used in patients with significant hypersensitivity to penicillins due to cross-reactivity.

From Dajani AS, Taubert KA, Wilson W, et al. Prevention of bacterial endocarditis. Recommendations by the American Heart Association. *Circulation* 1997;96:358–366, with permission.

Antibiotic prophylaxis regimens for genitourinary and nonesophageal gastrointestinal procedures

Situation	Drug	Dose
High-risk patients	Ampicillin plus gentamicin	Adult: ampicillin 2.0 g i.m. or i.v. plus gentamicin 1.5 mg/kg (limit 120 mg) within 30 min before procedure; 6 h later, ampicillin 1 g i.m./i.v. or amoxicillin 1 g p.o. Child: ampicillin 50 mg/kg i.m. or i.v. (limit 2.0 g) plus gentamicin 1.5 mg/kg within 30 min before procedure; 6 h later, ampicillin 25 mg/kg i.m./i.v. or amoxicillin 25 mg/kg p.o.
High-risk patients allergic to ampicillin/amoxicillin	Vancomycin plus gentamicin	Adult: vancomycin 1.0 g i.v. over 1–2 h plus gentamicin 1.5 mg/kg i.v./i.m.; complete within 30 min before procedure Child: vancomycin 20 mg/kg i.v. over 1–2 h plus gentamicin 1.5 mg/kg i.v./i.m.; complete within 30 min before procedure
Moderate-risk patients	Amoxicillin or ampicillin	Adult: 2.0 g p.o. 1 h before procedure or ampicillin 2.0 g i.m./i.v. within 30 min before procedure Child: amoxicillin 50 mg/kg p.o. 1 h before procedure or ampicillin 50 mg/kg i.m./i.v. within 30 min before procedure
Moderate-risk patients allergic to ampicillin or amoxicillin	Vancomycin	Adult: 1.0 g i.v. over 1–2 h; complete infusion within 30 min before procedure Child: vancomycin 20 mg/kg over 1–2 h; complete infusion within 30 min before procedure

From Dajani AS, Taubert KA, Wilson W, et al. Prevention of bacterial endocarditis. Recommendations by the American Heart Association. *Circulation* 1997;96:358–366, with permission.

Appendix 3

Usual Dosages of Drugs Commonly Used in Adults

Appendix 3. Usual dosages of drugs commonly used in adults

Drug	Representative Tradename	Oral	Intravenous
Acetaminophen	Tylenol	325–650 mg p.o. q 4–6 h; *limit* 4.0 g/24 h	—
Acyclovir	Zovirax	200 mg p.o. 5×/d × 10 d	5 mg/kg q 8 h × 7 d
Adenosine	Adenocard	—	6-mg rapid bolus; may repeat with 12 mg q 1–2 min × 2 doses
Amlodipine	Norvasc	5–10 mg q.d.	—
Amiloride (5 mg) and hydrochlorothiazide (50 mg)	Moduretic	1–2 tabs q.d.	—
Aminocaproic acid	Amicar	—	Load: 4–5 g; followed by 1-g/h infusion; *limit* 30 g/24 h[a]
Amiodarone	Cordarone; Pacerone	Load with 800–1,600 mg q.d. for 1–3 wks until response, then 200–600 mg q.d.[a]	For VF and pulseless VF: 300 mg × 1 For AF: 150 mg over 10 min, then 1 mg/min for 6 h, then 0.5 mg/min[a]
Amoxicillin	Amoxil; Trimox	250–500 mg q 8–12 h (see also *Appendix 1*)	—
Aprotinin	Trasylol	—	*See Table 3-9*
Aspirin	—	For pain/fever: 325–650 mg q 4 h; *limit* 4 g/24 h For prophylaxis: 81–325 mg q.d.	—

Continued

Appendix 3. *Continued*

Drug	Representative Tradename	Oral	Intravenous
Atenolol	Tenormin	50–100 mg q.d.	5 mg over 10 min, then 5 mg 10 min later; switch to p.o.
Atorvastatin	Lipitor	10–80 mg p.o. q.d.	—
Atropine sulfate	—	—	0.4 to 1.0-mg bolus
Azathioprine	Imuran	1–3 mg/kg q.d.[a]	1–3 mg/kg q.d.[a]
Bretylium tosylate	—	—	5 mg/kg over 1 min followed by 10 mg/kg q 5–30 min or infusion at 1–2 mg/min[a]
Bumetanide	Bumex	0.5–2.0 mg q.d.	0.5–1.0 mg q 2–3 h; *limit* 10 mg/24 h
Calcium chloride	—	—	8- to 16-mg/kg slow bolus (typical adult dose 0.5–1.0 g)
Calcium gluconate	—	—	1.0 to 2.0-g slow bolus
Captopril	Capoten	25–50 mg q 8 h	—
Cefazolin	Ancef; Kefzol	—	0.5–2.0 g q 6–8 h
Cefotaxime	Claforan	—	1–2 g q 8–12 h
Ceftriaxone	Rocephin	—	1–2 g q.d.
Cephalexin	Keflex	250–500 mg q 6 h	—
Chlorothiazide	Diuril	0.5–1.0 g q.d.	0.5–1.0 g q 6–12 h
Chlorpromazine	Thorazine	10–50 mg q 6–8 h	—

Chlorthalidone	—	50–100 mg q.d.	—
Cimetidine	Tagamet	300 mg q 6 h[a]	300 mg q 6 h[a]
Ciprofloxin	Cipro	250–750 mg q 12 h	200–400 mg q 12 h
Clarithromycin	Biaxin	500 mg q 8 or 12 h	—
Cyclophosphamide	Cytoxan	3–4 mg/kg/d for 4 d, then 1 mg/kg/d[a]	Same as oral
Cyclosporine	Sandimmune; Neoral	5–10 mg/kg/d, then decrease to maintenance dose[a]	5–6 mg/kg/d (begin prior to transplant)[a]
Diazepam	Valium	2–10 q 6–8 h	2–5 mg q 3–6 h p.r.n.
Digoxin	Lanoxin	Load: 0.5 mg, then 0.25 mg q 4–6 h for total of 1.0 mg; then 0.125–0.25 mg q.d.	Same as oral
Diltiazem	Cardizem	30–90 mg t.i.d. to q.i.d.	For arrhythmias: load with 0.25 mg/kg over 2 min, then infusion at 5–15 mg/h; adjust for SBP >90 mm Hg and HR 70–120 beats/min
Diphenhydramine hydrochloride	Benadryl	25–50 mg q 4–6 h	10–50 mg q 4–6 h
Dobutamine	Dobutrex	—	2.5–15.0 µg/kg/min
Dopamine	Intropin	—	2.5–15.0 µg/kg/min
Docusate	Colace	100–250 mg b.i.d.	—
Enalapril	Vasotec	2.5–40 mg q.d.	—
Enalaprilat	Vasotec IV	—	0.625–2.50 mg q 6 h

Continued

Appendix 3. ***Continued***

Drug	Representative Tradename	Oral	Intravenous
Epinephrine	Adrenalin	—	For cardiac arrest: 1.0 mg q 3–5 min Infusion: 1–10 μg/min
Esmolol	Brevibloc	—	Begin at 50 μg/kg/min; increase in 50-μg/kg/min increments q 5 min to max 200 μg/kg/min; maintain HR 70–120 beats/min and SBP > 90 mm Hg
Ethacrynic acid	Edecrin	50–100 mg q.d.	25–100 mg q.d.
Famotidine	Pepcid	20–40 mg q.h.s.	20 mg q 12 h
Fenoldopam mesylate	Corlopam	—	0.025–1.0 μg/kg/min
Fentanyl	Sublimaze	—	2–50 μg/kg
Furosemide	Lasix	20–80 mg q 6–24 h	Same as oral or constant infusion at 5–40 mg/h
Ganciclovir sodium	Cytovene	—	2.5–5.0 mg/kg i.v. q 12–24 h
Gentamicin	Garamycin	—	1.0–1.7 mg/kg q 8 h or 5–7 mg/kg/d; follow levels
Haloperidol	Haldol	0.5–5.0 mg b.i.d. or t.i.d.	0.5–5.0 mg q 4–8 h
Hydralazine	Apresoline	10–50 mg q.i.d.	10–40 mg q 4–6 h
Hydrochlorothiazide	Esidrix; HydroDIURIL	12.5–50 mg q.d.	—

Hydrochlorothiazide (50 mg) and triamterene (75 mg)	Maxzide	1–2 tabs q.d.	—
Hydrocodone (5 mg) with acetaminophen (500 mg)	Vicodin	1–2 tabs q 4–6 h p.r.n.; *limit* 8 tabs/ 24 h	—
Hydromorphone	Dilaudid	2–4 mg q 4–6 h p.r.n.	1–2 mg q 4–6 h
Ibuprofen	Advil; Motrin	200–400 q 4–6 h p.r.n.	—
Imipenem/cilastatin	Primaxin	—	250–500 mg q 6–8 h
Indomethacin	Indocin	25 mg b.i.d. or t.i.d.; *limit* 200 mg q.d.	—
Iron (ferrous sulfate)	—	325 mg b.i.d. to q.i.d.	—
Iron (i.v.)	Ferrlecit	—	125 mg over 10 min
Isoproterenol	Isuprel	—	0.01–2.0 μg/kg/min or 2–10 μg/min
Ketolorac	Toradol	10 mg q 6 h p.r.n.	15–30 mg q 6 h p.r.n.
Labetolol	Normodyne; Trandate	200–400 mg b.i.d.	Bolus: 10–20 mg followed by infusion at 1–2 mg/min
Lansoprazole	Prevacid	15–30 mg q.d. to b.i.d.	—
Levofloxacin	Levaquin	250–500 mg q.d.	Same as oral
Lidocaine	Xylocaine	—	Bolus: 1.0–1.5 mg/kg followed by 1- to 4-mg/min infusion
Lisinopril	Prinivil; Zestril	10–40 mg q.d.	—
Lorazepam	Ativan	0.5–2.0 mg q 6–8 h	0.5–2.0 mg q 2–4 h

Continued

Appendix 3. ***Continued***

Drug	Representative Tradename	Oral	Intravenous
Mannitol	Osmitrol	—	12.5 to 100-g slow bolus or as infusion
Meperidine	Demerol	50–100 mg q 4–6 h p.r.n.	12.5–100 mg q 4–6 h p.r.n.
Methylprednisolone succinate	Solu-Medrol	—	10–250 mg g 4 h
Metoclopramide	Reglan	5–10 mg q 6–8 h	Same as oral
Metolazone	Zaroxolyn	2.5–20 mg q.d.	—
Metoprolol	Lopressor; Toprol XL	12.5–100 mg b.i.d.	Load: 5 mg q 2 min × 3, then switch to oral
Midazolam	Versed	—	Bolus: 0.20–0.35 mg/kg or infusion 0.02–0.10 mg/kg/h (on ventilator)
Milrinone	Primacor	—	Load: 50 μg/kg over 10 min, then infusion at 0.375–0.75 μg/kg/min
Montelukast	Singulair	10 mg q.h.s.	—
Morphine sulfate	—	30–60 mg q 4–6 h p.r.n.	1–10 mg i.v. q 1–2 h p.r.n.
Mycophenolate mofetil	CellCept	1.5 mg b.i.d.	Same as oral
Nicardipine	Cardene	20–40 t.i.d.	2.5 to 15-mg/h infusion
Nifedipine	Adalat; Procardia	10–30 mg t.i.d. to q.i.d.	—
Nitroglycerin	NitroQuick; Nitrostat; Tridil	0.3–0.6 mg sublingual q 5 min; max 3 doses	5 to 300-μg/min infusion

Nitroprusside	Nipride	—	0.10 to 10.0-μg/kg/min infusion
Norepinephrine	Levophed	—	0.5 to 30.0-μg/min infusion
Nystatin	Mycostatin	0.5 million U swish and swallow q.i.d.	—
Omeprazole	Prilosec	20–40 mg q.d.	—
Ondansetron	Zofran	4–8 mg q 6 h p.r.n.	4 mg q 6 h p.r.n.
Oxycodone and acetaminophen	Roxicodone	5–15 mg q 3–4 h p.r.n.	—
Oxycodone and aspirin	Percodan	1 tab q 6 h p.r.n.	—
Oxycodone hydrochloride	Percocet	1 tab q 6 h p.r.n.	—
Oxymorphone	Numorphan	—	0.2–0.5 mg q 1–3 h
Pancuronium bromide	Pavulon	—	0.04 to 0.10-mg/kg initial paralyzing dose
Pantoprazole	Protonix	40 mg q.d. to b.i.d.	80-mg load, then 8-mg/h infusion
Phenylephrine hydrochloride	Neo-Synephrine	—	40–200 μg/min; adjust for effect
Phytonadione	Aqua-Mephyton	2.5–5.0 mg p.r.n.	0.5–10 mg p.r.n.
Pravastatin	Pravachol	10–80 mg q.d.	—
Prednisone	Deltasone	5–60 mg q.d.	—
Procainamide	Procan SR (p.o.); Pronestyl (i.v., p.o.)	250–500 mg q 3–4 h; 500–1,000 mg q 6–8 h (slow release)	Load: 500–1,000 mg over 20 min; maintenance dose 1–4 mg/min; follow levels

Continued

Appendix 3. ***Continued***

Drug	Representative Tradename	Oral	Intravenous
Prochlorperazione	Compazine	5–10 mg q 3–4 h; *limit* 40 mg/24 h	2.5 to 10.0-mg slow injection (over 2–5 min); *limit* 40 mg/24 h
Propoxyphene	Darvon	65 mg q 4 h p.r.n.	—
Propoxyphene napsylate (100 mg) and acetaminophen (650 mg)	Darvocet-N-100	1–2 tabs q 6 h p.r.n.	—
Propranolol	Inderal	40–240 mg b.i.d.	0.5–2 mg q 5 min up to 5 mg total
Ranitidine	Zantac	150 mg b.i.d.[a]	50 mg q 8 h
Simvastatin	Zocor	5–80 mg q p.r.n.	—
Sotalol	Betapace	80–160 mg q 12 h	—
Spironolactone	Aldactone	25–100 mg q.d. to b.i.d.	—
Sucralfate	Carafate	1 g b.i.d. to q.i.d.	—

Sulfamethoxazole	Gantanol	1,000 mg b.i.d.	—
Temazapam	Restoril	15 mg q.h.s.; may repeat 1×	—
Theophylline	Theo-Dur	100–200 p.o. b.i.d. to t.i.d.[a]	—
Vancomycin	Vancocin	—	1g q 12 h; follow levels
Vasopressin	Pitressin	—	For VT: bolus 40 U × 1 For hypotension: 0.04–0.06 U/min
Vecuronium	Norcuron	—	0.08–0.10 mg/kg (paralyzing dose)
Warfarin	Coumadin	Typical first dose 5 mg; subsequent daily doses per laboratory test (INR) results	Same as oral
Zafirlukast	Accolat	20 mg b.i.d.	—

AF, atrial fibrillation; HR, heart rate; INR, international normalized ratio; SBP, systolic blood pressure; VF, ventricular fibrillation; VT, ventricular tachycardia.

[a] Other dosage schedules are used. See text and/or product information.

Usual Dosages of Drugs Commonly Used in Infants and Children

Intravenous cardiovascular medications	
Pressors	
Amrinone	0.75–1.50 mg/kg bolus, then 5–10 mg/kg/min
Dopamine	2–5 μg/kg/min (renal effect); 5–20 μg/kg/min (cardiac effect)
Dobutamine	5–20 μg/kg/min
Epinephrine	0.1 μg/kg/min starting dose; titrate to effect
Isoproterenol	0.1 μg/kg/min starting dose; titrate to effect, keeping HR <200
Milrinone	50 μg/kg bolus 0.5–1.0μg/kg/min
Norepinephrine	0.1 μg/kg/min starting dose; titrate to effect
Phenylephrine	0.1 μg/kg/min starting dose; titrate to effect
Vasodilators	
Nitroglycerin	1 μg/kg/min starting dose; titrate to effect
Nitroprusside	1 μg/kg/min starting dose; titrate to effect; monitor BP and cyanide level
Prostaglandin E_1 (PGE_1)	0.05–0.20 μg/kg/min starting dose; when effect noted, decrease to lowest effective dose which may be as low as 0.01 μg/kg/min
Analgesics/narcotics	
Aspirin/ Acetaminophen	10 mg/kg/dose PO/PG/PR q4hr
Demerol	1 mg/kg/dose IM/IV q2–4hr
Fentanyl	2–10 μg/kg/dose IV q2–3hr; 5–40 μg/kg/hr continuous IV infusion for deep sedation
Morphine	0.1 mg/kg/dose IM/IV/SC q2–4hr; 0.1 mg/kg/hr continuous IV infusion for deep sedation
Narcotic reversal	
Naloxone	0.1 mg/kg/dose, repeat prn
Muscle relaxants	
Atracurium	0.5 mg/kg/dose VI, repeat q20–40min prn
Pancuronium	0.1 mg/kg/dose IV, repeat q1–2hr prn or 0.1 mg/kg/min continuous IV infusion
Succinylcholine	<1 yr: 2mg/kg/dose IV; >1 yr: 1 mg/kg/dose IV; 4 mg/kg/dose IM
Tubocurarine	0.5 mg/kg/dose IV, q2–3hr
Vecuronium	0.1 mg/kg/dose IV, repeat q20–40min prn
Muscle relaxant reversal (except succinylcholine)	
Atropine	0.02 mg/kg IV
Neostigmine	0.06 mg/kg IV (always precede with atropine)

Anticonvulsants	
Diazepam	0.1–0.3 mg/kg slow IV administration; contraindicated in hyperbilirubinemia
Lorazepam	0.1 mg/kg slow IV
Phenobarbital	10 mg/kg IV load × 2 (may repeat to total 40 mg/kg); maintenance 5 mg/kg/day ÷ bid; therapeutic level 20–40 µg/mL
Phenytoin	15–20 mg/kg IV (slow administration ≤1 mg/kg/min); maintenance 5 mg/kg/day ÷ bid; therapeutic level 10–25 µg/mL

Antihypertensives	
Captopril	1 mg/kg/day PO ÷ tid
Hydralazine	0.1–0.2 mg/kg/dose IM/IV q4–6hr
Labetalol	0.25 mg/kg slow over 2 min (pt. supine). Repeat prn
Nifedipine	0.25 mg/kg SL/PO q4–6hr
Nitroprusside	1 µg/kg/min starting dose; titrate to effect; monitor BP and cyanide level
Propranolol	0.05–0.10 mg/kg/dose IV 21–3hr; 0.5–1.0 mg/kg/day PO ÷ tid-qid

Sedatives/anesthetics	
Chloral hydrate	50–75 mg/kg/dose PO/PR q4–8hr
Diphenhydramine	0.25–0.50 mg/kg/dose IV q4–6hr; 5 mg/kg/day PO ÷ qid
Ketamine	1–2 mg/kg IV (useful for shock, asthma)
Lorazepam	0.1 mg/kg IV
Methohexital	1.0 mg/kg IV; 20 mg/kg PR
Midazolam	0.05 mg/kg IV
Pentobarbital	2 mg/kg/dose IV; "Barbiturate coma": load 5–10 mg/kg IV, maintenance 1–2 mg/kg/hr IV infusion
Thiopental	3–5 mg/kg IV

Diuretics	
Chlorthiazide	20–30 mg/kg/day PO ÷ bid
Furosemide	1–2 mg/kg/dose PO/IM/IV
Mannitol	0.25–1.00 g/kg/dose; repeat q2–4hr
Spironolactone	2.0–3.5 mg/kg/day PO

Antibiotics (IV)	**1st week of life**	**1–4 weeks**	**4+ weeks**
Ampicillin	100–200 mg/kg/d ÷ q12hr	200 mg/kg/d ÷ q8hr	200–300 mg/kg/d ÷ q4–6hr
Cefotaxime	100 mg/kg/d ÷ q12hr	150 mg/kg/d ÷ q6–8hr	200 mg/kg/d ÷ q4–6hr
Cefuroxime	—	—	75–150 mg/kg/d ÷ q8hr
Clindamycin	15 mg/kg/d ÷ q12hr	15 mg/kg/d ÷ q12hr	20 mg/kg/d ÷ q8hr
Gentamicin*	5 mg/kg/d ÷ q12hr	5.0–7.5 mg/kg/d ÷ q8hr	6 mg/kg/d ÷ q8hr

Nafcillin	50 mg/kg/d ÷ q12hr	100 mg/kg/d ÷ q6–8hr	200 mg/kg/d ÷ q4–6hr
Penicillin G	100,000 U/ kg/d ÷ q12hr	200,000 U/ kg/d ÷ q6–8hr	200,000–300,000 U/ kg/d ÷ q4–6hr
Ticarcillin	150 mg/ kg/d ÷ q12hr	200–300 mg/ kg/d ÷ q6–8hr	300–400 mg/ kg/d ÷ q4–6hr
Tobramycin*	4 mg/kg/d ÷ q12hr	6 mg/kg/d ÷ q8hr	6 mg/kg/d ÷ q8hr
Vancomycin*	20–30 mg/ kg/d ÷ q12hr	30–45 mg/ kg/d ÷ q8hr	30–45 mg/ kg/d ÷ q8hr

*Monitoring of blood levels required

Gastrointestinal/nutrition/metabolic

Calcium	Maintenance = 50 mg elemental Ca++/kg/day
Cimetidine	5 mg/kg/dose q6hr
Glucose	5 mg/kg/min
Insulin	0.1 U/kg/hr SC/IV drip. When blood sugar reaches ≥300, begin infusion of D_5W
Intralipid	1 mg/kg/d; increase by 1 gm/kg/d to maximum 4 gm/kg/d
Kayexalate	1 gm/kg/dose PO; 1.5–2.0 gm/kg/dose in 20% sorbitol PR (1 g removes 1 mEq K+)
Calories	Term neonate: 100–120 kcal/kg/d, increased following surgery
Fluids	Full-term newborn, Day 1: $D_{10}W$ @ 60 mL/kg/d; Day 2: D10W @ 80 mL/kg/d ± electrolytes; Day 3: D10W + (Na+ 2–3 mEq/kg/d) + (K+1–3 mEq/kg/d) @ 100 mL/kg/d. Decrease rate 20% if on ventilator Older infants and children: 4 mL/kg/hr for first 10 kg; 2 mL/kg/hr for next 10 kg; 1 mL/kg/hr for every kg over 20 kg

Resuscitation

Fluid bolus	10–20 mL/kg IV bolus (saline, Ringer's lactate, colloid)
Oxygen	100% O_2
Cardioversion	SVT/V Tach = 0.5 watt-sec/kg (synchronous), repeat at 2 watt-sec/kg
Defibrillation	V Fib/V Tach = 2 watt-sec/kg (asynchronous), repeat at 4-watt-sec/kg
Atropine	0.02 mg/kg IM/IV/ETT; min 0.1 mg, max 1.0 mg
Bicarbonate	1–23 mEq/kg IV; repeat according to blood gas determinations
Bretylium	5 mg/kg IV (repeat × 1)

Calcium	10 mg/kg elemental Ca++ IV slow push; 0.3 mL/kg 10% $CaCl_2$ or 1.0 mL/kg 10% calcium gluconate
Epinephrine	0.1 mL/kg (1:10,000) IV/(4 × Dose for ETT instillation)
Glucose	1 gm/kg = 4 mL/kg $D_{25}W$ IV push
Lidocaine	1 mg/kg IV bolus, then 20–50 μg/kg/min IV infusion

ETT, endotracheal tube.

Note: Page numbers followed by f refer to figures and those followed by t refer to tables.

A

Abciximab (ReoPro), 5, 172t, 173–174
Abiomed biventricular assist device, 258, 259t
Acetaminophen
for cardiac transplantation, 283
codeine and, for pain control, 100, 101t
usual dosage of
in adults, 301, 305, 307–308
in combination drugs, 305, 307–308
in infants and children, 310
Acid-base balance
in cardiac arrest, 133
in infants and children, 228–229, 237, 240, 240t
Acidosis, postoperative management of, 88–90, 89t, 239–241
Activated clotting time (ACT)
during cardiopulmonary bypass, 40–41
in postoperative bleeding, 175–176, 178f, 179
Activated partial thromboplastin time (aPTT), 168, 175–177, 178f, 179
Acute respiratory distress syndrome (ARDS), 157
Acyclovir, usual dosage of, 301
Adenosine, 137t, 141, 301
β-Adrenergic agonists, for low cardiac output, 122t–123t, 124
β-Adrenergic blocking agents
for arrhythmias, 136t, 141–142, 145, 147, 149
for cardiopulmonary bypass weaning, 50, 53
for hypertension, 75t, 76, 245
preoperative evaluation of, 4, 15, 17, 84
β-Adrenergic bronchodilators, 153–154
α-Adrenergic vasoconstrictor agents, 41, 73
Adult drug dosages, common, 301–309
Afterload, postoperative management of, 69–71
in infants and children, 233–234, 237–238
in low cardiac output, 118f, 119, 128, 130
Air emboli, 27, 72
with cardiopulmonary bypass, 48–49, 130
neurologic manifestations of, 191–193
Albumin, for hypotension, 73, 85
Albuterol, for bronchospasm, 154
Alkalosis, postoperative management of, 88, 89t, 90–91
Allen test, of radial circulation, 7, 25, 26f, 35, 196
Allograft coronary artery disease, in cardiac transplantation, 285–286
Alveolar-arterial (A-a) gradient, postoperative, 155–156
Ambulation, postoperative initiation of, 208–209
Amiloride, usual dosage of, 301
Aminocaproic acid, 99, 176, 301
Amiodarone, 4, 50, 78, 133, 301
for arrhythmias, 137t, 141, 145–147, 146t, 149
Amlodipine, usual dosage of, 301
Amoxicillin, 188, 298–299, 301
Ampicillin, 298–299, 311
Analgesics, usual dosage of, 301, 305, 307–308
Anastomoses, in cardiac transplantation, 279–280, 279f–280f
Anemia, with cardiac transplantation, 283–284
Anesthesia
for infants and children, 311
operative management of, 34–35
preoperative evaluation of, 14–15
Angina pectoris, Canadian Cardiovascular Society functional classification of, 1, 2t
Angiotensin-converting enzyme (ACE) inhibitors, 4, 73–74, 75t, 77, 104
Angiotensin II receptor antagonists, preoperative, 4
Ankle-brachial index, preoperative, 7
Antacids, renal failure and, 182
Antibiotics
prophylactic
for bacterial endocarditis, 211–212, 298–299
preoperative, 18, 184
for ventricular assist devices, 266, 266t
usual dosages for. *See* specific drug

Anticoagulation. *See also* specific agent
for cardiopulmonary bypass, 39–42
for prosthetic valves, 214, 215t, 216, 248
for thromboemboli prevention, 197–198
Anticonvulsant agents, usual dosage of, 303, 305, 311
Antihypertensive agents, 4, 304–308, 311
Antithymocyte globulin, for cardiac transplant rejection, 285
Aorta
ascending, cannulation for extracorporeal circulation, 42, 43f
coarctation of, 226–227, 243
paradoxical hypertension after repair of, 245–246
Aortic dissection, ascending, with cardiopulmonary bypass, 44, 46f
Aortic valve stenosis, 10–11, 16–17, 227
Aprotinin, operative use of, 37, 40, 192
dosing regimens for, 97, 98t, 301
for postoperative bleeding control, 97–99, 176
Arginine-vasopressin, 74, 99, 129
Arrhythmias
during cardiopulmonary bypass weaning, 49–51, 51f
operative management of, 34
postoperative, 134, 135t–136t
in cardiac arrest, 130–134
with electrolyte imbalances, 85–86, 88
in low cardiac output, 118f, 119
treatment of, 134, 135t–138t, 139–149
Arterial blood gas
for acid-base balance interpretation, 88–91, 89t, 246
in pulmonary care, 65, 81, 155
Arterial pressure monitoring
in infants and children, 230–232
intraoperative, 25, 26f
postoperative, 69, 71t, 117, 121
Arteriography, coronary. *See* Cardiac catheterization
Aspirin
for cardiac transplantation, 283–284
as platelet-inhibiting drug, 171, 172t
postoperative management of
for graft patency, 209–210
for prosthetic valves, 214, 215t, 216
renal failure and, 182
preoperative evaluation of, 5, 15, 18
usual dosage of, 301, 307, 310
Assist-control ventilation, in pulmonary care, 80
Asystole, postoperative, 134
Atelectasis, postoperative, 152–153
Atenolol, 147, 245, 302
Atherosclerosis, postoperative graft management of, 210
Atorvastatin, usual dosage of, 302
Atracurium, usual dosage of, 310
Atrial catheters. *See* Left atrial catheter; Right atrial catheter
Atrial electrode tracings, for atrial arrhythmias, 143, 144f
Atrial fibrillation/flutter
during cardiopulmonary bypass weaning, 49–50
characteristics of, 143, 144f
postoperative management of, 136t–138t, 143–147, 146t
prevention of, 147–148
Atrial overdrive pacing, for atrial flutter, 144–145, 148
Atrial sensing, during cardiopulmonary bypass weaning, 50–51
Atrioventricular canal, complete, 224–225
Atrioventricular dissociation, postoperative, 148
Atropine sulfate, 135t, 139, 302, 310, 312
Autologous blood donations, 93, 96–97
Autotransfusions, postoperative, 99
Axillary artery, cannulation for extracorporeal circulation, 42, 45f
Azathioprine, 282–283, 302
Azithromycin, prophylactic, 298

B

Bacterial endocarditis, 16, 211, 298–299
Bacterial infections, from blood transfusions, 91–92, 92t
Bacterial mediastinitis, 183–184
Behavioral disturbances, postoperative, 194
Benzodiazepines, 35, 103
Bicarbonate (HCO_3), in postoperative acid-base balance, 88–91, 89t
Bicaval cardiac implant, 278f, 279–280, 280f
Bioprosthetic valves, deterioration of, 212–213
Biopsy grading scale, for cardiac transplant rejection, 284–285, 284t
Biventricular implantation, of ventricular assist devices, 261, 261f, 267, 267f

Bleeding
perioperative
drugs to reduce, 97–99, 98t
measures to reduce, 3, 93, 96–97
from right pulmonary artery, 27, 70
postoperative, 168–180
clotting factors and, 174–175
determinants of excessive, 168–170
disseminated, 176
fibrinogen and, 174–175
fibrinolysis and, 176, 178f
in gastrointestinal tract, 188–189
heparin and, 175–176
management of, 55, 72, 168, 176–179, 178f
microvascular, 169, 177, 178f, 179
platelets and, 170–174, 172t
tamponade with, 179–180
preoperative evaluation of, 3, 93, 168
with ventricular assist devices, 262, 270
Bleomycin, preoperative, 4
Blood pressure
cardiopulmonary bypass impact on, 40–41, 52
operative monitoring of, 25, 26f
postoperative management of, 66, 68–69, 73–78, 75t
preoperative evaluation of, 4, 15–16
Blood products
perioperative use of, 91–99
autologous strategies for, 93, 96–97, 99
for cardiac transplantation, 270, 281
indications for, 85, 87, 92–93, 94t–95t
measures to reduce, 93, 96–99, 98t
risks of, 91–92, 92t
postoperative indications for, 85, 87, 92, 94t, 99, 181, 242–243
Blood pumps, mechanical, 256–257, 259t. *See also* Ventricular assist device (VAD)
Body surface area, preoperative evaluation of, 7, 295–296
Body temperature, 29, 120
in critically ill neonates, 229, 246
Body weight
for postoperative management, 85, 104
preoperative evaluation of, 7, 273, 295–296
Bradycardia, 34, 134, 135t, 139–140
Bretylium tosylate, usual dosage of, 302, 312
Bridge to transplantation, ventricular assist devices as, 256, 264–270
device selection for, 259t, 264–265
explantation of, 269–270
long-term issues with, 269
operative management of, 266–268, 267f
patient selection for, 265–266, 266t
postoperative care of, 268–269
Bronchoscopy, for postoperative respiratory insufficiency, 155–157
Bronchospasm, postoperative, 153–154
Bumetanide, usual dosage of, 302

C

Calcium
elemental, for infants and children, 312–313
serum, postoperative management of, 87–88, 244
Calcium carbonate, for cardiac transplantation, 284
Calcium channel blocking agents
for arrhythmias, 137t, 141, 145, 147
for hypertension, 75t, 77
preoperative, 4
Calcium chloride
postoperative indications for, 88, 127, 134
usual dosage of, 302, 312–313
Calcium gluconate, 88, 302, 312–313
Calorie intake, postoperative, 106–107, 312
Canadian Cardiovascular Society, functional classification of angina pectoris, 1, 2t
Cancer(s), 3–4, 56, 285
Cannulation
for cardiopulmonary bypass
arterial techniques, 42, 43f, 44, 45f–46f
in cardiac transplantation, 277–278, 278f
venous techniques, 42, 44
operative, of femoral artery, 37–38
Captopril, usual dosage of, 302, 311
Carbon dioxide (PCO_2), in postoperative acid-base balance, 88–91, 89t, 240
Cardiac arrest. *See also* Circulatory arrest
postoperative, 130–134
Cardiac catheterization
postoperative indications for, 119
preoperative, 10–11, 224
Cardiac enzymes, for myocardial infarction, 133, 150

Cardiac index (CI)
as mechanical assist device criteria, 253, 260t
postoperative management of, 70, 71t, 72
with low cardiac output, 116, 118f, 129
Cardiac massage, for cardiac arrest, 131–132
Cardiac output (CO)
low postoperative, 116–130
in infants and children, 119, 233–234
inotropic drugs for, 118f, 121–128, 122t–123t
left ventricular function and, 116–117, 118f, 120–121, 120f
management algorithm for, 117, 118f, 119
preoperative recognition of, 116–117
right ventricular failure and, 118f, 129–130
vasoactive drugs for, 118f, 128–129
postoperative management of, 66, 69–70, 71t, 72–73, 85
Cardiac pacing. *See* Pacemakers and pacing
Cardiac rehabilitation, postoperative, 208–209
Cardiac transplantation, 270–286
allograft coronary artery disease in, 285–286
blood products for, 270, 281
cardiopulmonary bypass for, 277–278, 281
chronotropic agents for, 280–281
donor cardiectomy for, 274–276, 275f
donor exclusion criteria, 272–274, 273t
donor management for, 274
donor selection criteria, 272–274, 273t
echocardiography for, 274–275, 285–286
hemodynamics with, 271, 272t, 273–274, 280–281, 283
immunosuppression for, 277, 282–283, 285
infections with, 281–283, 285
long-term problems with, 284–286, 284t
malignancies with, 285
panel-reactive antibody screen for, 274, 276
postoperative management for, 281–284
recipient cardiectomy for, 278–279, 278f–280f
recipient exclusion criteria, 271–272, 271t
recipient management for, 276–281
operative, 277–281, 278f–280f
preparation, 276–277
timing of operations, 277
recipient selection criteria, 271–272, 271t
recipient status level, 272, 272t
rejection of, 284–285, 284t
Cardiectomy
for heart donor, 274–276, 275f
for heart recipient, 278–279, 278f–280f
Cardiogenic shock. *See* Post-cardiotomy cardiogenic shock
Cardioplegia
for cardiopulmonary bypass, 46–47, 72
for donor cardiectomy, 275–276, 275f
Cardiopulmonary bypass (CPB)
arterial cannulation techniques for, 42, 43f, 44, 45f–46f
for cardiac transplantation, 277–278, 281
impact on fluid and electrolyte balance, 83–88, 153
inflammatory response to, 40–41, 53, 97, 157, 169
treatment of, 177, 178f, 179
microvascular bleeding with, 169, 177, 178f, 179
myocardial protection during, 46–48
operative management with, 37
anticoagulation for, 39–42
extracorporeal techniques for, 42–53
operative management without, 53–56
plaque detection with, 42, 43f–44f
preoperative evaluation for, 6–7, 15, 18
profound hypothermia and circulatory arrest with, 48
separation from, 48–53
decannulation with, 53
preparation for, 48–49
rhythm maintenance during, 49–51, 51f
weaning process, 51–53, 51f
venous cannulation techniques for, 42, 44
Cardiopulmonary resuscitation (CPR), postoperative, 131–132, 134, 177
Cardioversion, synchronized, 50, 143, 149, 312
Carotid occlusive disease, preoperative evaluation of, 3, 7

Catheter sepsis, postoperative, 186–187
Cefadroxil, prophylactic, 298
Cefazolin, 18, 184, 298, 302
Cefotaxime, usual dosage of, 302, 311
Ceftriaxone, usual dosage of, 302
Cefuroxime, 18, 184, 311
Central venous catheters, 186–187, 230
Central venous pressure (CVP)
  in cardiac transplantation, 281
  operative management of, 25, 27, 28f, 33
  with ventricular assist devices, 260–262, 260t
Cephalexin, 298, 302
Cerebral dysfunction, postoperative, 191–192
Chest radiograph, preoperative, 8t, 9–10, 13
Chest tubes, 82, 84f, 158, 159f
Chloral hydrate, usual dosage of, 311
Chlorothiazide, usual dosage of, 302, 311
Chlorpromazine, 191, 302
Chlorthalidone, usual dosage of, 303
Cholecystitis, acute postoperative, 189–190
Cholesterol emboli, postoperative, 189, 192–193
Chronotropic agents, for cardiac transplantation, 280–281
Chylothorax, postoperative, 158, 160
Cimetidine, 283, 303, 312
Ciprofloxin, usual dosage of, 303
Circulatory arrest
  during cardiopulmonary bypass, 46–48, 72
  in infants and children, 246
Clarithromycin, 188, 298, 303
Clindamycin, 298, 311
Clonidine, preoperative, 4
Clopidogrel (Plavix), 5, 18, 171, 172t, 173
Closed chest cardiac massage, for cardiac arrest, 131
Clotting factors
  in postoperative bleeding, 169, 174–175
    restoration of, 176–179, 178f
  preoperative evaluation of, 8t, 9, 168
Coagulation studies
  postoperative
    for bleeding control, 174–177, 178f, 179
    for infants and children, 245
  preoperative, 8t, 9, 168–169
Coarctation of aorta, 245–246
Codeine, and acetaminophen, 100, 101t
Cognitive impairments, postoperative, 191–192, 194, 246–247
Complete atrioventricular canal, 224–225
Complete blood count, preoperative evaluation of, 8, 8t
Complete heart block, 135t, 139–140
Computed tomography
  for neurologic complications, 194, 247
  surgical indications for, 12, 185, 197
Conduits, 3, 7, 36
Congenital heart anomalies
  ductus-dependent lesions, 229, 229t
  residual postsurgery, 234–235
  review of common, 224–228
Congestive heart failure
  in infants and children, 68, 232–233
  preoperative evaluation of, 11, 14–15, 106
Cooling, postoperative, arrhythmias and, 148
Coronary artery bypass graft (CABG)
  graft patency after, 209–210
  operative management of, 25–57
  postoperative management of, 65–108
    late, 208–219
  preoperative evaluation for, 5, 8–11, 13, 15, 17–18
Coronary artery disease
  allograft, 285–286
  preoperative evaluation of, 10, 15–16
  risk factors for, 2, 3t
Coronary artery spasm, in perioperative infarction, 150, 152
Creatine kinase-myocardial band (CK-MB) isoenzyme, in myocardial infarction, 150–151
Cromolyn sodium, for bronchospasm, 154
Cross-clamping
  for cardiac transplantation, 277, 280–281
  during cardiopulmonary bypass, 46–47, 53, 130
Cryoprecipitate, for postoperative bleeding, 95t, 178f, 179
Crystalloid fluids, postoperative
  for hypotension, 73, 84–85
  for infants and children, 242–243
  for low cardiac output, 118f, 121
Cyclic adenosine monophosphate (cAMP), in low cardiac output, 124, 126
Cyclophosphamide, usual dosage of, 303

Cyclosporine, 282–285, 303
Cytolytic induction protocol, for cardiac transplantation, 282–283
Cytomegalovirus (CMV), in cardiac transplantation, 282

D

D-Dimer, in postoperative bleeding, 8f, 176
Deep venous thrombosis, postoperative, 197–198
Defibrillation
  for cardiopulmonary bypass weaning, 49–50
  operative management of, 34, 36, 312
  for postoperative cardiac arrest, 131–132, 149
Desmopressin. *See* Arginine-vasopressin
Destination therapy, ventricular assist devices as, 256–257, 270
Dexamethasone, for extubation of infants and children, 241
Dextrose infusion, postoperative
  for diabetes management, 104–105, 105f
  for infants and children, 242
  for low cardiac output, 127–128
Diabetes mellitus
  postoperative management of, 104–106
    infection risks and, 184, 197
  preoperative consideration of, 3, 104
Diagnostic studies, preoperative, 10–12
Dialysis, postoperative renal, 180, 182
Diaphragm, in pulmonary complications, 154, 158
Diastolic function, normal, 10, 14, 117
Diazepam, 103, 247, 303, 311
Digoxin, 4, 303
  postoperative indications for, 127, 137t, 145–147
Diltiazem, 137t, 303
Diphenhydramine hydrochloride, 283, 303, 311
Discharge planning, preoperative initiation of, 15
Disseminated intravascular coagulation (DIC), 176
Diuretic therapy
  postoperative management of, 86, 103–104
    for pulmonary complications, 154, 157
    for renal failure, 181–182
  usual dosage of, 4, 302, 304, 306, 308, 311
Dobutamine
  for low cardiac output, 118f, 122t, 124–125, 129, 233
  usual dosage of, 303, 310
Docusate, usual dosage of, 303
Donor management. *See* Cardiac transplantation
Dopamine
  for hypotension, 73, 129
  for low cardiac output, 118f, 122, 124, 126, 129, 233
  usual dosage of, 303, 310
Drug dosages, common
  for adults, 301–309
  for infants and children, 310–313
Ductus-dependent lesions, congenital, 229, 229t
Duodenal ulcers, 188–189
Dysphagia, postoperative, 190–191

E

Echocardiography
  for cardiac transplantation, 274–275, 285–286
  postoperative
    indications for, 119, 180, 212, 214, 219
    for infants and children, 119, 234–235, 248–249
  in preoperative evaluation, 10–11, 17
    for infants and children, 224–227
  transesophageal. *See* Transesophageal echocardiography
  transthoracic, for infants, 119, 249
Edema, interstitial, 40–41, 53, 84–85
Effusions, postoperative
  pericardial, 218–219
  pleural, 158, 160
Eisenmenger syndrome, 237
Ejection fraction (EF), 116–117, 151–152
Electrocardiogram (ECG)
  for perioperative myocardial infarction, 150–152, 151t
  preoperative, 8t, 9–10, 13, 274
Electrocautery, impact on pacemakers, 34
Electrolytes, serum
  postoperative management of, 83–88, 242–245
  preoperative evaluation of, 8–9, 8t
Embolization
  intraoperative monitoring for, 42, 44f, 46
  postoperative, 27, 72
    in infants and children, 246–247
    neurologic manifestations of, 191–193

with prosthetic valves, 212–214, 215t, 216
pulmonary, 78, 197–198
Enalapril, usual dosage of, 303
Enalaprilat, 75t, 77, 303
Encephalopathy, postoperative metabolic, 193–194
Endocarditis
bacterial, 16, 211, 298–299
fungal, 212
prosthetic valve, 211–212
Endoscopy, for gastrointestinal tract bleeding, 188–189
Endotracheal intubation
for cardiac arrest, 131
for infants and children, 235–236, 235t, 240–241
End-stage heart failure, ventricular assist device for, 256–257, 264–270
Enteral nutrition, postoperative, 106–107
Epinephrine
for bronchospasm, 154
for cardiac arrest, 131–134
for cardiopulmonary bypass complications, 41
for low cardiac output, 118f, 122t, 125, 129, 234
racemic inhalation for extubation, 241
usual dosage of, 304, 310, 313
Eptifibatide (Integrilin), 5, 16, 172t, 174
Erythropoietin, recombinant, for red blood cells, 93
Esmolol, 304
for arrhythmias, 137t, 142
for hypertension, 75t, 76, 177, 245
Esophageal procedures, prophylactic antibiotics for, 298
Ethacrynic acid, usual dosage of, 304
Exercise stress test, 10, 209
Extracorporeal circulation, operative, 42–53, 96. *See also* Cardiopulmonary bypass (CPB)
Extubation, postoperative management of, 78, 81–83, 82t–83t

F

Famotidine, 188, 304
Femoral artery
arterial blood pressure monitoring in, 25
cannulation for extracorporeal circulation, 42
intraaortic balloon pump insertion technique, 253, 254f, 255
operative cannulation of, 37–38
Femoral vein, cannulation for extracorporeal circulation, 42, 44
Fenoldopam mesylate, 75t, 77–78, 304
Fentanyl, 236, 304, 310
Ferrous sulfate, usual dosage of, 305
Fibrate agents, for postoperative graft patency, 210
Fibrillation arrest
during cardiopulmonary bypass, 46–47
postoperative, 130–131, 133
Fibrinogen, in postoperative bleeding, 174–175, 177, 179
Fibrinolysis, in postoperative bleeding, 176, 178f
Fingertip ischemia, postoperative, 196
First-degree heart block, 135t, 139–140
Flow-directed pulmonary catheter. *See* Swan-Ganz catheter
Fluid management, postoperative, 83–85
for infants and children, 242–243, 312
for low cardiac output, 118f, 121
for renal failure, 181–182
Fluid resuscitation, for infants and children, 233, 312
Fontan procedure, pulmonary care for, 235, 237, 241
Fresh frozen plasma
for bleeding, 85, 178f, 179
guidelines for, 95t, 242, 245
Fungal endocarditis, postoperative, 212
Furosemide
for cardiac transplantation, 283
for postoperative management, 85, 103–104, 181
usual dosage of, 304, 311

G

Ganciclovir sodium, usual dosage of, 304
Gas exchange, pulmonary
alveolar-arterial gradient in, 155–156
in infants and children, 238–241, 240t
postoperative complications of, 152–153
Gastric drainage, operative monitoring of, 29, 106
Gastric ulcers, 188–189
Gastrointestinal bleeding, postoperative, 188–189
Gastrointestinal (GI) complications, postoperative, 187–194
Gastrointestinal ischemia, postoperative, 189
Gastrointestinal procedures, prophylactic antibiotics for, 299

Genitourinary procedures, prophylactic antibiotics for, 299
Gentamicin, 299, 304, 311
GIK (glucose, insulin, potassium), for low cardiac output, 127–128
Glucose, serum, postoperative management of, 104–106, 243–244
Glucose supplements, for infants and children, 243–244, 312–313
Glycoprotein IIb/IIIa inhibitors
  postoperative indications for, 171, 172t, 173–174
  preoperative evaluation of, 5, 15, 18
Graft patency, postoperative management of, 151, 209–210

H

Haloperidol, 103, 304
Heart anomalies, congenital
  ductus-dependent lesions, 229, 229t
  residual postsurgery, 234–235
  review of common, 224–228
Heart blocks, 135t, 139–140
Heart complications, postoperative, 116–152. *See also* Cardiac entries
Heart failure
  end-stage, ventricular assist devices for, 256–257, 264–270
  New York Heart Association classification of, 1, 2t, 270–271, 271t
  postoperative, 116–130, 118f, 122t–123t
HeartMate ventricular assist devices, 265, 267–268, 270
Heart rate/rhythm
  complications of. *See* Arrhythmias
  in low cardiac output, 118f, 119
  stable, for cardiopulmonary bypass weaning, 49–51
Heart valve regurgitation, management of, 10–11, 16–17
Heart valve stenosis, management of, 10–11, 16–17, 227
Hemodilution, intraoperative, 69, 83–85
Hemodynamics
  in cardiac transplantation, 271, 272t, 273–274, 280–281, 283
  during cardiopulmonary bypass, 40–41, 49, 52–53
  in critically ill neonates, 228–230, 229t
  postoperative management of, 66, 68–78
    blood pressure, 73–78, 75t
    cardiac output, 72–73
    complications with, 116–130, 118f, 122t–123t
    evaluation and monitoring for, 66–72, 71t
    renal failure and, 181–182
  preoperative evaluation of, 10–11, 14, 16, 18, 116–117
  with ventricular assist devices, 260–262, 260t
Hemolytic reactions, 92, 92t, 214
Heparin
  for cardiopulmonary bypass, 39–42
  for off-pump surgery, 54
  postoperative complications and, 175–176, 198
  preoperative evaluation of, 5, 15, 17–18
Heparin-bonded surfaces, for extracorporeal circulation, 96
Heparin-induced thrombocytopenia (HIT), 41–42, 170
Heparin resistance, during cardiopulmonary bypass, 41
Hepatic failure, acute postoperative, 190
"Herald" bleed, 27, 70
Herbal supplements, preoperative, 6, 6t
Hetastarch, for hypotension, 73
Hiccups, postoperative, 191
High-density lipoprotein (HDL), postoperative graft patency and, 210
"High-output" hypotension, 129
Histamine blockers, 41, 188
Histology grading scale, for cardiac transplant rejection, 284–285, 284t
Homocysteine, 210
Hydralazine, 304, 311
Hydration status, preoperative evaluation of, 8–9, 8t
Hydrochlorothiazide, 104, 301, 304–305, 311
Hydrocodone, 100, 101t, 305
Hydromorphone, 100, 102t, 305
Hyperalimentation, postoperative, 107, 243
Hyperbaric oxygen therapy, for air embolism stroke, 193
Hyperglycemia, postoperative management of, 104–106, 243–244
Hyperkalemia, postoperative management of, 86, 244–245
Hyperkalemic cardioplegia solutions, 46, 86
Hyperlipidemia, postoperative graft patency and, 210
Hypernatremia, postoperative management of, 87
Hypertension
  postoperative management of, 74, 75t, 76–78
    after coarctation repair, 245–246

pulmonary, in infants and children, 237–238
Hypocalcemia, postoperative management of, 87–88, 244
Hypoglycemia, postoperative management of, 106, 243–244
Hypokalemia, postoperative management of, 85–86, 244
diuretic therapy and, 103–104
Hypomagnesemia, postoperative management of, 87, 244
Hyponatremia, postoperative management of, 87
Hypoplastic left heart syndrome, 228
Hypotension
during cardiopulmonary bypass, 40–41, 52
postoperative management of, 73–74, 129
preoperative evaluation of, 4, 15–16
Hypothermia
for cardiopulmonary bypass, 47–48, 246
postoperative management of, 68, 229, 246
Hypovolemia, in critically ill neonates, 228–230, 229t
postoperative, 233–234

I

Ibuprofen, usual dosage of, 305
Ibutilide, 146–147
Ice slush, topical, 154, 158, 276
Ileus, postoperative intestinal, 187–188
Iliac artery, external, cannulation for extracorporeal circulation, 42
Imipenem/cilastatin, usual dosage of, 305
Immunosuppression, for cardiac transplantation, 277, 282–283, 285
Incentive spirometer, for pulmonary care, 78, 79f
Indomethacin, usual dosage of, 305
Infants and children
cardiopulmonary resuscitation technique for, 132
congestive heart failure in, 68, 232–233
drug dosages, common, 310–313
intravenous lines for, 229–232, 231f
mechanical ventilation for, 235–241
critically ill neonates, 228–229
endotracheal intubation for, 235–236, 235t
extubation requirements, 241
parameter guidelines for, 236–237, 237t
pulmonary blood flow factors with, 238–241, 240t
pulmonary hypertension and, 237–238
tracheostomy for, 241
monitoring lines for, 229–232, 231f
postoperative care for, 232–249
cardiovascular assessment, 232–233
coagulation disorders, 245
echocardiography indications, 119, 234–235, 248–249
fluids and electrolytes, 242–245, 312
low cardiac output, 119, 233–234
neurologic complications, 246–247
nutritional management, 243–244
paradoxical hypertension, 245–246
phrenic nerve injury, 154
pulmonary management, 235–241, 235t, 237t, 240t
renal failure, 181–182, 247
residual lesions, 234–235
rhythm management, 241–242
sepsis, 247–248
tamponade physiology, 234
temperature regulation, 246, 249
valve replacement, 248
prostaglandin E_1 for ductus-dependent lesions in, 228–229, 229t
prosthetic valves for, 248
surgical management of, 224–249
common indications for, 224–228
operative considerations with, 229–232
postoperative care for, 232–249
postoperative complications with, 119, 154, 181–182
preoperative preparation for, 228–229
synchronized cardioversion for, 312
transthoracic echocardiography for, 119, 249
Infections
from blood transfusions, 91–92, 92t
with cardiac transplantation, 281–283, 285
postoperative, 56, 183–187
in infants and children, 247–248
with prosthetic valves, 211–212
preoperative, 8
with ventricular assist devices, 266, 266t, 269
Inflammatory response, to cardiopulmonary bypass, 40–41, 53, 97, 157, 169
treatment of, 177, 178f, 179

Inhalation agents, 35, 78, 82
Inotropic agents
for cardiopulmonary bypass weaning, 50, 53
for postoperative management, 72–74
of low cardiac output, 116, 118f, 121–128, 122t–123t, 130
Inspiration/expiration ratio (I/E ratio), in pulmonary care, 79–80, 80t
for infants and children, 237, 240, 240t
Insulin
postoperative
for diabetes management, 104–105, 105f
for infants and children, 243–244, 312
for low cardiac output, 127–128
preoperative, 4–5
Intensive care unit (ICU)
immediate postoperative care in, 65–66, 66f–68f, 78, 108
transfer out of, 66, 67f, 82
Interleukin-2 receptor antibodies, for cardiac transplantation, 283
Intermittent mandatory ventilation (IMV), in pulmonary care, 80, 80t, 237
Internal mammary artery
complications related to mobilization of, 158, 196–197
sternotomy consideration of, 37, 37f, 39
International normalized ratio (INR), 214, 215t, 216–219
International Society for Heart and Lung Transplantation (ISHLT), on cardiac transplant rejection, 284–285, 284t
Interstitial edema, 40–41, 53, 84–85
Intestinal ileus, postoperative, 187–188
Intraaortic balloon pump (IABP), 253–255
complications of, 255
contraindications for, 253, 255
indications for, 253, 255
for low cardiac output, 116–117, 129–130, 133
percutaneous insertion of, 253, 254f
preoperative evaluation for, 8, 15–18, 255
transthoracic insertion of, 255, 256f
Intralipids, usual dosage of, 312
Intraventricular hemorrhage, postoperative, 247
Iron supplements, 283, 305
Ischemia
fingertip, postoperative, 196
gastrointestinal, postoperative, 189
leg, with intraaortic balloon pump, 253
myocardial, perioperative, 149–152, 151t
Isoproterenol
for bradycardia, 135t, 139
for cardiac transplantation, 280–281
for low cardiac output, 118f, 122t, 126, 130
usual dosage of, 305, 310

J

Jugular vein, internal
cannulation for extracorporeal circulation, 42
pulmonary artery catheter insertion via, 25, 27, 28f
Junctional rhythms, 135t, 139–140, 148

K

Kallikrein inactivator units (KIU), 37, 97–98
Kayexalate, usual dosage of, 245, 312
Ketamine, 35, 311
Ketolorac, 305
codeine and, 100, 101t

L

Labetalol
for postoperative hypertension, 75t, 76–77, 245
usual dosage of, 305, 311
Laboratory testing, preoperative, 8–10, 8t
Lactate dehydrogenase, paravalvular leaks impact on, 214
Lansoprazole, 188, 283, 305
Latex allergy, 6
Left atrial catheter
for operative transthoracic monitoring, 29, 32f
postoperative management of, 71–72, 121
Left atrial pressure, postoperative changes in, 130
Left main coronary artery disease, preoperative management of, 10, 15–16
Left ventricular assist device (LVAD), for cardiogenic shock, 255–270, 259t, 261f, 264t
Left ventricular function
during cardiopulmonary bypass weaning, 52–53
depressed
preoperative management of, 10–11, 15
ventricular assist device for, 259–261, 259t, 261f, 263–264, 264t

postoperative
in low cardiac output, 116–117, 118f, 120–121, 120f
management of, 70, 71t
Leg ischemia, with intraaortic balloon pump, 253
Levofloxacin, usual dosage of, 305
Lidocaine
postoperative indications for, 133, 138t, 149
usual dosage of, 305, 313
Lipid emboli, postoperative, 189, 192–193
Lipid-lowering agents, for postoperative graft patency, 210
Lisinopril, usual dosage of, 305
Lorazepam, usual dosage of, 305, 311
Low molecular weight heparin (LMWH), postoperative bleeding and, 175–176
Lung complications. *See also* Pulmonary entries
postoperative, 152–160

M

Magnesium, serum, postoperative management of, 88, 244
Magnesium sulfate, postoperative, 133, 138t, 147, 182
Magnetic resonance imaging, in preoperative evaluation, 12
Malignancies, 3–4, 56, 285
Mandatory minute ventilation (MMV), in pulmonary care, 80, 80t
Mannitol, usual dosage of, 306, 311
Mean airway pressure, in infants and children, 235, 237, 240, 240t
Mechanical blood pumps, 256–257, 259t. *See also* Ventricular assist device (VAD)
Mechanical cardiac support
intraaortic balloon pump as, 253–255
applications of, 116–117, 129–130, 133
preoperative evaluation of, 8, 15–18
ventricular assist devices as, 255–270
for acute myocarditis, 257
as bridge to transplantation, 256, 264–270
as destination therapy, 256–257, 270
indications for, 255–256, 259t
for postcardiotomy cardiogenic shock, 256–264
Mechanical ventilation
for infants and children, 235–241
critically ill, 228–229
endotracheal intubation for, 235–236, 235t
extubation requirements, 241
parameter guidelines for, 236–237, 237t
pulmonary blood flow factors with, 238–241, 240t
pulmonary hypertension and, 237–238
tracheostomy for, 241
postoperative
for acute respiratory distress syndrome, 157
for infants and children, 228–229, 235–241
pain control and, 100, 103
prolonged, 155–157
for pulmonary care, 78–81, 80t
weaning guidelines, 81–83
Mediastinal tubes, routine postoperative, 55, 55f, 82, 169
Mediastinitis, postoperative, 56, 183–186
Medical history, in preoperative evaluation, 1–4, 12–13
Medication review, preoperative, 4–6
MedMath program, for body measurements, 7
Meperidine (Demerol), usual dosage of, 306, 310
Meralgia paresthetica, 195
Mesenteric arteritis, after coarctation of aorta repair, 246
Mesenteric ischemia, postoperative, 189
Metabolic acidosis, postoperative management of, 89–90, 89t
Metabolic alkalosis, postoperative management of, 89t, 91
Metabolic encephalopathy, postoperative, 193–194
Metformin, preoperative, 4
Methohexital, usual dosage of, 311
Methotrexate, for cardiac transplant rejection, 285
Methylprednisolone, 41, 306
for cardiac transplantation, 282–283, 285
Metoclopramide, 107, 187–188, 190, 306
Metolazone, usual dosage of, 306
Metoprolol, usual dosage of, 306
Microvascular bleeding, postoperative, 169, 177, 178f, 179
Midazolam, 100, 103, 306, 311
Milrinone, 53, 238, 306, 310
for low cardiac output, 118f, 123t, 126–128, 233
Mitral valve regurgitation, preoperative management of, 10–11, 16

Mixed venous oxygen saturation (SVO_2), 33, 71, 233
Monitoring techniques, operative
basic, 25–33
for cardiac transplantation, 276–277
for infants and children, 229–232, 231f
other, 33–34
Monoclonal antibodies, interleukin-2 specific, in cardiac transplantation, 283
Montelukast, 154, 306
Morphine sulfate
for postoperative pain control, 100, 102t
usual dosage of, 306, 310
for ventilatory control, in infants and children, 236
Muromonab-CD3, for cardiac transplantation, 282–283
Muscle relaxant reversal, 310
Muscle relaxants, 35, 103, 307, 309–310
Mycophenolate mofetil, usual dosage of, 306
Myocardial contractility, in low cardiac output, 118f, 119, 130
Myocardial infarction (MI), perioperative, 133, 149–152, 151t
Myocardial ischemia, perioperative, 149–152, 151t
Myocardial perfusion imaging, preoperative, 10
Myocardial protection, during cardiopulmonary bypass, 46–48
Myocardial viability, preoperative, 11–12

N

Nafcillin, usual dosage of, 312
Naloxone, usual dosage of, 310
Narcotic agents
for anesthesia induction, 34–35
mechanical ventilation weaning and, 82
for postoperative pain control, 100, 101t–102t
usual dosage of, 304, 306, 310
Narcotic reversal, 310
Narrow QRS-complex tachycardia, 136t–137t, 141
Nasogastric tube, indications for, 29, 106–107
Nausea, postoperative, 190
Neostigmine, usual dosage of, 310
Nerve injury, perioperative, 154, 194–195
Neurobehavioral disturbances, postoperative, 194
Neurologic complications, postoperative, 191–194
New York Heart Association, functional classification of heart failure, 1, 2t, 270–271, 271t
Niacin, for postoperative graft patency, 210
Nicardipine, 75t, 77, 306
Nifedipine, usual dosage of, 306, 311
Nitrate therapy, preoperative, 4, 15
Nitric oxide, for pulmonary hypertension, 238, 281
Nitroglycerin
for afterload reduction, 238
for hypertension, 74, 75t, 177
for low cardiac output, 118f, 128–129, 234
usual dosage of, 306, 310
Nitroprusside
for afterload reduction, 238
for hypertension, 75t, 76, 177, 245
for low cardiac output, 128–130, 234
usual dosage of, 307, 310–311
Nitrous oxide, for operative anesthesia, 35
Nodal rhythms, 135t, 139–140, 148
Nomograms, for body measurements, 7, 295–296
Nonoliguric renal failure, postoperative, 182
Nonsustained ventricular tachycardia (NSVT), 149
Norepinephrine
for hypotension, 73–74
for low cardiac output, 118f, 123t, 125–126, 129
usual dosage of, 307, 310
Norwood procedure, pulmonary care for, 238–240
Nutrition
postoperative management of, 106–107
with complications, 190–191
for infants and children, 243–245
warfarin and, 216–218, 217t
Nystatin, 191, 307

O

Obesity, surgical consideration of, 7, 56, 295–296
Off-pump surgery
cognitive advantages of, 191–194
operative management of, 53–56, 170
postoperative management of, 83, 96
OKT3, for cardiac transplantation, 282–283, 285
Oliguria, postoperative, 182, 247
Omeprazole, 188, 307
Ondansetron, 190, 307

Open chest cardiac massage, for cardiac arrest, 131
Operative management, 25–57
  anesthesia for, 34–35
  arrhythmias and, 34
  with cardiopulmonary bypass, 37, 39–42
  without cardiopulmonary bypass, 53–56
  conduct during procedure, 35–39
  extracorporeal circulation techniques for, 42–53
  for infants and children, 229–232
  monitoring techniques for
    basic, 25–33
    other, 33–34
  pacemakers for, 33–34
  transport of patient, 56–57
Oral hypoglycemic agents, preoperative, 4
Oral procedures, prophylactic antibiotics for, 298
Organ Procurement Organization (OPO), 273–274
Organ transplants. *See* Cardiac transplantation
Oscillating saw, for redo sternotomy, 38, 39f
Oxycodone hydrochloride, usual dosage of, 307
Oxygen, supplemental, in pulmonary care, 82–83, 156
  for infants and children, 237–240, 237t, 312
  with prolonged ventilatory support, 156
Oxygen saturation, monitoring of, 29, 33, 35–36, 71
Oxymorphone, usual dosage of, 307

P

Pacemakers and pacing
  for cardiac transplantation, 280
  for cardiopulmonary bypass weaning, 49–51, 51f
  mode abbreviations for, 140
  operative management of, 33–34
  postoperative
    for asystole, 134
    for atrial flutter, 144–145, 148
    for bradycardias, 134, 135t, 139–140
    for low cardiac output, 118f, 119
Pain control, postoperative, 99–103, 101t–102t
Pancreatitis, acute postoperative, 190
Pancuronium bromide, 103, 307, 310
Panel-reactive antibody (PRA) screen, for cardiac transplantation, 274, 276
Pantoprazole, 188, 307
Paradoxical hypertension, after coarctation of aorta repair, 245–246
Parallel circulations, postoperative, in infants and children, 238–241, 240t
Paravalvular leaks, postoperative management of, 213–214
Parenteral nutrition, postoperative, 107
Partial sternotomy, 36, 37f–38f
Partial thromboplastin time, activated (aPTT), 168, 175–177, 178f, 179
Patent ductus arteriosus, 227, 229, 229t
Patient positioning
  for cardiopulmonary bypass weaning, 48–49
  operative, 35–36
Peak airway pressure, in pulmonary care, 79, 81
Pediatric surgery. *See* Infants and children
Penicillin G, usual dosage of, 312
Pentobarbital, usual dosage of, 311
Percutaneous coronary interventions, failed, preoperative management of, 15–18
Perfusion, operative management of. *See* Cardiopulmonary bypass (CPB)
Perfusion imaging, myocardial, 10
Pericardial constriction, 219
Pericardial effusions, postoperative, 218–219
Pericardiectomy, 219
Pericarditis, postoperative management of, 218–219
Pericardium
  in off-pump surgery, 54–55
  postoperative complications of, 218–219
Peripheral nerve injury, perioperative, 194–195
Peripheral vascular disease, preoperative evaluation of, 7–8
Peritoneal dialysis, for renal failure, 182, 247
pH, in postoperative acid-base balance, 88–91, 89t, 240, 246
Phenobarbital, 247, 311
Phenylephrine hydrochloride (Neo-Synephrine)
  for hypotension, 73, 129
  for low cardiac output, 118f, 123t, 129
  usual dosage of, 307, 310
Phenytoin, 247, 311
Phrenic nerve injury, postoperative, 154

Physical examination
in postoperative management, 65–66, 66f, 68–69, 117
for infants and children, 232–233
in preoperative evaluation, 7–8, 12–13, 224
Phytonadione, 307. *See also* Vitamin K
Plaque detection, during cardiopulmonary bypass, 42, 43f–44f
Platelet dysfunction
drugs that cause, 171, 172t, 173–174
postoperative, 170–171, 176–179, 178f
Platelet-inhibitor agents
postoperative indications for, 171, 172t, 173–174
preoperative evaluation of, 5, 15, 18
Platelet transfusions, postoperative guidelines for, 93, 94t–95t, 245
Pleural effusions, postoperative, 158, 160
Pneumonia, postoperative, 183, 263, 283
Pneumothorax, postoperative, 157–158
Porcine bioprosthetic valves, deterioration of, 212–213
Positive end-expiratory pressure (PEEP), in pulmonary care, 79, 80t, 81, 154, 157
for infants and children, 237, 240–241, 240t
prolonged need for, 155–157
Postcardiotomy cardiogenic shock, ventricular assist device for, 256–264
biventricular implantation technique for, 261, 261f
device selection, 258–261, 259t
hemodynamics following termination of, 260–262
hemodynamic status during, 260, 260t
left ventricular failure definition, 259, 259t
patient selection for, 257–258
postoperative care for, 262–263
right ventricular failure with, 259t, 262
ventricular function recovery indicators for, 264, 264t
weaning from, 263–264
Postoperative complications
acute respiratory distress syndrome, 157
arrhythmias, 134, 135t–138t, 139–149
atelectasis, 152–153
bleeding, 55, 72, 168–180, 178f
bronchospasm, 153–154
cardiac arrest, 130–134
deep venous thrombosis, 197–198
of gastrointestinal tract, 187–194
of heart, 116–152
in infants and children, 119, 154, 181–182
infections, 183–187
of internal mammary artery mobilization, 196–197
low cardiac output, 116–130, 118f, 122t–123t
of lungs, 152–160
myocardial ischemia and infarction, 149–152, 151t
nerve injury, 154, 194–195
of neurologic system, 191–194
pleural effusions, 158, 160
pneumothorax, 157–158
preoperative discussion of, 13
prolonged respiratory insufficiency, 155–157
pulmonary embolism, 78, 197–198
of radial artery use, 196
renal failure, 180–183
of saphenous vein harvesting, 195–196
Postoperative management, 65–108
acid-base balance in, 81, 88–91, 89t
blood products in, 85, 91–99, 94t–95t
cardiac rehabilitation, 208–209
diabetes management in, 104–106
diuretic therapy in, 103–104
fluid and electrolytes in, 83–88
of graft patency, 209–210
of hemodynamics, 66, 68–78, 71t
immediate intensive care, 65–66, 66f–68f, 78, 108
for infants and children, 232–249
late, 208–219
nutritional support in, 106–107
pain control in, 99–103, 101t–102t
of pericarditis, 218–219
of prosthetic valves, 211–216, 215t
pulmonary care in, 78–84
of radial artery harvest site, 107–108
of tamponade, 218–219
of ventricular assist devices, 262–263, 268–269
warfarin issues in, 216–218, 217t
Postoperative orders, typical preprinted, 66, 67f
Potassium, serum, postoperative management of, 85–86, 244–245
diuretic therapy and, 103–104
Potassium supplements, postoperative, 127–128, 182, 244–245
Pravastatin, 284, 307

Prednisone, 4, 284–285, 307
Pregnancy, cautions with, 18, 218
Preload
postoperative complications of
acute respiratory distress syndrome, 157
in infants and children, 233–234
in low cardiac output, 118f, 119–121, 128, 130
postoperative management of, 69–70, 85
Premature ventricular contractions (PVCs), 135t, 148–149
Preoperative evaluation, 1–19
for antibiotic prophylaxis, 18
diagnostic studies in, 10–12
final presurgery visit elements, 12–15, 12t
of infants and children, 224–229
laboratory testing in, 8–10, 8t, 168
management of special problems, 15–18
medical history in, 1–4
medication review, 4–6
physical examination in, 7–8
skin preparation, 18
Preoperative teaching, 13
Pressure support (PS), in pulmonary care, 80, 80t
Procainamide, 133, 307
for arrhythmias, 138t, 141, 146–149
Prochlorperazine, 190, 308
Propafenone, 146–147
Prophylactic antibiotics
for bacterial endocarditis, 298–299
preoperative, 18, 184
for ventricular assist devices, 266, 266t
Propoxyphene napsylate, usual dosage of, 308
Propranolol, 138t, 308, 311
Prostaglandin E_1 (PGE_1), 310
postoperative, for low cardiac output, 118f, 128, 130, 234
preoperative, for ductus-dependent congenital lesions, 228–229, 229t
Prosthetic valve endocarditis (PVE), 211–212
Prosthetic valves
for infants and children, 248
infection of, 211–212
leaks with, 213–214
malfunction of, 213
postoperative management of, 211–216, 215t
preoperative management of, 16–17
thromboembolism with, 212, 214, 215t, 216
tissue deterioration with, 212–213
Protamine
for cardiopulmonary bypass, 40–41, 53
for postoperative bleeding, 178f, 179
preoperative, 5
Prothrombin time (PT), 168, 174, 177, 178f, 179
Proton pump inhibitors, 188
Pulmonary artery catheter. *See* Swan-Ganz catheter
Pulmonary artery (PA) pressures
in infants and children, 237–239
operative management of, 25, 33–34
postoperative management of, 69–70, 117, 119, 129–130
Pulmonary artery rupture, 27, 70
Pulmonary atresia, with/without ventricular septal defect, 226
Pulmonary blood flow, postoperative, in infants and children, 237–241, 240t
Pulmonary capillary wedge pressure (PCWP), postoperative, 181
in low cardiac output, 117, 118f, 120–121, 128, 130
Pulmonary embolism, postoperative, 78, 197–198
Pulmonary function
postoperative management of, 78–84
complications with, 152–160, 197
for infants and children, 235–241, 235t, 237t, 240t
preoperative testing of, 12
Pulmonary hypertension, in infants and children, 237–238
Pulmonary vascular resistance (PVR)
in cardiac transplantation, 280–281
postoperative management of, 71, 71t
acid-base balance impact on, 89–90
in low cardiac output, 118f, 119, 126, 128
Pulseless electrical activity (PEA), 134
Pulse oximetry, with mechanical ventilation, 155
Pulses, preoperative evaluation of, 7–8

Q

Quinidine, 146–147

R

Radial artery
circulatory evaluation of, 7, 14, 25, 26f, 35
harvesting of, 36, 107–108, 196

Radial artery catheter, for blood pressure monitoring, 25, 26f, 69
Radial nerve injury, 195
Ranitidine, usual dosage of, 308
Recombinant erythropoietin, for red blood cell stimulation, 93
Red blood cell (RBC) transfusion
autologous donations of, 93, 96
for postoperative management, 85, 87, 92, 94t, 181, 242
risks of, 92, 92t
Redo sternotomy, 36–38, 39f
Rejection, of cardiac transplantation, 284–285, 284t
Renal failure, postoperative, 180–183
in infants and children, 181–182, 247
Renal function, preoperative evaluation of, 8t, 9
Respiratory acidosis, postoperative management of, 89t, 90, 237
Respiratory alkalosis, postoperative management of, 89t, 91
Respiratory insufficiency, prolonged postoperative, 155–157, 197
Right atrial catheter, for operative transthoracic monitoring, 29, 33f, 230
Right atrial pressure, postoperative changes in, 130
Right ventricular assist device (RVAD), 259t, 261–262, 261f
Right ventricular failure, postoperative
in low cardiac output, 118f, 129–130
mechanical support for, 259t, 261–262, 261f, 264t
Risk, surgical, preoperative evaluation of, 13–14, 14t

S
Saphenous nerve injury, 195
Saphenous veins, harvesting of, 8, 195–196
Second-degree heart block, 135t, 139–140
Sedatives, usual dosage of, 303, 305–306, 311
Seizures, postoperative, 247
Sepsis, postoperative, 186–187, 247–248
Septal defects, as common anomaly, 224, 226
Shivering, postoperative, 120
Shunting, cardiopulmonary
in congenital heart anomalies, 224–228
intentional maintenance of, 229, 229t
residual postsurgery, 233, 235
operative management of, 33
postoperative management of, 71, 81, 119, 129, 233
ventricular assist devices and, 253, 260
Simvastatin, usual dosage of, 308
Sinus tachycardia, 136t, 141–142
Skin preparation
operative, 36
preoperative, 8, 18
Skin temperature, in infants and children, 232, 246
Sodium, serum, postoperative management of, 87, 103, 107
Sodium bicarbonate (HCO_3), 133, 312
Sodium polystyrene sulfonate, for postoperative hyperkalemia, 86
Sotalol, 147, 308
Spironolactone, 86, 104, 308, 311
Staphylococcus spp.
in endocarditis, 211–212
in postoperative infections, 184–185, 247
Statin therapy, 210, 284, 302, 307–308
Sternotomy
partial, 36, 37f–38f
postoperative complications of, 56, 184–185
redo, 36–38, 39f
Sternum
in off-pump surgery, 54–55
postoperative infections of, 183–186
Steroids, 4, 41, 154
for cardiac transplantation, 282–285
Streptococcus spp., in postoperative infections, 247
Stress echocardiography, preoperative, 10
Stroke, postoperative, 192–194
Stroke volume (SV), postoperative management of, 70, 71t
Succinylcholine, usual dosage of, 310
Sucralfate, usual dosage of, 308
Sulfamethoxazole, usual dosage of, 309
Superior vena cava, cannulation for extracorporeal circulation, 42, 44
Supraventricular tachycardia (SVT), 136t–138t, 141–142, 144
Surgical risk, preoperative assessment of, 13–14, 14t

Sustained ventricular tachycardia (NSVT), 135t, 149
Swan-Ganz catheter
complications of, 27, 29
in operative management, 25, 27, 28f, 29, 30f–31f
pacing wires of, 33–34
in postoperative management, 69–70
in preoperative evaluation, 14
Synchronized mandatory ventilation (SIMV), in pulmonary care, 80, 80t
Systemic inflammatory response
to surgery, 40–41, 53, 97, 157, 169
treatment of, 177, 178f, 179
Systemic vascular resistance (SVR), postoperative management of, 70–71, 71t, 73
in infants and children, 238–241, 240t
in low cardiac output, 118f, 119–121, 124, 126, 128–129
Systolic function, normal, 10, 14, 116–117

T

Tachyarrhythmias, postoperative, 135t–138t, 140–149
Tamponade, postoperative pericardial, 55, 72
classic signs of, 179–180
in infants and children, 234
management of, 129, 180, 218–219
Temazapam, usual dosage of, 309
Temperature, patient. *See* Body temperature
Tension pneumothorax, postoperative, 157–158
Tetralogy of Fallot, 225–226
Theophylline, 154, 309
Thermodilution cardiac output, postoperative monitoring of, 70, 72
Thermoregulation, in critically ill neonates, 229, 246
Thiopental, usual dosage of, 311
Third-degree heart block, 135t, 139–140
Thoracentesis, for postoperative pleural effusions, 158
Thoracotomy, left lateral, for coronary artery bypass graft, 36
Thoratec biventricular assist device, 258, 259t, 264, 266–267, 267f
Thrombocytopenia, heparin-induced, 41–42, 170
Thromboembolism
deep venous, 197–198
in infants and children, 247
neurologic manifestations of, 191–193
with prosthetic valves, 212–214, 215t, 216
Thrush, oral, 191
Ticarcillin, usual dosage of, 312
Ticlopidine (Ticlid), 171, 173
Tidal volume (TD), in pulmonary care, 80–81, 99
for infants and children, 236–237, 240t, 240–241
Tirofiban (Aggrastat), 5, 15, 172t, 174
Tissue prostheses, valvular, deterioration of, 212–213
Tobramycin, usual dosage of, 312
Total anomalous pulmonary venous connection, 228
Toxoplasmosis gondii, in cardiac transplantation, 282
Tracheostomy, postoperative, 155–157, 184, 241
Tranexamic acid, for bleeding control, 99, 176
Transesophageal echocardiography
intraoperative, 33–34, 44, 44f, 53, 213
postoperative indications for, 119, 180
in infants and children, 234–235, 249
preoperative, 11, 14
for ventricular assist devices, 260, 263, 266t, 268
Transfer orders, typical preprinted, 66, 67f
Transplants. *See* Cardiac transplantation
Transposition of great arteries, 226
Transthoracic echocardiography, for infants, 119, 249
Transthoracic intraaortic balloon pump placement, 255, 256f
Transthoracic pressure monitoring, intraoperative, 29
Trendelenburg position, for cardiopulmonary bypass weaning, 48–49
Triamterene, 86, 104, 305
Tricuspid atresia, 227
Tri-iodothyronine, 127, 274
Tromethamine (THAM), for metabolic acidosis, 90
Troponin I, in myocardial infarction, 150
Truncus arteriosus, 228
Tube feedings, for postoperative nutrition, 106–107
Tubocurarine, usual dosage of, 310

U

Ultrasound, postoperative indications for, 181, 192, 247
Umbilical artery catheters, 230, 231f, 232
Umbilical vein catheters, 230, 231f, 232
United Network for Organ Sharing (UNOS), 272–273, 272t
Univentricular heart, congenital, 227
Urinalysis, preoperative, 8t, 9
Urine output, postoperative, 69, 84, 181–182

V

Valve disorders. *See* Heart valve entries
Vancomycin
  preoperative prophylactic, 18, 184, 299
  usual dosage of, 248, 309, 312
Varicosities, preoperative evaluation of, 3, 8
Vasodilator therapy
  for afterload reduction, 238
  for cardiopulmonary bypass complications, 41
  for low cardiac output, 118f, 128–129
  preoperative evaluation of, 4, 15–16
  usual dosage of, 306–307
Vasodilatory shock, postoperative management of, 73–74
Vasopressin, 309
  for cardiac arrest, 131, 133
  for cardiac transplantation, 274
  for low cardiac output, 74, 99, 129
Vasopressor therapy
  for low cardiac output, 118f, 128–130
  usual dosage of, 303–307, 310
Vecuronium, 103, 309–310
Venous duplex scan, for thromboemboli, 197
Venovenous hemofiltration, postoperative, 182, 281
Ventilation
  assessment in infants and children, 224, 232
  mechanical. *See* Mechanical ventilation
  postoperative complications of, 152–153
Ventilation-perfusion scan, for thromboemboli, 197
Ventricular assist device (VAD), 255–270
  for acute myocarditis, 257
  bleeding with, 262, 270
  as bridge to transplantation, 256, 259t, 264–270, 266t, 267f
  as destination therapy, 256–257, 270
  explantation of, 260–264, 269–270
  indications for, 255–256, 259t
  infections with, 266, 266t, 269
  for postcardiotomy cardiogenic shock, 256–264, 259t–260t, 261f, 264t
  transesophageal echocardiography for, 260, 263, 266t, 268
Ventricular fibrillation (VF), postoperative, 130–131, 133, 152
  management of, 137t–138t, 148–149
Ventricular filling pressure. *See* Preload
Ventricular function
  during cardiopulmonary bypass weaning, 50–53
  mechanical assist devices for. *See* Mechanical cardiac support
  postoperative management of, 70, 71t, 72, 116–117
  preoperative evaluation of, 10–11, 14–15
Ventricular septal defect (VSD), 17, 224, 226
Ventricular tachycardia (VT), postoperative, 131, 133, 152
  management of, 135t, 137t–138t, 148–149
Verapamil, 138t
Viral infections, from blood transfusions, 91–92, 92t
Visual deficits, postoperative, 193
Vitamin D, for cardiac transplantation, 284
Vitamin K, 6, 190
  warfarin interaction with, 216–218, 217t
Volume expansion, postoperative, 85

W

Warfarin, 309
  drug interactions with, 216, 217t
  postoperative management of
    for arrhythmias, 146–147
    endocarditis and, 212
    in infants and children, 248
    long-term issues with, 216–218
    pericardial effusions and, 218–219
    for prosthetic valves, 214, 215t, 216, 248
    for thromboemboli prevention, 197
  pregnancy cautions with, 218

preoperative evaluation of, 5–6, 168
vitamin K interaction with, 216–218, 217t
Weaning guidelines
for cardiopulmonary bypass, 52–53
cardiac pacing for, 49–51, 51f
for mechanical ventilation, 81–83
for ventricular assist device, 263–264
Wide QRS-complex tachycardia, 137t–138t, 141
Wolff-Parkinson-White syndrome, 142
Wound infections, postoperative, 56, 183–186

X

Xenograft bioprosthetic valves, deterioration of, 212–213

Z

Zafirlukast, 154, 309